K

CONCEIVING SPIRITS

DATE DUE

Smithsonian Series in Ethnographic Inquiry

William L. Merrill and Ivan Karp, Series Editors

Ethnography as fieldwork, analysis, and literary form is the distinguishing feature of modern anthropology. Guided by the assumption that anthropological theory and ethnography are inextricably linked, this series is devoted to exploring the ethnographic enterprise.

Jennifer W. Nourse

CONCEIVING SPIRITS

Birth Rituals and
Contested Identities
among Laujé
of Indonesia

Smithsonian Institution Press

Washington and London

Copy editor: Marsha A. Kunin
Production editor: Duke Johns
Designer: Chris Hotvedt

Library of Congress Cataloging-in-Publication Data
Nourse, Jennifer.
    Conceiving spirits : birth rituals and contested identities among Laujé of
Indonesia / Jennifer W. Nourse.
        p.   cm.
    Includes bibliographical references.
    ISBN 1-56098-875-4 (alk. paper). — ISBN 1-56098-850-9
(pbk. : alk. paper)
    1. Laujé (Indonesian people)—Rites and ceremonies.   2. Laujé
(Indonesian people)—Religion.   3. Laujé (Indonesian people)—Psychology.
4. Birth customs—Indonesia—Donggala (Kabupaten).   5. Childbirth—
Religious aspects.   6. Donggala (Indonesia : Kabupaten)—Religious life and
customs.   7. Donggala (Indonesia : Kabupaten)—Social life and customs.
I. Title.
DS632.L37N68   1999
306'.089'9922—dc21   99-19368

British Library Cataloguing-in-Publication Data available

Manufactured in the United States of America
06 05 04 03 02 01 00 99   5 4 3 2 1

⊚ The paper used in this publication meets the minimum requirements of
the American National Standard for Information Sciences—Permanence of
Paper for Printed Library Materials ANSI Z39.48-1984.

CONTENTS

PREFACE AND ACKNOWLEDGMENTS

Sulawesi is an exciting place to study. It lies at the crossroads of two geographic and culture areas, Inner and Outer Indonesia, which which were until recently considered distinct. Sulawesi's pivotal position thus defies neat categorization into typologically distinct areas. Scholars of Outer Indonesia have tended to approach their data using structuralist and symbolic theory (Fox 1989; Forth 1991; McKinnon 1991; Traube 1989), while Inner Indonesia's scholars have tended to use postmodern theory (Geertz 1995; Pemberton 1994; Steedly 1993; Tsing 1993). Though the scholarship of Indonesia can never be entirely fit into neat classifications, the bottom line is that Sulawesi's blurred ethnographic location invited me to incorporate disparate theories.

Indonesia's geographic and cultural diversity was divided into a three-part typology by Hildred Geertz (1963): (1) the hierarchical kingdoms with their wet-rice agriculture and elaborate court rituals, Islamic and Hindu-Buddhist, in interior regions of Inner Indonesia; (2) the remote hill tribes with their swidden agriculture, egalitarian politics, and animist religions that typify Outer Indonesia; and (3) the coastal trading towns with their polyglot multiethnic "culture," home to immigrants who settled along shores throughout Indonesia. Sulawesi, as Shelly Errington notes, is where hierarchical Inner meets egalitarian Outer Indonesia, but rarely have the "two Indonesias" been brought together in one study. My work, focusing on a variety of communities inhabited by one ethnic or linguistic group called Laujé, blurs the Inner/Outer boundaries while adding a third ingredient to the ethnological stew, the coastal trading town. I conclude that highland, lowland, and coastal Laujé living in communities that seem to conform to Hildred Geertz's typologies are not as distinct as one would think. Instead, Laujé from all three communities sometimes share and sometimes distinguish their ideas about birth spirits, identity, and religion and in the process create a complex and diverse mix of local and global ideas. To understand these complexities one needs to consider not only the classic structural and symbolic perspectives, focusing on broad social patterns, but also the postmodern approach, which addresses individuality, dissonance, and disagreement.

Never could I have come to these insights without the assistance of many people and institutions along the way. My initial two years of fieldwork research, from 1984 to 1986, were supported by the Fulbright-Hayes Doctoral Dissertation Program, Wenner-Gren Society for Anthropological Research, and the Institute for Intercultural Studies. I thank those organizations for their assistance. LIPI and Universitas Tadulako sponsored my research in Indonesia and I thank Doctor Mochtiar Buchori, Rektor Mattulada, and Ibu Naingollan of those organizations for their assistance. I also thank Greg Acciaioli for encouraging me to work in Central Sulawesi and introducing me to Bupati Jan Kaleb, who, in turn, pointed out the highland Laujé as potential people with whom I could conduct research. Locally, I thank Mayors Daeng Malondeng, K. P. Kiango, and Mawere Djumpeter, Pak Edi Rumambi, Pak Veki Borman, and Pak Udin Tombolotutu for their assistance while in the field. I would also like to thank Om Abdullah Bilhindi, Om Husin Makaramah, and Om A Peng Tho for assistance in settling into life in the Laujé land, as well as the New Tribe Missionary families—the Lees, Williamsons, and Whateleys—for their kind assistance.

This work began as a dissertation and slowly developed into a book. Along the way many people, too numerous to mention, have assisted me, though some advice is worth noting. For instance, Chris Crocker first pointed out Indonesia as a research site and continually encouraged me to reveal the human side of individuals so they never disappeared behind the screen of social structure. Roy Wagner nurtured my experimentation with new ways of understanding Laujé people and their ideas, and Richard Handler constantly worked with me to turn rough ideas into coherent written arguments, in the dissertation and beyond. Peter Metcalf provided insightful analysis of the relationship between prayer and speech, social structure, and human interpretation of that structure, and Greg Acciaioli offered thorough reading and suggestions throughout the last stages of the manuscripts' development. I also wish to thank readers of the present manuscript in its first preparatory stages, Peter Jacxsens, Holly Kerr, Emily Hill, Deborah Hopper, Laurie Linder, Sheila McKenna, Jason Meyler, Aditi Mehta, Susan Parker, and Amy Sette. Their insights and meticulous analyses were of immense aid.

Ivan Karp, as series editor of the Smithsonian Series in Ethnographic Inquiry, was an exacting and inspirational guide who facilitated my reformulation of ideas so that they encompassed a broader, yet deeper, scope. I am most sincerely grateful to his and Bob Lockhart's editorial input and to the three anonymous readers of the manuscript. I also thank Marsha A. Kunin for her precise copy editing. Many of the key ideas included in this book were developed during my sabbatical in 1997, provided by the University of Richmond, for which I am most appreciative.

As ever, from beginning to the end, one of my largest debts goes to Eric Gable, my husband and colleague. Eric's dazzling inquisitiveness and engaging personality attracted many Laujé during fieldwork. I benefited tremendously from Eric's tremendous talent as an ethnographer and analyst of anthropological material. His tireless efforts editing and reading, or watching our two children, Larsen and Grace, while I have worked, have carried this project to its completion. Thanks are not enough.

It is to the Laujé people that I am most deeply grateful. Though many of the people highlighted in this book are no longer alive, I will always remember that without them this book would never have been.

NOTE ON TRANSCRIPTION AND LANGUAGE

In transcribing the Laujé language, I have tried to follow modern Indonesian orthography wherever possible. This means the only diacritical mark I have used is to distinguish the mid-front /é/ from the unmarked /e/, which indicates a schwa.

A glossary of many of the Laujé words used here is provided after the text. I have provided the words just as they appear in the text, not separating the root word from the prefix, suffix, and infix. In Laujé, each verb can be written with various degrees of transitivity. Thus a verb is not merely transitive or intransitive. A prefix is added to a root word, say *lampa* (to walk), indicating the degree of transitivity. For instance, ma + root *lampa, malampa,* is intransitive and means walk. Me + root *lampa, melampa,* is more transitive and means to walk to. Mo + root *lampa, molampa,* is even more transitive and means walk toward a place. The infix in Laujé designates even more transitivity. For instance, the infix *po* is often added to *molampa* to become *mopolampa* and it would mean to make to walk somewhere (as in a child or a goat). But if the suffix *an* is added, as in *mopolampaan,* it would mean the place where it is made to walk (as in a schoolyard or a fenced yard). Laujé is a rather complicated language, in comparison to Indonesian. This is just one example of its complexity.

Much of the Laujé language does not really appear in this text, because I promised many people that the secret prayers they gave me would not be widely distributed. I have provided some Laujé for the cases when I did receive permission. The few chants I do provide here are broken into lines in order to highlight the quality of these chants as psalms or poems. Though it does require that I make the Laujé conform to a Western format for how poetry and psalms are written, the pauses uttered by the spirits possessing mediums do roughly correspond to the breaks in the lines where a western poem would have them.

INTRODUCTION: IN THE BEGINNING
Ethnography and Theory

"It's here!" shouted the breathless eight-year-old outside my window as the morning sun peeked over the mountain. "The baby came out. Father said I should fetch you as quickly as possible."

Fumbling through my precoffee haze I leaned out my bamboo window toward Saudara's daughter to hastily ask, "What is it? Boy or girl?"

"Girl. Father said to hurry."

"OK, I'm coming," my voice trailed off as I quickly hunted for my research tools, notepad, and pen. I turned to my husband, Eric, also an anthropologist, asking him to grab our camera. Not wanting to squander my first chance to witness the all important Laujé birth rituals, which my mentor, Siamae Sanji, had told me so much about, I frantically dug in my daypack for a baby gift. "Where did I put those cigarettes?" I muttered out loud to no one in particular.

Suddenly a voice from the front room interrupted my self-musing. "Who do you need cigarettes for?" I remembered that Sair, who was the son of Siamae Sanji, had decided to spend the night on our "living room" floor.

"Saudara's family," I told Sair. "Their baby has just arrived and I need a gift. I've also gotta go. I'll see you later," I announced, halfway out the house.

"Oh." I stopped in midstride. "I'll come get you at your house after the ritual for the baby is done. We can finish translating your father's tape this afternoon after everything with Saudara is finished."

Sair, his voice still husky from sleep, managed to collect his thoughts enough to reply, "I'll wait here. You'll be back in an hour. Saudara doesn't know much ritual. His ceremonies will be brief."

I didn't stop to question Sair, only minimally murmuring, "OK, fine," as I followed Saudara's eldest daughter down the back path. "It's not fine, though," I fumed as I ran down the hill. "That Sair, he's such a snob. Sair thinks only his father has full ritual knowledge about how to perform lengthy birth rites and that only Siamae Sanji and his children can talk at length about birth spirits."

Siamae Sanji, I thought, may have spent the last six months telling me how much he knows about birth spirits and childbirth rites, but surely everyone in the whole mountain village knows about birth. Afterall, this is Saudara's seventh daughter. By now he has to know this stuff.

My internal dialogue ended abruptly as we arrived at Saudara's house, a small ramshackle lean-to on stilts. Eric and I climbed inside the narrow doorway. All six girls gathered around us as their father, Saudara, nestled the baby close to his chest. "Very good," I said, not knowing any Laujé equivalent to congratulations. I knew Saudara had desired a son to take care of him in old age. Another girl was a bit of a disappointment, but as he cooed and held her, his disappointment seemed, from my perspective, to dissipate. I hoped to cheer Saudara with my gift of clove cigarettes. With his free hand he gave both packs to the children, who, to my chagrin, lit up immediately.

"Hey," he said "don't smoke them all! I'm busy with your new little sister now." Mesili, the new mother, climbed up the stairs from the garden and found a place to sit in the crowded lean-to.

"It's time," said Saudara, "to prepare her first bath and wash the placenta. Here, you hold her." Saudara gingerly handed the newborn to its mother, Mesili, who rather stiffly grabbed the swaddled bundle, holding it far from her body, as if, it seemed to me, the baby would contaminate her. Meanwhile, Saudara warmed water for washing the babe and the placenta. When it was time he gently unwrapped the babe and scrubbed the blood from her extremities, dabbing her eyes and cooing to her as she squirmed. Saudara carefully avoided the dried umbilical blood he had already dotted on her forehead and cheeks when he had cut the umbilical cord before we arrived. Finished, Saudara patted the babe dry and tightly swaddled her in layers of blankets. He nestled her closely to his chest, asking his oldest daughter to light him a cigarette as he gazed adoringly, so it seemed to me, down at the newborn. He smiled and sang the child a lullaby.

Hmmm, I thought. No difference here as far as I can see between what Siamae Sanji said and what Saudara was doing; fathers nurture and mothers neglect. This father may be sorry he didn't have a son, but he certainly seems to genuinely care for his daughter. His ritual actions are just as Siamae Sanji predicted. I asked the mother how she felt.

"Fine. Didn't you see me in the garden?"

"Yes, of course. I saw you working. What about the birth and labor?" I asked.

Mesili looked toward Saudara. Rather than the long, detailed narratives my friends in America had given of their experiences, Saudara preempted his wife and said matter of factly, "We were asleep and she woke up right before the cock crowed. The baby was out before sunrise. The placenta out at sunrise. That's when I sent my oldest up to your house. I'm so used to this I had the prayers for the umbilical cord uttered while she was at your house. The cord is wrapped up right there." Saudara pointed to the rafters. "Here," he said and handed the bundled baby to his wife who again rather awkwardly held her (see Figure 0.1). "I've got to clean this placenta before something bad happens."

Just as Siamae Sanji had told me, Saudara wiped all blood from the placenta. He patted the placenta dry (just as he had the baby), wrapped it in a banana leaf bundle, and placed it in a coconut shell cradle. He gently took the baby from its mother's arms and placed her in a cloth cradle—a stork's bundle hanging from the rafters. When finished Saudara looked at me as if embarrassed. "I'm going to hang this placenta [bundle] in the tree, but you shouldn't come. It's dangerous. Eric, he's a man, he can come."

Disappointed because I was unable to see the rest of the birth rites, I was simultaneously excited that gender played such a central role in this ritual and confirmed what Siamae Sanji had told me. Siamae Sanji had said that for the highland Laujé, the things of birth—placenta, blood, umbilicus, and fluids—were not merely substances, but homes for spiritual entities that, like persons, were gendered. If treated properly, nurtured by the father, they would aid the child's spirit. If neglected, however, as they inevitably were while the mother was giving birth, then the spirits could bring sickness and death. It was thus incumbent upon every father to propitiate the good placental spirit so it would protect the child from harm. Though I couldn't watch what Saudara did with the placenta, I knew I could rely on the pictures and meticulous notes Eric would take to tell me the rest of the story.

That afternoon when I read Eric's notes I was very pleased. The results were just as I had expected. Despite Sair's disparaging remarks

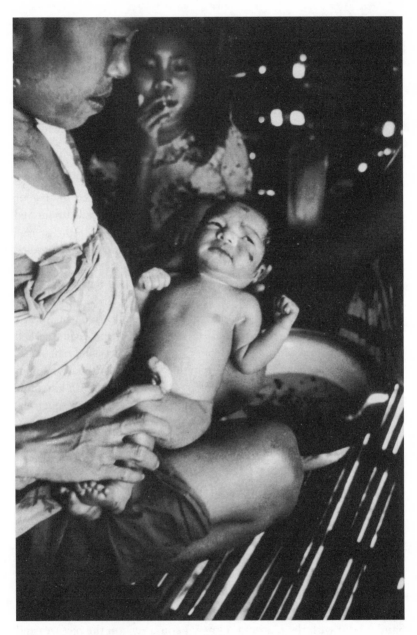

Figure 0.1. Mesili holding her newborn child

about Saudara's ritual knowledge, the ritual Saudara performed was almost exactly as Siamae Sanji said it should be. Moreover, what Saudara said about the ritual echoed, if in a more truncated form, what I was learning from Siamae Sanji. I took this as proof that one articulate, insightful informant's interpretation of the ritual—Siamae Sanji's—could represent everyone's understanding of what the ritual meant.

My theoretical assumptions at that time were loosely based upon Émile Durkheim's notion of a "collective representation."[1] I had been taught in the early eighties that a ritual like this one was a crystallization of Laujé thought. As one of my professors put it, with an ironic smile, "If two people say it, it's a collective representation." His intended joke was meant to spoof the anthropological tendency to weed out idiosyncrasies by using as few informants as possible, but it also spoke to a general truth in anthropological fieldwork: Using just a few informants and glossing over their differences allows the anthropologist to focus on collective ideas and draw general conclusions about what a whole culture thinks.[2] Following this and more complex lessons, I saw my task during fieldwork in Indonesia as an effort to collect and learn from the most knowledgeable members of the Laujé community, like Siamae Sanji, and to see how their ideas represented those of others, like Saudara, unable to articulate as effectively. From my fieldwork interviews I could rely on others to fill in the blanks left by key informants and then assemble an approximation of collective thought—the mind behind the external object—about the ritual's meaning. As such, then, I saw fieldwork as a kind of quest, an attempt to solve the mysteries of others' meanings, by finding the one or two people who could unlock the ultimate secret that would explain Laujé thought.

Very early on in fieldwork I was doubly sure I had followed my professors' lessons and unlocked the mysteries of highland Laujé life, because I had found a similarly articulate leader, an aristocrat in the lowland "court" of Dusunan. This other Laujé man, named Sumpitan,[3] explained, like Siamae Sanji, how central the secrets of the birth spirits called *umputé* were to his community of lowland Laujé.[4] Now, through what these two men told me, usually without my prompting them, I assumed I had come to understand how each group of Laujé, lowland aristocrats and highland commoners, constructed their own unique, but collective and systematic notions of self, world, and spirit in the two separate communities. Each man told me his own mystical, sometimes secret, stories about birth spirits that nurture fetuses in the womb, follow their soul-twins to heaven, and plague those soul-twins when neglected. They each spoke of good spirits and bad, healing and pestilent, and local and distant spirits.

Their ways of dividing and symbolizing spirits, while different from each other, nevertheless resonated with some of my training as a symbolic, structural anthropologist. Their categorized spirits also echoed what anthropologists of the late seventies and early eighties, studying other parts of Indonesia, had written following symbolic and structural theories.[5] Structuralism presumed that people think and collectively represent their world in categories that oppose one another. For instance good, white, and male may be opposed to bad, black, and female. The goal of a structuralist was to find what ideas or things were opposed in a culture, thereby enabling the theorist to understand the underlying logic of "native" thought. Symbolic anthropology built on this idea by presuming each "cultural system" used core, dominant, or key symbols that congealed thought about the mysteries of life.[6] Symbols, then, if decoded properly, were the master tropes through which the anthropologist sought to understand a particular "culture." These tropes explained the way locals understood the world. Structuralism aided in seeing how people classified those perceptions into neatly opposed categories.

What was exciting about my early fieldwork was that it so perfectly coincided with my structuralist/symbolic training and the other research conducted throughout the Indonesian archipelago. Not only were Sumpitan's and Siamae Sanji's views in and of themselves structured around core birth symbols, but they also formed perfect symbolic oppositions in ways that paralleled the opposition between lowlands and highlands, aristocrats and commoners. I was thrilled to find, so early in my fieldwork, articulate informants who provided the key to understanding the Laujé world in structural and symbolic terms. At the time I did not realize how wrong I was to presume, as many structural and symbolic theorists did, that others in each of their respective communities generally agreed with Siamae Sanji's and Sumpitan's structuralist interpretation of the symbolism of birth spirits.

Sadly, it was only through their deaths in 1985, each within a month of the other, that I came to understand how mistaken I was to have believed that their voices represented the most complete and encompassing explanations of the range of meanings the Laujé attributed to birth spirits. After these two men died, a number of people who had been reticent, women like Siinai Alasan, as well as men like the Haji, began to reveal to me their own versions of how and why these birth spirits nurture or plague humans. Some people, especially Siamae Balitangan, argued that spirits were not gendered or personlike. The spirit world was vast, mysterious, and nebulous. To interpret spirits otherwise was to misrepresent them. Besides revealing a sometimes confusing, but always intriguing assortment of ways to view the birth spirits, these people exposed my mistake of relying too strongly on Sumpitan and Siamae Sanji to speak for an entire culture.

I realized that it had been Laujé men who had first provided me with an articulate and all-encompassing exegesis about the "secrets" of birth spirits. Even though this philosophy did focus on things feminine—wombs, fetuses, placentas, and fluids—the way I first came to understand the Laujé philosophical universe was biased by the men who spoke about gender and birth spirits from their own perspectives. Once I understood that women as well as men, lower- as well as upper-class people had alternative perspectives, I found I could juxtapose their stories and interpretations to present on the one hand, a more fragmented picture, but on the other hand a more general picture of how Laujé of a particular class, religion, or gender looked at the world.

It is these juxtaposed stories and patterns of interpretations about birth spirits, overheard and elicited among mountain and lowland Laujé of Central Sulawesi, Indonesia, during my 1984–86 fieldwork,[7] that form the heart of this book (see Figure 0.2). The Laujé I studied live on the coast and in the mountains overlooking the Tomini Bay.[8] These Laujé communities are divided among seven riverine systems of which Tinombo is the largest. Along the Tinombo River and its branches live about 6,000 Laujé, almost half of whom reside in coastal communities. One coastal community, Dusunan, was at one time the royal court for the Laujé polity. Even today, its autochthonous leader, the *olongian,* continues to oversee important community rituals that are a mixture of Islamic and "animist" beliefs. Sumpitan claims this leader and all elite Laujé are devoutly Islamic and distinct from their highland, animist subjects. Highlanders such as Siamae Sanji, however, make broad claims to a longstanding Muslim heritage, and he and others are generally dismissive of lowlanders' pretensions to political sovereignty. Instead, men such as Siamae Sanji recognize, indeed em-

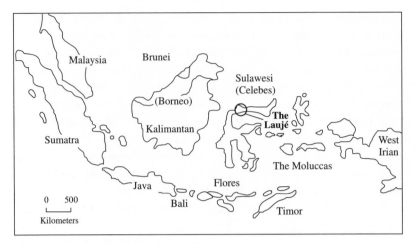

Figure 0.2. The Indonesian archipelago

phasize, highland *and* lowland incorporation as lowly subjects into foreign kingdoms, colonies, and states. Laujé from a number of "subject positions," therefore, articulate vastly divergent and constructed perspectives of their history and identity. The way these perspectives are revealed through contradictory and overlapping stories about birth spirits form the subject of this book.

By characterizing Laujé "subject positions" and by juxtaposing fragmentary stories, I am writing about the Laujé from a particular theoretical perspective, one that is sometimes labeled postmodernist. I learned about this set of perspectives when I returned from the field in 1986. At that time I thought this cutting-edge theory was, as it claimed, a radical break[9] from classic anthropology and could best explain various Laujé's representations of umputé. Now I realize that the best, most useful, conclusions of anthropology's postmodern movement deal with enduring ethnological questions. Differences between classic and new theory are more arbitrary than real. My anthropological training actually gave me the tools to analyze data in subtle and complex ways, but I was so enamored of this new theory's claims against older theory that I failed to recognize the virtues of my solid training. In hindsight I also recognize the limitations of postmodernism, especially if it ignores questions as old as anthropology and fieldwork itself. When I returned from the field, however, postmodernism offered fresh and exciting insights into the limitations of symbolic and structural approaches. I thus embraced it with open arms.

My shift toward the postmodern approach began when I tried to "write up" my Laujé experiences. I could not "get on top of the data" as one professor said I should, because I could not find one person to give me the skeleton key to cultural truth, the answer to what the Laujé thought rituals meant. I could not reconcile the ordered, symbolic data I had collected in conversations from Sumpitan and Siamae Sanji with the varied interpretations given me after Sumpitan and Siamae Sanji died. I took my problem of making sense of "the Laujé" as a problem with the theory I had been using, a problem with my fieldwork methods steeped in the search for key informants who could offer collective representations. I knew it was wrong to assume (as I had in the birth scenario above) that one person's actions corroborated another's interpretations, and that both could provide the sound bites and images from which I could construct a picture of Laujé thought. But until I learned about postmodern theory, I did not know any other way to frame a narrative without losing its essential coherence.

Similar problems plagued scholars in other fields. In literary criticism, postmodernists such as Lyotard (1984) and Bakhtin (1981) taught that even novels obviously authored by a single person comprised, in fact, an essential multivocality. Novels were "dialogic"— they spawned conflicting interpretations, offered conflicting exegeses or explanations. Scholars such as Jameson (1984) and Rorty (1979)[10] questioned whether the scholarly tendency to create ordered systems and unifying categories describing natural patterns were real or merely constructed representations of reality. Such questions began to percolate into anthropologists' conversations. Two such anthropologists, George Marcus and Michael Fischer, along with James Clifford, a pioneer in cultural studies of anthropology as a literature, took this "corridor talk" and made it theoretically central to anthropology by publishing two books interweaving postmodern ideas into anthropological concerns about culture and ethnographic writing. *Anthropology as Cultural Critique: An Experimental Moment in the Human Sciences* was published by Marcus and Fischer in 1986 and *Writing Culture: The Poetics and Politics of Writing Ethnography,* an edited volume with essays by Tyler, Clifford, Pratt, Rosaldo, and others, was published in 1986 by Clifford and Marcus. Together the two books had a profound impact on my work and that of others trying to reconcile the concept of a collective culture with the chaos of their field research.

One central theme was that culture was not whole, or static. Culture was contested and constantly created by a variety of individuals. As Clifford said in his own 1997 summary of his 1986 book: "I worried about culture's propensity to assert holism and aesthetic form, its tendency to privilege value, hierarchy and historical continuity in notions of common 'life.' I argued that these inclinations neglected, and at times actively repressed, many impure, unruly processes of collective invention and survival" (1997:2). Clifford as well as other postmodernists critiqued symbolic and structural anthropology for its preoccupation with the perfectly coherent depictions of culture, because such "systemic" views ignored the reality of individual voices, contest, difference, and chaos. "If 'culture' is not an object to be described," said Clifford, "neither is it a unified corpus of symbols and meanings that can be definitively interpreted" (1986:19).

Though authors in the Clifford and Marcus, and Marcus and Fischer volumes criticized symbolism and structuralism for highlighting coherence, most of their criticisms focused on older, "classic anthropological texts." Marcus and Fischer, for instance, suggested that anthropologists should expose hidden colonialist agendas[11] of earlier anthropological texts to point out their egregiously racist mistakes, but also to turn those mistakes into more positive goals for an activist discipline. Marcus and Fischer, then, wanted to "repatriate anthropology as a cultural critique," to work multiple voices into their texts or, at least, multiple points of view, which reflect the actual research process and constructive task of writing ethnography" (1986:164). Their point was that classic anthropology avoided the contests between people, the resistance to authority, the general chaos of life because classic anthropology emphasized order, structure, and consensus.

Postmodern anthropology, then, saw itself in opposition to classic anthropologists such as Malinowski (1929), Evans-Pritchard (1940), Mead (1928), Firth (1936), and Benedict (1932; 1934) whom they criticized as writer/agents erasing the messiness of life in the field, denying individuals a major role in creating diverse and contested perspectives of the world. These classic anthropologists, said postmodern critics, believed they alone could explain "native" life, because they alone could give objective, scientific explanations of "natives'" odd customs and practices (Clifford and Marcus 1986:23).

Tyler claimed that the reason the early anthropologist's voice drowned out the locals was because most anthropologists used the authoritative tone of science:

> The urge to conform to the canons of scientific rhetoric has made the easy realism of natural history the dominant mode of ethnographic prose, but it has been an illusory realism, promoting, on the one hand, the absurdity of "describing" nonentities such as "culture" or "society" as if they were fully observable, though somewhat ungainly, bugs, and, on the other hand, the equally ridiculous behavioral pretense of "describing" repetitive patterns of action in isolation from the discourse that actors use in constituting and situating their action. (1986a:131)

Pratt too believed the older ethnographies were too objective, erasing the subjective from the ethnography. Pratt wondered how anthropologists, who were "such interesting people doing such interesting things [could] produce such dull books" (Pratt 1986:33). She concluded that contemporary anthropologists should include their own thoughts, subjective desires, and motivations in ethnographies so that the fragmentary dialogues of fieldwork could be more faithfully evoked. By making anthropologists less authoritative, Pratt believed that local interlocutors, in all their diversity, could finally have their say.

An implicit, often explicit theme in such critiques of older ethnographies was that everyone's interpretations, the anthropologists' and the locals', were subjective and thus not reflections of the whole truth. They were merely "partial truths" (Clifford 1986). Clifford's phrase "partial truth" subverted "classic" assumptions that empirical data was collected objectively, that there was an observable reality that could be summarized in systemic and structural terms. In making such claims about the constructed quality of knowledge, Clifford implied that postmodern approaches were superior to those of earlier anthropologists because they erased bias and false unity, allowing locals to speak for themselves.

I certainly agreed with Clifford, Tyler, Pratt, Marcus, and Fischer when I rushed to adopt their theories and drop my own structural symbolic assumptions. Now, however, I realize that some postmodern assumptions may have been too extreme. In their effort to let other voices speak, to knock the anthropologist off his or her authoritative pedestal, postmodernists unwittingly emphasized a contrived equality or multivocality. For instance, Tyler, borrowing his dialogic theory from the Russian theorist Bakhtin, claimed ethnographies should be filled only with dialogues. By erasing the anthropologist from the text, Tyler avoided the troublesome problem of an anthropologist deciphering "native" motivations and allowed the speakers to speak for themselves. Tyler claimed good ethnographic writing is: "a denial of the metaphor of surface vs. depth in which our deciphering 'penetrates' the hymenal surface of the text fathoming its underlying real meaning and reveling in the revelations of orgasmic mystery" (1986b:25). Tyler confidently eradicated all anthropological explanations from his work, rejecting "writing which forms a picture of reality . . . in favor of a writing that 'evokes' or 'calls to mind,' not by completion and similarity but by suggestion and difference. The function of the text is not to depict or reveal within itself what it says. The text is 'seen through'" (ibid.:45).

Though Tyler's approach seemed to sidestep the problems of anthropological, colonialist bias and collective conclusions about culture, it created confusion in many readers' minds. Part of the problem was that Tyler's "dialogic" approach did not originate in anthropological circles, but in literary criticism where the readers understood the same subtle linguistic and cultural cues as the speaker. Ethnographic readers, however, have different needs. Readers of ethnographies not only desire, but require some sort of explanation. The cross-cultural reader needs to be told, for instance, what particular cultural nuances mean, what the social position of the speaker is, and what the political and historical contexts are that frame the speech act. Ethnographic readers have no embedded references to the linguistic and visual cues that signal those meanings within their own (and studied) languages. Ethnographic readers are thus completely dependent upon the anthropologist to act as cultural broker and translator.

Without this analytical "guidance," ethnographic readers can make even more egregiously hegemonic and ethnocentric assumptions than a biased anthropologist might make.[12] When, for instance, Marjorie Shostak's Nisa, Story of a !Kung Woman (1981) was selected as one of the books to be taught in a freshman core course at my university, some of the humanities professors complained that Shostak's cultural analysis of Nisa intruded on Nisa's own words. Thus they taught Nisa by deleting Marjorie Shostak's commentary. After the course was over I was appalled to hear from students that they and the professors had deduced from their readings that "All !Kung women and probably all

African women are promiscuous," "The !Kung have no family values," and "Sexual promiscuity always leads to violence." Even when
readers did not draw such dreadful conclusions, in almost every other
case, readers assumed Nisa represented all of !Kung culture. Though
Shostak's representation of !Kung culture may be, as her critics sometimes note, ahistorical, circumscribed, and overly idealized, Shostak at
least provides a context for Nisa's idiosyncrasies within a broader pattern of !Kung culture (Pratt 1986:43; Behar 1995:79; Vail and White
1991). Certainly Shostak's portrayal is more sensitive and subtle than
the dangerous assumptions that the educated core-course readers
made on their own. If the core-course reading of Nisa is any indication
of how "raw" dialogue is interpreted, the anthropologist's voice is not
only better than nothing, it is absolutely necessary for a nuanced understanding of an ethnographic text. In retrospect, then, I can only
conclude that Tyler's approach of avoiding anthropological commentary, which he borrows too naively from another discipline, under-
mines his own goal: to fairly represent the speaker's words.

To avoid similar theoretical mistakes, I think it imperative to be
aware of anthropologists' unique circumstances as cultural brokers.
Moreover, it is best not to reject the answers past anthropologists have
proffered in response to questions of how to represent the native
voice, how to analyze the field experience in nonintrusive and fair
ways. Granted, until recently many anthropologists wrote their ethnographies in a way that glossed over the individuals they interviewed,
making those individuals anonymous, using their words as the raw
material from which to construct "culture" or "thought." But anthropologists are a diverse group. Despite "new theorists'" claims otherwise, anthropology's focus on the individual in the life-history ethnographies of Radin (1926), Parsons (1936), T. Kroeber (1961), Sapir
(1938), Griaule (1948), Briggs (1970), and Casagrande (1960) and its
attempt to integrate subjective perspectives and context in ethnographies by Geertz (1968 and 1976), E. Turner (1992), Sapir (1924), and
Bohannan (1954) have been at the heart of the discipline. And even
some of the most egregious emphasizers of culture as a collective representation, Benedict (1934) and Mead (1928), have considered individuals and how to present those individuals in a non-ethnocentric
manner.

The point is that the goals and aims of classic anthropology and
postmodern anthropology, while not always accomplished, have been

roughly the same. The dividing line between the two is less defined
than postmodernism portrays it. Both perspectives want to present local interlocutors in as fair and unbiased a manner as possible. How to
do this, though, is not as simple as it would seem. Some of the same
dilemmas facing postmodernists about the complexity of representing
local voices were noted by Edward Sapir back in 1938 in an article
called "Two Crows Denies It." Sapir highlighted the basic dilemma in
anthropology then and now. "Respectable anthropology," on one
hand, believes it must "assay source material" to find cultural patterns
and discern "truth from error." Otherwise it believes it "passes the
buck to the reader," making the reader do the job the anthropologist
should do. On the other hand, Sapir points out that anthropologists
"ahead of their time" recognize that in any society humans give themselves the "privilege of differing from one another." The dilemma that
Sapir noted in 1938 is the same one highlighted in the cutting edge
theory of the 1980s and 1990s: Does the reader draw conclusions
from the material or does the authoritative voice draw those conclusions for the reader?

In a similarly prescient manner Victor Turner's work demonstrated
the postmodernist point: It is through personal, subjective interactions
between anthropologist and informant that conclusions are drawn. In
"Muchona the Hornet, Interpreter of Religion" (1967), Turner describes Muchona, an eloquent philosopher and healer, and the various
personas he undertakes to deal with his outsider status in Ndembu
land. In this poignant article, Turner explains that he chose Muchona,
like many other anthropologists chose their informants (Shostak 1981;
Behar 1993; Crapanzano 1980) because Muchona was articulate and
able to philosophize about his own culture from the margins. Despite
Muchona's outsider status, Turner finds Muchona's philosophical interpretations the ideal key to an understanding of Ndembu ritual.
Turner emphasizes, however, that Muchona's view is not the only one.
Others in the community have competing voices. Muchona's views are
expressed in, and perhaps constructed during, conversations with
Turner.

Like postmodernists, Turner's classic study of society depended
upon dialogues with an individual who was an articulate outsider.
Turner's training in the Manchester school emphasized rebellion and
dissension just as postmodernists emphasized the same thing thirty
years later.[13] Members of the Manchester school recognized that indi-

viduals act as agents to construct their own views of themselves and their world, which may be at odds with mainstream beliefs, an idea that coincides with some postmodernists'.[14] And most important, like the postmodernists, Turner recognizes his friend Muchona as an equal. Muchona's and Turner's ideas develop in reaction to each other through dialogues (a process Turner calls reflexivity). Muchona does not merely interpret and Turner does not merely provide questions. Their views and perspectives are intimately intertwined. Turner's example directly and indirectly inspired a whole subdiscipline of anthropology, often called reflexivity (Myerhoff 1978; Karp and Kendall 1982; Crapanzano 1980; Lacoste-Dujardin 1977; Shostak 1981), which in many respects resembles the postmodern quest.

Fabian explicitly defined the reflexive method in 1971 and later in 1983. "It is imperative for anthropology to recognize the subjects of research as equal" (he called the process coevalness). Rather than placing the anthropologists' view above the "natives'," rather than dividing the "West from the Rest" or the rational/logical beings from the metaphoric/symbolic ones, Fabian maintained that the "project of dismantling anthropology's intellectual imperialism must begin with alternatives to positivist conceptions of ethnography. . . . I want language and communication to be understood as a kind of praxis in which the Knower cannot claim ascendancy over the Known" (Fabian 1971). Karp and Kendall's "Reflexivity in Fieldwork" article (1982) takes Fabian's notion one step further, arguing that equality and interaction with locals goes "beyond just the notion that 'natives' construct reality along with the anthropologist" (254): "The interpretive procedures through which natives render their experiences intelligible are just that, interpretive procedures. They no more provide actors with true statements about the internal states of others than they provide anthropologists with true pictures of 'what the natives really think'" (1982:266).

Thus, prior to the postmodern movement, especially in the reflexive school, but also in other arenas, anthropologists had been trying to resolve the dilemma between relying solely on what people say they think and conveying in a nonintrusive, nonimperialist way what the anthropologist thinks. There has always been a recognition, at least in some anthropological corners, that partial truths, approximations of "native" thought, are all that sensitive anthropologists can hope to reveal to Western-educated audiences unfamiliar with the context evoked in local dialogues. The said is never the real. Moreover, there has always been a recognition, in some circles, that contest, rebellion, and dissension are the stuff of life in other communities. Anthropologists can convey that contest and dissension through their unique role as cultural brokers.

When in the past anthropologists have talked about "culture" in rather holistic terms, it has often been to speak about the constructed quality of "culture," not, as postmodernists claim, about its "static" quality. For instance, Roy Wagner, one of my professors, wrote *The Invention of Culture* in 1975. His ideas presaged postmodernists' thinking, discussing the processes through which people constantly create and change their ideas about the world. Three of my other professors, David Sapir and Chris Crocker in *The Social Use of Metaphor* (1977), and Victor Turner in *Dramas, Fields, and Metaphors* (1974), discussed the complex and contradictory ways in which metaphor and symbols could be used instrumentally by individuals or social groups. In other words, my own professors as well as other prominent anthropologists were not as guilty of collective-static structural sins as I had presumed when I jumped onto the postmodern bandwagon.

In dredging up past approaches to ethnographic issues I am not merely using this as an opportunity to enhance my own professors' reputations, nor merely to show that classic goals (in the hands of thoughtful analysts) are similar to those embraced by the postmodern critique. Nor am I merely urging postmodernists to recognize their debt to theoretical ancestors. I hope to also demonstrate that in their attempt to sever ties to historic theories and claim their own innovations, the postmodernists have at best drawn the same conclusions as older theorists, sometimes with less profound insights, and at worst have ignored the insights past anthropologists have gained when analyzing the same set of issues. As a result, postmodern claims have often been self-defeating and contradictory. For instance, in their introduction to *Writing Culture*, Clifford and Marcus characterize reflexive methodology as both "sophisticated and naive" (1986:14). They criticize this classic approach because it merely "stages dialogues" and merely narrates interpersonal confrontations. They contrast reflexivity with Tyler's dialogic approach, saying Tyler goes "well beyond the more or less artful presentation of 'actual' encounters" (ibid.:14–15), by providing actual, not artfully constructed, dialogues. As I said earlier, however, by advocating dialogue over analysis, postmodernists make the local voice even more obscure than necessary, defeating their own goal of presenting the untainted local voice. Moreover, when the dialogic approach denies anthropologists a role as analysts, it is ultimately at odds with Marcus and Fischer's call to repatriate anthropology as critique. One cannot use anthropology as critique if one silences the anthropologist.

This contradiction I have noted in the first postmodernists' critiques of anthropology had been realized ten years later by one author, Clifford. In looking back at his earlier work, Clifford recently critiqued his (and Tyler's) naïveté: "My own attempt to multiply the hands and discourses involved in 'writing culture' aims *not to assert a naive democracy of plural authorship* [my italics], but to loosen at least somewhat the monological control of the executive writer/ anthropologist and to open up for discussion ethnography's hierarchy and negotiation of discourse in power-charged unequal situations" (1997:23). Clifford now recognizes that his own and others' postmodern approach to the anthropological task was naive.

Despite Clifford's desire to bring postmodern literary criticism in line with the anthropological task, given past problems in joining the two theoretical perspectives, I think it is best to resolve the dilemma in another way. Classic anthropological questions and answers, as they relate to the postmodern critique, must be repatriated into contemporary anthropological theory. The point Clifford made above, in the nineties, as well as points Sapir made in the thirties; Turner in the fifties through the eighties; and Fabian, Wagner, Sapir, Crocker, and Karp in the seventies and eighties are that the ethnographic writer must always make clear how various perspectives differ and how the anthropologists' desire to explain that variety involves negotiation, interpretation, and power differentials. Past anthropologists have dealt with these issues by making the anthropologists' voices equal to the locals', not as Tyler advocates in dialogics (1986a, 1986b, 1992), by denying the anthropologist any voice at all.

I believe equal, though not naively idealized, time for the anthropologists' perspective is the only way the discipline can move forward if it wants, as Clifford *now* says, to avoid asserting a "naive democracy of plural authors" and if it wants, as Marcus and Fischer (1986) say, to critique our own society. Rather than presuming that the locals' perspective is more "real" and more unbiased than the anthropologists' (Obeyesekere 1990), it might be more fruitful to see both in

equal terms: Both the anthropologists' and the locals' views are constructed and biased.[15] To allow for the constructed quality of both
voices, the ethnographer must outline how and why she chooses some
voices over others and how and why others in the community listen to
particular voices. Karp and Kendall allude to such a method in their
reflexivity and fieldwork article:

> Actors' constructions of their own behaviors are not irrelevant data, no
> matter how curious or beside the point they may seem. Even if they are not
> true reflections of interior states, or full explanations of action, they have
> to be examined critically. This is so because there is always the chance that
> other actors will take such reports at face value and act upon them. "Un-
> true" interpretations may become true by virtue of their consequences.
> (1982:265)

By observing and recording who reacts to whom in a community, the
anthropologist can document what locals regard as important and
thus avoid naive assumptions that all utterances deserve an equal hearing. Individual agents, particular leaders, particular informants can
have a profound impact on the way local ideas are accepted or rejected. In short, some voices, some informants' interpretations are
more important than others. Some people speak more strongly, com-
pellingly, than others. They are the agents of social and political
change. Words, rituals, exegeses, then, are not merely commentary after the fact. They are the stuff of political and religious action. The
words of theorists like Turner, Sapir, Clifford, or Marcus have compelled some anthropologists to change the way they write and talk
about culture, agency, and society. Likewise, the words of Laujé like
Sumpitan and Siamae Sanji, have compelled their consociates and descendants to talk about birth spirits and to carry out birth rituals in
particular ways. These people acted not only as self-interested agents,
but also as visionaries creating and describing key cultural notions
that resonated with others' ideas of how the world did or did not
work as a system. They were not just creating their view of the world
from "scratch." These informants were compelling because they went
beyond their own self-interests to address a self-less, moral vision that
touched some fundamental (dare I say cultural) chord. There were basic cultural ingredients, the fundamental building blocks, which they
used to erect their own visionary structures. It is imperative that the
anthropologist document these fundamental features for the reader.

In this Laujé case, Sumpitan and Siamae Sanji erected visionary structures of umputé, which they divided into binary opposites (umputé was either white or black, male or female, native or foreign). These men expressed their visions structurally not just because that particular approach fit the questions I asked them, nor only because I was predisposed (through graduate training) to hear their answers in structural and symbolic terms. Seeing the world through a categorically opposed lens *also* resonated with and appealed to perceptions of the world they and others in the community already shared. As Errington (1989) notes, it is no accident that structuralism was first discovered in island Southeast Asia (by van Wouden in 1935). The profusion of binary oppositions, which often line up in two clear columns in these Austronesian societies, is ineluctable (see Fox 1980; Traube 1986; Forth 1981; Hicks 1972, 1973; Kuipers 1990; Hoskins 1988a).[16] Thus, Sumpitan and Siamae Sanji created their own notions of the world through the lens of their own particular experiences, but the way they connected those experiences was circumscribed by shared notions that the world is structurally ordered. Granted, I may have noticed their structural and symbolic answers more than others because I was trained in structuralism and symbolism, but these ideas were floating around the community and shared in repeated conversations when I was a mere listener, not a solicitor of information.

In making claims that Laujé share notions about structure, I am not returning to a modernist or a structuralist theoretical model, nor am I claiming that the world is essentially structured in binary categories. I presume that there are cultural themes floating around in any community, which in the case of the Laujé (and others throughout Austronesia) happen to be structured. In conversations, some people highlight these cultural themes while others leave them dormant. Individuals use the bits and pieces, the fragments of these ideas, to construct their own views of the world, their own truths. These constructed truths are not random, nor can they be created into an infinite array of possibilities. These "truths" are limited by the ideas people have shared with each other for generations. These ideas change and vary from person to person. Some people build a bigger, more coherent collective structure than do others. Some people tie the "culture" together into a coherent theme, while others play around with its loose ends, its fragments. Some people believe what others say about these themes, while more cynical others focus on the self-interested quality of agents' political agendas and challenge the moral selflessness of the visionary's statements.

The bottom line here, at least theoretically, is that the anthropologist must explain to the reader why one person's, one agent's, construction of reality is more important than another's. Why, for instance, were Sumpitan's and Siamae Sanji's perspectives more highly regarded in the community than Siamae Balitangan's? The simple answer is that these men said something that resonated with shared notions in the community, while the more complex answer has to be explained in the ethnographic context. To provide the simple and the complex answers, the anthropologist must move beyond an unreflective attempt to make all voices equal. Readers have to recognize the contests, the chaos, and the dissension in a community, but also whose voice counts more. We can move beyond Clifford's 1986 claim that all perspectives are partial truths and Tyler's 1986 assumption that the anthropologist should not analyze what she observes for fear of imposing her own cultural perspective on another. Anthropologists can and should present their own analytical interpretations (indeed, as Wolf (1992) says, it is our responsibility to do so) as long as we avoid claiming ours is the final, the only, and the most objective truth. We can assume that some informants, some narrators, speak not only as self-interested agents, but as persuasive cultural spokespersons whose ideas represent, at least in some cases, a collective vision of what the world should or should not be like. In other cases and at other times, there may be no visionary spokesperson, only marginal analysts like Nisa, Muchona the Hornet, or Siamae Balitangan. The reader, however, needs the anthropologist to listen to various people's fragmentary views and tell us how they fit. Whose voice is really central, whose is marginal? We must know if people with similar backgrounds have similar responses to events and experiences. If so, these patterns deserve to be noted too.

In what follows, I show that despite the conflicting, idiosyncratic quality of individual interpreters' views, there are consistent patterns in the ways groups of people talk about birth spirits they call umputé, and there are certain eloquent figures whose visions stimulate others to think about umputé and act upon those thoughts in similar ways. On one hand, these ideas are enduring, in that many people speak of umputé as though it is divided into pairs, into structural oppositions. On the other hand, not all people speak this way. But even when people do not speak structurally, they do tend to speak as others like them do, their words shaped by political, economic, and religious events that similarly affect marginal people throughout Indonesia. Thus their ideas about umputé are intimately intertwined with their perceptions of themselves and others in local and global contexts.

As elsewhere in the Indonesian archipelago, many Laujé perceive themselves to be only marginal citizens of the Indonesian state and only partially integrated into the hierarchy of Islam as a world religion.[17] These persistently fluid notions of marginality, in turn, can modulate how people come to understand their social, political, and spiritual worlds. If a particularly eloquent person like Sumpitan or Siamae Sanji can describe these factors in such a way (usually moralistic) as to strike a chord in people's hearts and minds, then the speaker's words are more representative, more collective, and thus more ascendant than others'.

In sum, then, in this book I take a common theme stressed in books about marginal peoples in Indonesia and I highlight the varieties these themes take when individual Laujé creatively situate themselves vis-à-vis the state or global religion. I presume that locals actively create and reconstitute their own political, religious, and economic identity, not as passive victims of state intervention nor as one unified cultural group, but as assertive thinkers, as agents. Some people create their visions of the world not only according to their interests narrowly defined and clearly perceived, but also according to more altruistic, broadly shared notions of what counts as morality and inequity. It is these people's visions, and their voices, that deserve more attention. At the same time, though, it should never be assumed that the eloquent orators speak for everyone. Contest, chaos, and dissension do exist. Some people even view the world through partial, fragmentary perspectives. In the end, though, and this is the crucial point, whether people are systematic, fragmentary, or resistant to analysis matters less than that all the people with whom I spoke during the 1984–86 period, all of whom claimed to be Laujé, shared an assumption that umputé was *the* central concept defining all "Laujé." In this book I delineate the subtle nuances of these many definitions of umputé.

In the first chapter I introduce individual people who have their own perspectives of umputé, and the way I came to know them. I also discuss my own romantic quest to find an isolated field site and the choices that led me to eventually conduct research in two places, one

more remote, and the other at the center of Laujé ritual life. More important than the place, though, are the people who explained it to me.
I describe how I came to understand the two areas, the lowland village
of Dusunan and the highland village of Taipaobal, through the eyes of
my two key informants, Sumpitan and Siamae Sanji.[18] In Chapter 2 I
go into greater detail outlining Sumpitan's and Siamae Sanji's persuasive arguments about history and the impact the perceptions had on
how each man talked about birth spirits. Sumpitan divided historical
and contemporary life into good and bad, Laujé, and all other ethnic
groups (whom he called foreigners). In later chapters we will see how
he also divided the world of birth spirits into good and bad, Laujé,
and foreign. Using a different perspective of history, but similarly
structured logic, Siamae Sanji divided the social and historical world
into those who maintained connections to the past, males, and those
who neglected connections, females. Siamae Sanji's historical divisions
between good males and bad females had a direct impact on the way
he defined birth spirits in rituals, which are the subject of Chapter 3.
Here we learn how Siamae Sanji defined umputé in rituals, pregnancy,
and birth. Siamae Sanji delineated the good, white spirits of the placenta, which are like the fathers who nurture them, and he juxtaposed
these good spirits with the black spirits of childbirth blood that are
like the mothers who neglect children while working. We see how similar, yet idiosyncratic, Siamae Sanji's views are to structuralist writings
on Eastern Indonesia and anthropology in general. In Chapter 4 we
turn to Sumpitan's ritual divisions of spirits, which are reminiscent of
Siamae Sanji's divisions. In Sumpitan's household-curing rites he divided various umputé spirits into good and bad in the same way as he
divided social history. Good spirits are like the good Laujé, bad spirits
like the bad immigrants (who he called foreigners). Chapter 5 provides
Sumpitan's visions of the communitywide rite for umputé spirits, the
momasoro of 1985. We see how Sumpitan choreographed the rite so
that his antiimmigrant, pro-Laujé message prevailed. He delineated
bad umputé spirits bringing red and black sicknesses from non-Laujé
territories, on the one hand, and, on the other hand, good umputé
spirits bringing human and plant fertility from Laujé areas. In the
ritual, Sumpitan choreographed it so that the bad foreign spirits were
invited in for a week, given enough offerings so they would not bother
the Laujé for a whole year, and then cast out to sea in boats. By con-

trast, the good (i.e., Laujé) spirits were retained at the "center" of the Laujé universe at the ritual leader's, the olongian's, house.

Sadly, it was before the next rite that Sumpitan, and coincidentally Siamae Sanji, died. Chapter 6 describes what happens to the momasoro of 1986 without Sumpitan's masterful vision. Here the interpretations of the Haji and the olongian's wife, who are elite elaborators of umputé's message, prevailed, but somehow their visions were not as persuasive as Sumpitan's. They advocated bringing together the spirits Sumpitan had divided, but few people in the community listened to this message as they had to Sumpitan's. Chapter 7 analyzes commoners', mediums', and *sando*'s interpretations of umputé spirits in the momasoro of 1985. It especially focuses on the perspectives of people like Siamae Balitangan and Siinai Alasan, who "refused" to interpret the spirit world in terms of the social world. It concludes that commoners and female mediums are the groups who most often take this perspective, while elites tend to elaborate upon umputé by dividing it into parts, by metaphorizing it, and by relating its parts to the social world. Chapter 8 summarizes everyone's perspectives and discusses how these differences among interpreters advance anthropological study of ritual and symbolization. It reminds us that thorough ethnographies should always allow locals to speak for themselves and the anthropologist to comment on whose voice is more important and whose voice, if any, reflects general patterns and trends.

One

CONCEIVING THE PAST THROUGH SPIRITS IN THE PRESENT

1

MEETING "THE" LAUJÉ

My reasons for studying the Laujé were partially inspired by the first anthropological texts I had read by Malinowski (1929) and Radcliffe-Brown (1922). From these classic ethnographies I absorbed rather old-fashioned, romantic ideas about working with "primitive" people practicing indigenous religion in relative isolation. By the time I began fieldwork, I was more theoretically and ethnographically sophisticated, but the romance of finding an isolated community in which to work was still with me. Moreover, Elizabeth Traube's work on the Mambai in nearby East Timor provided a wonderful inspiration that tied into my earlier training.[1] Traube worked with Mambai men and women of power, shamans, who shared her quest to understand the Mambai's complex cosmology. I, too, sought such key informants and a seemingly "intact" religious system, but finding for my own fieldwork the same circumstances Traube had found in the early 1970s was not going to be easy.

First Contact

I chose the northern district of Central Sulawesi, Kabupaten Donggala, because this region was renowned for its "primitive" mountain dwellers.[2] At the time, in the early eighties, the New Tribes missionaries had just begun their work with highland Laujé and no anthropologists had yet conducted research there. Looking at a map, it was easy to see why the area remained isolated. Stretching up along a north-south axis, and traversed by a steep spine of mountains framed on both sides by rough seas, here, mountain peaks cut by rivers flowing into the sea and the Tomini Bay were separated from each other by sharp valleys, making transportation over the mountains on the east-

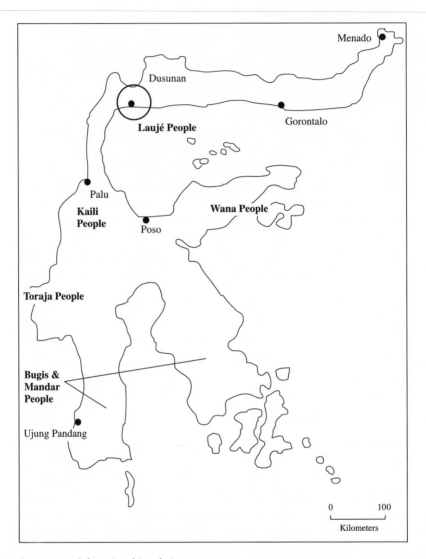

Figure 1.1. Sulawesi and its ethnic groups

west axis very arduous (see Figure 1.1). Indonesian officials told me
the Laujé living in the mountains would be a perfect "pure" "tribe"
(suku terasing) to work with because the rough terrain kept them separated from other mountain tribes and lowland religion (cf. Mashyuda
1979). Government officials told me the highland Laujé were totally

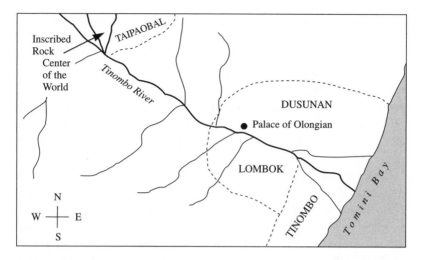

Figure 1.2.   Laujé fieldwork sites

unrelated to any other people in the lowlands, they were a "foreign-like" tribe. "Pure" highland Laujé never married lowlanders who were immigrants from ethnic groups throughout Sulawesi and beyond. The coastal was distinct from the highland "culture."

Though I could see through the thin veneer of prejudiced claims that "primitive" highlanders were a cultural "other,"[3] I mistakenly began fieldwork in May 1984 with the government-inspired notion that highlanders and lowlanders had very little influence over one another. For this reason I was still unaware I would eventually include lowland Laujé in my research. I settled in the town of Tinombo, situated at the mouth of the river flowing down from highland Laujé villages. My sole purpose there, or so I thought, was to study the Laujé language through an Indonesian interpreter. Once I became more proficient, my plan was to move to a "pure Laujé" village in the isolated mountains (see Figure 1.2).

My first impression of the region corroborated the government officials' assumption that highland Laujé were "untouched" by the "modern" world even though they were only 15–20 kilometers from the coast.[4] Every evening, Tinombo, a town of 3,000 or so people, with its lighted cafés, bustling warehouses, and nightly traffic, seemed to be festive, brightly lit, and noisy. The public address system at the freshly painted mosque loudly called community members to prayer. It reminded everyone, five times a day, that most people in Tinombo, like Indonesia at large, were Muslims. Adding to the cacophony were the constant shouts and groans from Tinombo's port and harbor where "foreign"[5] products entered and Laujé mountain products exited the region. Similarly the Trans-Sulawesi highway brought in and took out rumbling truckloads of goods for the stores and businesses in Tinombo. Its all-night restaurants and bus stops formed the night-life nucleus for importers and exporters traveling through in a town that never seemed to sleep.

By contrast, Laujé villages hidden in the velvety steep mountains above the Tinombo River or in the lush green coconut groves across from Tinombo were eerily silent and dark. Even in the daylight when farmers punctuated the silence by shouting from one swidden field across the mountains to another or when lowland children yelped playfully while scattering smoldering copra husks in nearby house-yards, the deep silence soon absorbed the pranksters' high-pitched din. In Laujé villages the distance from motorcycles, trucks, and loudspeaker calls to mosque impressed upon me the notion that the Laujé communities were more "traditional," more harmonious, less cacophonous.

It was only later that I learned that the sharp divisions between highlands and lowlands were more indistinct than government officials and lowland dwellers had led me to believe. For instance, the government said animism was the highlanders' religion, Islam the lowlanders', but I quickly observed that Islam had crept into all the nooks and crannies of highland life while various magical and healing beliefs prevailed in Tinombo. Moreover, contrary to government depictions of boundaries between the two areas, I found that peoples from highlands and lowlands exchanged forest products, religious ideas, magic, and vows of friendship. Some even married. Government officials said highlanders were swidden cultivators, lowlanders wet-rice farmers.[6] Though officials had valid reasons for recognizing these ecological divisions, nevertheless, even here, the contrast was more blurred than the government reports led me to believe. For instance, some lowlanders from the villages of Lombok and Dusunan did farm swidden plots in the high foothills while some highlanders from Taipaobal and Polumelee farmed irrigated plots near their lowland spouses.[7]

Other divisions were even more murky. When I looked closely at economic data, the greatest differences between community wealth were not between highlands and lowlands, as the government predicted, but between Tinombo and every other community. In lowland and highland Laujé villages, people made a living as best they could, by mixing subsistence farming, cash cropping, intermittent wage-labor or buying and selling (from and to highlanders). In Tinombo, however, almost all the people lived off the cash economy, as wage-earners. The main reason was that they, unlike residents in Lombok and Dusunan, were immigrants with economic ties to other regions. One second generation Tinomboer explained it thusly:

> We here in Tinombo are not like the people all around us who farm and the Laujé up in the mountains without religion. . . . We weren't born here. We brought our religion and our work with us. Most ancestors stopped here as traders. They liked it and stayed. . . . Now [in Tinombo] we have Protestants, Catholics, orthodox Muslims and reform Muslims all living together in harmony [in Tinombo] because we have chosen this place as our home.

Though this person's claims to religious and ethnic tolerance were a bit idealistic, they did reveal the polyglot ethos of Tinombo. Most of Tinombo's inhabitants reckoned ethnic identity through ties to other communities. Most of the people or their parents came to Tinombo during the Dutch colonial period (1912–1953)[8] when the Bugis/Mandar raja[9] was installed to oversee colonial plantations created by the Dutch. Bugis and Mandar immigrated from South Sulawesi, Kaili from Central Sulawesi, and Gorontalese from North Sulawesi (see Figure 1.1). Chinese and Middle Eastern immigrants also moved to Tinombo during the colonial period. Descendants of these Chinese and Arab traders owned almost all of Tinombo's stores and businesses.

In addition to its cosmopolitan flavor, Tinombo also had its own aristocrats, descendants of the last raja, Kuti Tombolotutu (see Figure 1.3). Most of his descendants occupied positions in the regional government, while a few still lived in Raja Kuti's former palace.[10] The palace, an anachronistic Dutch structure now surrounded by modern tin-roofed bungalows, harkened back to the colonial period. Its wide veranda and neatly manicured yard filled with bougainvillaea shrubs, once hosted scores of Laujé from the highlands who gathered to seek an audience with the raja or pay him their respects. It was this immigrant raja who taught highland Laujé, like Siamae Sanji, about Islam. It was the immigrant raja who hired highlanders to gather rattan, ebony, and damar resin. Thus, even though government officials and

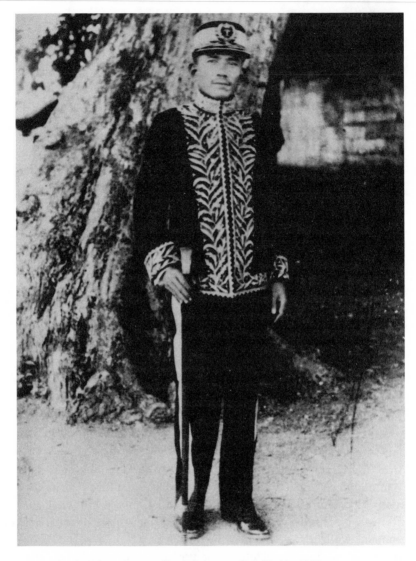

Figure 1.3.   Raja Datu Pamusu Tombolotutu, or Raja Kuti in 1935

descendants of this raja liked to characterize the differences between, and isolation of, Laujé from immigrants, it was actually these Tinom-boers who helped to penetrate highland and lowland boundaries.

Such fluid interchanges between Tinombo, Dusunan, Lombok, and highland Laujé villages like Taipaobal were still a mystery to me when

I first settled in Tinombo. Eric and I began research by renting a modern Tinombo house from a Chinese store owner in the middle of town. The house was equipped with a pump in the courtyard, a Turkish toilet, screens on the bedroom windows, and a concrete floor. I knew this modern Dutch-style bungalow would differ greatly from our bamboo house once we moved to the mountains. For now, though, I enjoyed "modern" life. Our house was located next to the doctor's house on Tinombo's main street, which descends straight through town from the Laujé mountains all the way to the nearby port and marketplace. From here I could watch, twice a week, the mountain Laujé who would make the long trek down the mountains and across the swelling Tinombo River to bring their products to market or to visit the doctor.

The mountain Laujé always stood out in sharp contrast to lowlanders. Both men and women were shorter and stockier than lowlanders. Their gait, bent at the knees from walking in the mountains, was made even more awkward because some of them donned shoes to appear presentable in "the city." The men with their long hair, dressed in cheap, brightly colored shorts and T-shirts gone muddy with age, the women with their tattoos, their eyebrows plucked, their lips colored, in an outmoded 1920s style, were the subject of subtle and not-so-subtle snickers as they placed their machetes on the fence of the doctor's house next door.[11] None of the Laujé responded to these jeers and snickers, but I always felt indignant for them. Partly out of pity, but also to establish a relationship with Laujé, I would ask them into my "modern" bungalow for a glass of water and a chat. To my chagrin someone would invariably spit betel juice onto my concrete floor. Then my neighbors in Tinombo, always seeking reasons to prove how much more polite and cosmopolitan they were than these hillbillies, would use the betel stains as an excuse to tell me, yet again, how crude the mountain Laujé were.

This prejudice, of course, only reinforced my own growing unease around lowlanders, who seemed unnecessarily snobbish and callous. Some people, I later found out, at least had a motivation for their callousness. Many of the immigrants had Laujé wives, mothers, or grandmothers. Thus they desperately wanted to differentiate themselves from their "hillbilly" relatives. In fact, it was primarily "pure" Laujé in coastal villages like Dusunan, just across the river from Tinombo, who jeered and snickered at the mountain Laujé when they came to market, because they, more than those claiming immigrant status, wanted to distance themselves from mountain Laujé who were animists.

Initially I believed the Laujé in Dusunan were just like the Laujé in Tinombo—typical lowlanders. Thus I had no interest in Dusunan or its people.[12] Nevertheless my language teacher in Tinombo, Pak Husin Makaramah, insisted I meet an important "Laujé" leader who lived in Dusunan, named Sumpitan. Though I believed this had no ultimate relevance to my eventual research, I was anxious to do anything in the initial months of my field research that might allow me to speak the Laujé language.[13] Thus I traveled over the river to Sumpitan's house in Dusunan amidst the dark coconut trees and far from the noisy din of Tinombo.

Sumpitan was one of the most well-respected people in Dusunan— talkative, friendly, and obviously intelligent. Moreover, Sumpitan was the descendant of the olongian. Olongian were the indigenous Laujé leaders.[14] Thus, Sumpitan, as he was quick to tell me, was a Laujé aristocrat. He was anxious to set the record straight about the history of the Laujé's rulers. Every visit, he promised that if I came again he would show me something "special": the genealogy chart of the olongian (lontar). He described it as an ancient artifact that charted the marriages of olongian and family members for more than seven generations. I envisioned a scroll, perhaps on bark-cloth or some sort of parchment. It took several visits before Sumpitan finally produced the promised chart, which proved to be rather disappointing. I felt as if Sumpitan had tricked me, but I now realize he was just naively fervent about the chart's authenticity. The "ancient" artifact turned out to be an oddly childish document, drawn in colored pencil on manila school paper, scotch-taped together, rolled and stored in a cardboard tube once used to sell badminton birdies. Under the chart's circles and triangles depicting male and female ancestors were names written using Dutch orthography. I was to learn later, that this "ancient document" had been produced in the early 1950s to impress upon the Dutch that the Laujé had the right to succeed to the throne. Sumpitan complained that the Dutch ignored the chart because "foreigners" (his term for the Tinombo immigrants), family members of the raja, had deceived the Dutch and won the throne. The ineffective chart was saved and stored with the heirlooms of the olongian.

Despite the less than ancient genealogy chart, Sumpitan's obvious love for his community and its lore, his charm as a humane person and

as a raconteur had me hooked. Though Sumpitan's versions were obviously biased, he described Laujé history, colonialism, and the raja in
Tinombo as no one else had. His stories were obviously contrary to
"official histories" I had heard in Tinombo and in government
archives, and I was eager to learn about any history that added depth
to the thinly disguised elitist promotions Tinombo officials seemed to
offer as colonial history. Sumpitan's descriptions were so vivid and eloquently drawn that I came again and again to hear them. Sumpitan
struck me as a showman, eager for an audience. I knew he had an antiimmigrant, antiraja, anti-Tinombo axe to grind and he was delighted
I might immortalize his words in a book so he could promote Laujé
ritual and the Laujé olongian, because he felt the history about the immigrant raja had drowned out this more important news. I thought it
worthwhile to hear his version of the truth and then sort it out later.

Sumpitan emphasized that the Laujé in Dusunan were Muslims, but
they also were the keepers of Laujé regalia and philosophy centered on
birth spirits. In Sumpitan's rendition of history, the Laujé had lost their
power during the colonial period. All that remained were the regalia,
rituals, and philosophy of birth spirits, which were protected by the
olongian. All else, said Sumpitan, had been "stolen" by immigrant
"foreigners," the rajas from South Sulawesi, under the auspices of
Dutch colonialism beginning in 1905.[15]

Sumpitan taught me about the Laujé's original sovereign, the olongian (see Figure 1.4). The olongian had once offered spiritual and political protection for a string of subcourts on the river mouths to the
north and south of Dusunan. Sumpitan and others living near him in
Dusunan were descendants of officers in the once-flourishing olongian
court. Sumpitan and some of his neighbors were descendants of *tadulako*, a samurai-like warrior-prince. Other neighbors were descendants
of *jogugu*, the spokesperson and judge for the court. Still others were
descendants of the *kapitau dagaté*, the sea captain whose job it was
to interact with foreigners. Sumpitan said this once flourishing kingdom had been lost because of immigrant treachery. The olongian
should have become raja in the 1910s, and later again in the 1950s,
not outsiders.

Though today there is no raja, the last one having died in 1963,
there is still an olongian who carries out ritual duties in Dusunan, ostensibly for all Laujé. When I compared the former raja's palace in
Tinombo[16] to the olongian's in Dusunan, Sumpitan's point about the

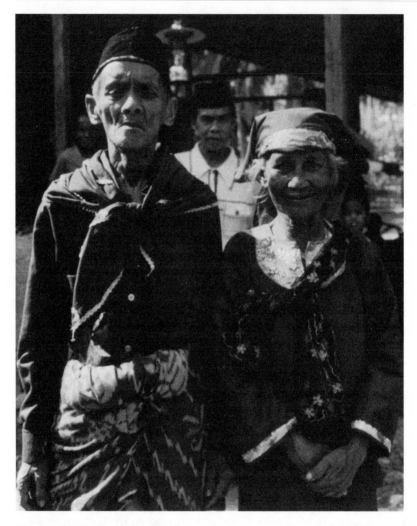

Figure 1.4.   Olongian and wife

two was clear. Though the olongian was the Laujé leader, his house
was no palace, as Sumpitan claimed it should be. Instead it was a half-
finished brick and cement structure with a tin roof and a partial wall.
The rest of his house was a roofed open-air porch. The olongian could
not afford to buy sufficient bricks to enclose the "parlor."[17] Ritual pro-
scriptions prohibit the olongian's family from farming or working the

fields given to them in office. They live through "tribute" given to them by their subjects, but this tribute is dwindling.[18] Sumpitan blamed descendants of the raja for stopping the tribute. He also blamed "foreigners" (the immigrant rajas) for confiscating other aristocrats' coconut trees and land, thereby preventing them from gaining the surplus needed to pay tribute to the olongian.

As Sumpitan portrayed history, the tensions between the Laujé of Dusunan and the immigrants of Tinombo were not just remote incidents in the past, but recent, divisive events. In 1982 two rather zealous bureaucrats from Tinombo had the audacity to ban an ancient curing ritual, the Laujé's main rite called the momasoro.[19] The Tinombo bureaucrats stated the rite undermined Islamic ideals in the community. Sumpitan was infuriated with the ban, viewing it as just one more immigrant plot designed to weaken the power of the olongian, since the olongian was the chief officiant of this ritual.[20] Sumpitan, uneducated in Islamic law, did not understand the complex religious and political motivations behind these reformist bureaucrats' dictates. Thus Sumpitan translated their actions in familiar terms: Immigrants or foreigners are enemies of the Laujé people.

When I met Sumpitan in June 1984, the immigrants had just instituted the ban eighteen months before. When I asked Sumpitan questions about the banned ceremony and the circumstances that led up to the ban, he could not recount the story in a calm, detached manner. This normally kind and collected man would begin to yell and swing his arms, venting his anger against the immigrants and the now dead raja. The more questions I asked about the rite, the more galvanized he became to reinstate it. In August 1984 Sumpitan, as a spokesperson for the Laujé, began to lobby the highest bureaucratic officials in Tinombo, asking for permission to enact the momasoro. Eventually the permission was granted.

A triumphant Sumpitan invited me to a reinstated momasoro beginning December 1984 and lasting through January 1985. By that time I had already begun fieldwork in the highland village of Taipaobal, but I eagerly accepted, even though I initially thought it tangential to my focus on mountain Laujé. I did not want to miss the "last opportunity" to see the rite that had created so much controversy. Little did I know I would discover that its emphasis on birth spirits was ultimately the same as I was studying in the mountains with "isolated" Laujé.

Under Sumpitan's leadership, the momasoro became a rite defining birth spirits in relation to his view about immigrant treachery against the Laujé people. As he explained it, the rite invited good Laujé birth spirits (umputé) and bad "foreign" or immigrant birth spirits into the house of the olongian for a weeklong ritual. Sumpitan choreographed the rite so that healing, "Laujé" spirits were in the most sacred ritual space, while pestilent "foreign" (immigrant) spirits were in another, more public arena. After feasting and praising the spirits for a week, the Laujé birth spirits were asked to stay in the community to heal people, making the animals, rivers, and fields fertile. The "foreign" spirits were asked to leave the community to rid it of illness and pestilence. Symbolic offerings to these "foreign" spirits were placed in a boat and sent out to sea. By casting out the boat with the pestilent "foreigners," Sumpitan's version of the ritual rectified the wrongs in his everyday world. Metaphorically, Sumpitan rid the Laujé community of the immigrants who had usurped power from the olongian. I later found out that this same kind of social delineation between "us" and "them" figured in Siamae Sanji's depictions of the highland world of birth spirits (see George 1996).[21]

Meeting the Mountain Laujé: Siamae Sanji and His Kin

As I said before, my initial goal was colored by the romance of finding an "untouched community." I wanted to find a highland fieldwork site and leave the lowlands as soon as possible. I worked for several months in Tinombo with my Laujé language instructor, Pak Husin, but also made attempts to meet highlanders who came down to the weekly markets.[22] Having arrived in Tinombo in May, I had to wait until August before the rains stopped and I could cross the flooded streams leading to the mountains. Through discussions with missionaries and a few brief encounters with highlanders at market and at the doctor's house, I decided I would visit Sinalutan and Taipaobal and any villages in between, making my decision about a highland research spot after my visits.[23]

Toward the end of August, Pak Husin, Eric, and I set out for Taipaobal. Taipaobal is about fifteen very steep kilometers from the coast. The trail follows the course of the river that divides Tinombo from Dusunan, crossing it a dozen times. From the last river crossing to Taipaobal, the trail reaches almost straight up. As it rises, it wends through forests and then into a grasslands area (called the bald *gio*).[24] Taipaobal is above the grasslands, comprised of a string of bamboo stilt-houses situated on the spine and flanks of a sharp ridgeline stretching for two or three miles. Taipaobal ends at the forest's edge.

Like Tinombo, Taipaobal is a frontier of sorts. It is the westernmost (and therefore the farthest inland) community of the nominally Islamic Laujé. As an Islamic community, Taipaobal is oriented to the lowlands. I was told it was one of the few highland communities that is directly under the sphere of influence of the Indonesian government. (I later found out there were many communities that had more recently come under the protective umbrella of the government, but Taipaobal was the first mountain community to do so). Taipaobal's community spokesperson reports directly to the lowland mayor of Lombok, who serves as the leader for all the mountain communities. Taipaobal reaps some benefits from this association with the lowland government. Aside from a school built in 1983 and a bamboo mosque built in 1970, it is the beneficiary of occasional government "money-making" or "development schemes."[25] These may or may not have a lasting effect on the community's prosperity.[26] Like the mosque, such schemes usually generate considerable initial enthusiasm and are proudly discussed by the villagers, only to dwindle in popularity after a few months or years.

Taipaobal is arguably the most "modern" highland community, but despite community members' willingness to "progress," many Taipaobal Laujé are still somewhat hesitant about completely embracing lowland life and people. When I decided Taipaobal could be a potential field site, Pak Husin felt it his duty to guide us into the mountains, afraid the Taipaobal Laujé would be too reticent toward strangers such as us, despite their contact with lowlanders. We hiked the first day to Polumelee, spent the night there with an imam Pak Husin knew, and woke up early the next morning to hike up to Taipaobal. When we arrived, I realized Pak Husin had been right, for no one spoke to us. In fact all doors were shut to our questions about where we could find water for our parched throats. Luckily, someone recognized Pak Husin and began speaking to him through the neatly woven bamboo walls of a tall hut on stilts perched on the edge of a cliff. The person, Siamae Sanji, was a friend of Husin's father and had known Husin (who was sixty-eight years old) when Husin was a young boy. We were invited into Siamae Sanji's house and formally introduced to the oldest living man of the mountains. Siamae Sanji had no teeth, was intermittently deaf, could barely walk, but his mind was still sharp (see Atkinson 1989).

Husin told us that Siamae Sanji was one of the most renowned healers in the Laujé mountains. As a contemporary of Husin's father, he must have been roughly 100 years old. Siamae Sanji had been one of the first highlanders to convert to Islam, having learned his Islam from the immigrant raja in Tinombo. Siamae Sanji also had acted as a community leader, convincing many people to stay in Taipaobal and accept colonial authority in the 1920s rather than run off in fear to the mountains of Sinalutan.[27] His Islamic beliefs did not conflict with his power as a sando, or shaman; in fact, those beliefs allowed him to travel in two worlds: He was a healer for many of the lowland Muslims and for the animist highlanders. Four of Siamae Sanji's adult children by his second wife were still unmarried and at home, learning their father's animist prayers and cures that continued despite his Muslim faith. Sair, Larsen, Zhairudden, and Idola were excited that we were considering moving to Taipaobal, and we felt excited by their intelligence and enthusiasm, and the knowledge of traditional culture they had gained from their father. They all knew a little Indonesian, something unusual for highlanders, so when my embryonic Laujé failed I could work out a translation with them through Indonesian.

Despite these promising aspects, I still had some misgivings about Taipaobal as a field site. One misgiving was a practical one: Water was scarce. More important, though, Taipaobal seemed a little less "primitive" than I had imagined my field site to be. Though lowlanders had told me that Taipaobalers were only "shallow Muslims," they did have a new imam, who had moved up from the lowlands. I feared that this new reform imam might introduce more strict adherence to Muslim ideals such as observing fasting and relinquishing traditional rites. Moreover, the men and boys scattered around the schoolyard seemed vaguely similar to the lowland Laujé. Many wore long polyester pants just like lowlanders, and most had short-cropped hair. A few even carried boom boxes, radios they had bought from profits selling goats on the west coast of the peninsula. In short, these were not the long-haired, isolated, and blowgun-carrying animists with whom I had planned to work. We left, but Eric and I made plans to return and visit Sinalutan deeper into the mountains. Siamae Sanji's son Sair agreed to be our guide.

A week later, Eric and I returned, but we found Sair reluctant to make definite plans for our trip to Sinalutan. He finally admitted he thought it dangerous. He and his siblings said the Sinalutan dwellers were *bela,* a term first translated to me in positive terms as meaning trade partner. Later I learned it meant many pejorative things like hillbilly, animist, uncouth, and primitive.[28] They said Sinalutan dwellers were "wild," as likely to kill and maim as to be friendly. Since I had heard Tinomboers call the people of Taipaobal bela, and since they seemed quite sedate and modern to me, I was not dissuaded by Sair, Larsen, and Idola's assertions. I had learned from lowlanders that the Sinalutan leader, Siamae Tubag, was a distant cousin of Siamae Sanji's. He had moved to Sinalutan from Taipaobal in the 1920s when the colonial government forced all highland Laujé to resettle in the lowlands. People who lived in Sinalutan thus represented the defiant separatists, those in Taipaobal the acquiescent joiners. I was anxious to see if I could find more "authentic" Laujé in Sinalutan than I had in Taipaobal, but I couldn't go there without Sair as my guide. Sair feared the "radical" separatists in Sinalutan would harm me or him and worried when I insisted I would go on my own to visit Siamae Tubag. Reluctantly, Sair accompanied Eric and me to "dangerous Sinalutan." Eric and I planned to spend the night and be welcomed into Siamae Tubag's house as guests of Siamae Sanji. Sair's plan was a bit different. My notes on the experience are as follows:

> Somewhere in the middle of the path when we were finally nearing our destination, Sair stopped in mid-stride. . . . A young man with just a loin cloth on, several tattoos on his cheeks and upper lip,[29] a cloth headband around his long black hair hanging to his lower back, and a very long blowgun in hand stepped out of the bush. Sair still didn't move. Eric and I followed Sair's stony cues. The young man with the blowgun circled us, saying nothing. I said "Siamae Tubag." Finally the young man replied "follow me."
>
> Sair was frightened and though I sensed that the fellow with the blowgun had been frightened himself, he seemed to have accepted us as unthreatening, curious "objects" to bring to the village and ogle with his buddies. But Sair's fear and prejudice were contagious. Through Sair's eyes, I also saw them as he did: savage and dangerous, human, but barely. We entered a cleared knoll alive with music, *tadeko* music, a locally made wooden xylophone. The houses were totally different from those in Taipaobal. Here were only lean-to's, houses made from scraps of fallen palm leaves, matted and propped up against a stump. Some "houses" looked like squirrel's nests perched among the trees on bamboo poles.

The children came to us first. Many of them were bald, or had thin strands of red, not black, hair. Some had cloudy eyes. Their diet must have very little fruit in it, I thought. All had the symptoms of worms, bloated stomachs. Their faces were decorated with blue and red tattoos, a few wore geometric tattoos as moustaches. In my broken Laujé I asked them where their fields were. Sair, crouched in a corner, smoking a cigarette and far from the curiosity seekers. He replied in his broken Indonesian, unintelligible to these people "they don't plant here, they just gather root crops." I saw a few scraggly corn plants here and there, so doubted Sair's prejudiced explanation.[30] Soon we were hustled into a mud and palm lean-to, the home of Siamae Tubag. I offered Siamae Tubag tobacco and watched as his young wife roasted an ear of corn in a fire in the dirt. I looked around for cooking utensils. I saw not a single metal spoon or cooking pot in the whole room. The cloths the women wore were the same cheap batik so popular in Taipaobal, but the bright pink and green patterns were dulled to a solid muddy green from the filth and grime of constant use. These people are really far away from the lowland markets, I thought. They don't grow cash crops to buy the commodities the Taipaobalers do. These people are truly isolated. They'd be great to work with if I could handle the logistics. I looked over at Sair who was unusually quiet and sulking. I found myself irritated with him, he's letting his prejudices against the bela get in the way of introducing us. He's shirking his duties now when I need him most. I began to speak to Siamae Tubag instead of relying on Sair. I tried to say that we had come to visit him because we had heard he was an important and respected man. We wanted to sit at his knees and would be honored if he would teach us something. I don't know what he heard since I was still far from proficient in the Laujé language. It seemed as if he responded in a harsh manner for a Laujé host. "Your language is the language of foreigners of the lowlands. I will not speak with you." All eyes turned toward me. I wasn't sure I had heard right. Siamae Tubag sat there with his palms pointed skyward, a gesture of conciliation, asking forgiveness from Allah or the gods. His gesture was apologetic, but his words, as I understood them, were far from conciliatory. I looked at Sair. Sair was reaching into my day pack to search for another wad of tobacco. He hurriedly placed it in front of Siamae Tubag and stood up, as best he could in the lean-to, and began to make apologies for leaving. I followed suit. I nodded and smiled, using my most honorific Laujé to say goodbye (again, probably a mistake since this was the language of the olongian in the lowlands and not of the highlands) and followed Sair backing out, the polite way to exit a hut. Siamae Tubag called after us "when you speak like a human, then we can talk." I wondered if that was what he had said before and wished I could trust Sair to give me an unbiased translation. Sair, though, was already down the knoll and into the dark forest. The three of us dog-trotted down the ridgeline, too breathless to speak. It was not until a remarkably speedy three hours later, when we arrived at Siamae Sanji's house, that we relaxed somewhat, ate, and fell into an exhausted sleep. When we woke up the next day, Sair told his version of our misadventures in Sinalutan to his siblings. As Sair told it, the threats of Siamae Tubag and the blowgun seemed more ominous than I remembered. Sair retold Siamae Tubag's parting words thusly: "Your language is the language of the foreigners of the lowlands. It is the language of animals. We kill animals and eat them."

The room was silent. Sair's sister Idola broke the silent tension with a joke. "Remember it's not *Sina*lutan, it's *Ghina*lutan." Her imitation of the lispy dialect difference just two peaks over from Taipaobal made everybody laugh. Zhairuddin, Sair's younger brother, expressed the opinion most people in the room held. In a venomous snarl, almost spitting out the words, Zhairuddin said: "They're bela. They're cannibals. They're dirty and eat pig that's rotten with maggots. The people who live in Babong and Gianang marry bela women . . . but we don't! Their women are lazy and dirty. They don't know how to cook rice. . . . You can't trust bela, they lie; they practice sorcery. You are better off here."

It was this experience and the contagious prejudice against bela that determined I would work in Taipaobal, not in a bela community. It was not until a year later that I came to understand the experience in Sinalutan. The man with the blowgun showed up at my house one day. My notes are as follows:

The short tattooed man from Sinalutan, the man with the blowgun, coughed at my door today [a cough is a Laujé version of a knock]. I walked out expecting a neighbor requesting aspirin or worm medicine. To my surprise it was that same man. I looked at him from my veranda, he still tentatively on the ground waiting to be invited in. I nodded my head [a friendly gesture]. He nodded back and said, "do you remember me?" "Yes." I invited him up on the porch. He removed his machete and climbed up. The man (I never found out his name) asked again. "Do you remember me? From Sinalutan?" "Yes" I said. I remember. We both chuckled nervously. "I almost killed you," he said. A long pregnant pause ensued. "I was really scared. I thought you all were Dutch." Another pause. "I've heard from my sister-in-law who lives over there (he pointed to a nearby house) that you give medicine and speak mountain Laujé. My wife has malaria. . . ."

I gave him medicine, a cup of coffee, some leftover rice and taro and shared some cigarettes with him. Afterwards I asked him about that day in

Sinalutan. "What did Siamae Tubag say to me?" "He said you spoke like a lowlander and he couldn't understand you. (Long pause). Now you speak a little better. We can understand you like we understand a child. (Long pause). You don't sound like *them*."

In this encounter I realized several things about my first meeting in Sinalutan. Though I had convinced myself otherwise, I had been subtly persuaded by Sair's prejudice that the bela would aggressively harm me for no reason. Now that I understood that they had feared me and had their own prejudices about Westerners, I knew they might have harmed me had I been aggressive myself, but not without provocation. I learned that I was extremely susceptible to local prejudices and that the anthropologist is not the only one who has stereotypes about the other. Moreover, the divisions I believed existed between the bela community of Sinalutan and this community were less obvious than they were that first day. Not only did this fellow speak without a distinct lisp (as Sair's sister had implied), but he had close kin who lived in Taipaobal. I had wanted a "primitive" "untouched" community to work in because my classic anthropological training taught me each community would be culturally distinct from the other. In retrospect I know there are no cultural boundaries. Ideas, products, and people flow in and out of a variety of communities. Now I know the boundaries between Sinalutan and Taipaobal were just as blurred as between highlands and lowlands.

When I first returned from Sinalutan, though, Sair and his siblings' comments about the "cannibals" in Sinalutan bothered me, but logistically I knew I could not easily work in a place like Sinalutan. I was already a friend of Siamae Sanji's family and Siamae Sanji himself was the kind of informant I had always fantasized (rather romantically) about finding. Here was the true wise old man of the mountains. I decided, then and there, I would sacrifice one of my romantic notions, that of living in the bush with truly isolated highlanders, for the romance of working with the oldest sando, or healer, in the hills. I would live here and learn as much as I could from this wonderfully kind (to me at least) family.

When Eric and I asked permission to build a house in Taipaobal, lowlanders seemed relieved that I was definitely going to settle in Taipaobal. They thought it was safer there, the people more civilized, saying that some of their ancestors had come from Taipaobal. I knew they were right, but at the time this still nagged me. Lowlanders have too much influence over the people in Taipaobal, I thought, and it will be difficult to distinguish what is Laujé and what is coastal Indonesian since Taipaobalers seem to copy lowland style of dress and covet the same material objects—radios, lipsticks, watches, and long pants—as they do. At that time I still thought the lowland Laujé "culture," totally Islamic and likely to overwhelm highland animist culture. I thought, wrongly, that highland "culture" was more passive. It could be distinguished from lowland "culture," which would actively annihilate highland belief. Eric's journal notes concerning our return to Taipaobal with the village chief from Lombok, Pak Kiango (under whose jurisdiction were all the mountain Laujé), conveys the ambivalences and prejudices we both had at that time.

The first day we returned, resting at the Taipaobal school I was struck by how much Taipaobal felt like an Native American reservation.[31] The school yard was a crown of polished packed brown earth high above the village, looking both to the sea in the eastern distance and the high mountains in the west. Beyond lay row upon row of mountains, clouds pouring over them, pushed by a strong wind. The mountains, dark, cold, reassuring like rocks washed by waves on the seashore. It was late afternoon, the children gathered in silent clumps, hair blowing across a cheek in the wind. Standing like statues keeping their distance, each wrapped in a colored cloth as rich in possibility as the mountains beyond. Floral patterns, bright pinks and iridescent greens. The visual complement to the pewter, deep cobalt and grey of the mountains and cold sky. The school looked solid. White. A modern structure reminding us that this was a reservation and that the ceremonies that have flattened and polished the earth in front of it are imported and new—the *modero*[32] dances from the Bare'e of Lake Poso area, the *takra* games from the Bugis of South Sulawesi, the *kongtau* martial arts from Java and the kickball of Indonesian school children. It is not the ancestors' feet that have packed and smoothed this earth, it's the feet of the modern Laujé.

There was a certain passivity in the way the children stared at us yet kept their distance. This was their turf, yet they made no moves to assert their claim on it. We were there; they moved out of our way and took up places at some distance quietly watching, waiting passively for us to leave so they could continue their games on the cleared crown of earth. The passivity of a stereotypical reservation Indian, I thought. We already knew that Taipaobal was more "modern" than most of the mountain Laujé communities. It had a school and a mosque. We expected it to be sort of like a reservation with the wild Indians still living in the forests in the mountains below the clouds.

. . . Passivity. We've noticed how the people here take government de-
cree with passive acceptance. Little or no resistance. Jennifer and I came to
Taipaobal with the lowland chief. He decreed that a house should be built
for us "near the school"; near the path to Gianang and Babong further in
the hills (we had told him we wanted to be as centrally located as possible).
We squatted with him and twenty or so of the heads of households in Taipaobal. All were silent, but the chief who talked and talked. He had a sore
tooth and asked us for aspirin which we duly gave. The chief was exercis-
ing his prerogatives. A young man with a prince valiant haircut passed by
and the chief called out to him, "Isn't that your field over above the
school?" The young man nodded, his body frozen in mid-stride. "These
people want to build a house in your field is that okay?" He nodded again
and was allowed to go. The chief chatted on. "Well, its settled. You'll build
your house in that field. It's a perfect spot." He looked at the other men
and received unanimous nods of assent.

A week later, when we returned without the chief, Sair, Larsen and
Zhairuddin, who would help us build the house, "suggested" we might
build "closer to them." "It's better here; you'll be close to us; we can help
you fetch water and we are your friends. Up by the school we'll hardly
have a chance to visit you." Later they let it be known that the young man
with the prince valiant haircut had wanted to plant corn in his field. A
house would get in the way. But who was he to publicly turn down the request of the chief?

So our house in Taipaobal (see Figure 1.5) was built right next to Siamae Sanji's. We settled in our little bamboo hut with stilts on October
5, 1984, right after Siamae Sanji consecrated it with a house-blessing
ceremony (see Figure 1.6). At night, as adopted members of Siamae
Sanji's family, we gathered at his house (since he was too old to walk
to ours) huddled around the low glow of flickering oil lamps. We listened as Siamae Sanji talked about the past and about umputé spirits.

Like Sumpitan, Siamae Sanji viewed the umputé spirits through the
lens of his social, historical narratives. In Siamae Sanji's narratives,
though, he did not mention evil immigrants; he focused on women as
the evil "other." In narrative after narrative, Siamae Sanji told how
bela women had caused Taipaobal men to neglect their families and
move away. He also felt that Taipaobal women who married lowlanders were bad. In one narrative, a Taipaobal woman, the niece of the
olongian seven generations ago, married a lowland immigrant. She
took the regalia of the olongian with her when she converted to Islam.
From this time until the present, Siamae Sanji lamented that the office

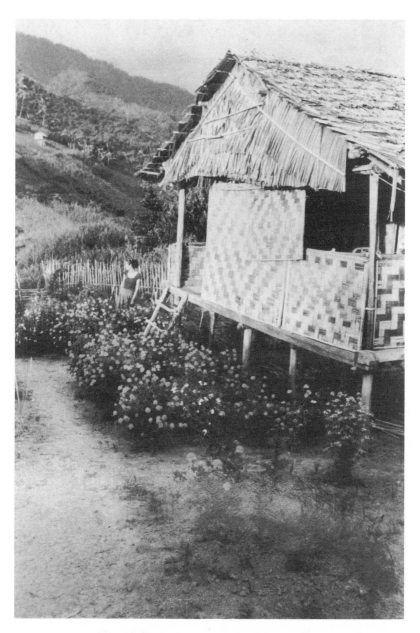

Figure 1.5. Our house in Taipaobal

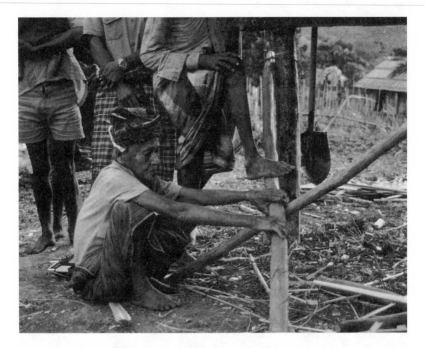

Figure 1.6.   Siamae Sanji at our house-blessing ceremony

of the olongian was traced through the female line rather than the
male line.[33] The lowlanders refused to send their daughters to marry
highland men, because lowlanders were now Islamic and highlanders
were not. Siamae Sanji complained that the descendants of the olongian, related to Taipaobalers through the female (uterine) line, had
never reforged the unity engendered by the split.

Besides narrating histories, Siamae Sanji also performed rituals and
taught me and his children how to present the offerings and to utter
prayers to the umputé spirits. In various rituals Siamae Sanji divided
into structurally opposed categories the disease-bearing "black" spirits from the healing "white" spirits. He characterized the illness-
causing spirits as female, "neglectful," "wild and unpredictable," "like
bela." He opposed these spirits to the healing spirits he characterized
as "male," "gentle and nurturing," "like a father." As I came to understand the spiritual world populated with two kinds of umputé spirits, I began to understand how the spirits' characteristics coincided
with the characteristics of Siamae Sanji's social world.

Siamae Sanji believed one kind of birth spirit (black umputé) caused illness. He characterized this spirit as female. Siamae Sanji carried the offerings symbolizing female birth spirits out of the house to cure the people in the house from disease. This was similar to the way Sumpitan had cast out the so-called foreign birth spirits (red and black umputé) in boats so as to rid the lowlands of disease. Both men's interpretations of spiritual illness were analogies of their cures for social illness. Their interpretations of umputé spirits referred to social history and the problems engendered by social fission (see George 1996).

A Year Later: Death and Community Response

My research with Siamae Sanji as my mentor continued alongside my research with Sumpitan. Though I had initially intended to focus my research on the highlands, we never gave up the lease on the house in Tinombo, using it as a lowland base to replenish supplies, receive mail, maintain contacts with government officials, find out what was happening with my friends in Tinombo and Dusunan, and ask Sumpitan about the interesting parallels and oppositions between his ideas and those of Siamae Sanji. Eric and I had become fairly good hikers, making the trek from Tinombo to Taipaobal, which once took two days in only four hours. We traveled back and forth between communities, even receiving permission from Sumpitan to carry cassette recordings of possessed spirits in the momasoro ritual to the highlands so Siamae Sanji and his children (see Figure 1.7) could help us transcribe them. Since Siamae Sanji and his children were so fluent in the antiquated spirits' language spoken on the tapes, they were perfect assistants. Their knowledge of spirit speech, of who the mediums were who were possessed by spirits, and of who audience members were whose voices appeared on the tape, indicated how open the communication of ideas was between highlands and lowlands.

It was a full six months after the first spirit possession rite, the momasoro, during the beginning of the month of Muslim fasting, Ramadan, that Siamae Sanji fell into a coma after a stroke. He died three days later. His death was a sad event—he was greatly loved—but it was not a tragedy, considering his age and the suffering brought on by his failing health. Because Siamae Sanji died an old man, locals say his long life meant he was blessed by the spirits. His children continued to practice what he had preached and even though soon after Siamae

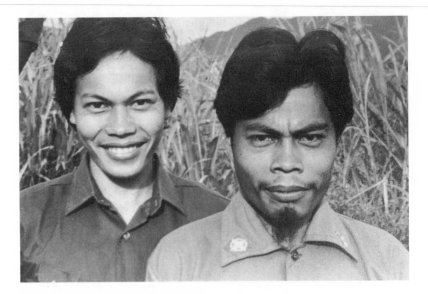

Figure 1.7.   Larsen and Sair, two of Siamae Sanji's sons

Sanji's death, another well-respected healer, Siamae Balitangan, came to pay his respects to the children. Balitangan told us that the olongian had always been female. His statement unwittingly contradicted Siamae Sanji, yet Siamae Sanji's children never interpreted the alternative explanation as a threat to their father's visionary legacy.

Not so with Sumpitan; Sumpitan died suddenly a week after Siamae Sanji. Sumpitan's death was a shocking tragedy. He had repaired his fence that morning and gone to mosque that night, keeling over with what the doctor said was a heart attack. Sumpitan, seemingly in good health, died prematurely in his fifties. Many people interpreted his death as a negative omen sent by the spirits. Sumpitan also died childless. After his death there was no one able or willing to convince people that Sumpitan's version of "the truth" was right. Thus many in the community distanced themselves from Sumpitan's eloquent arguments, even though these same people had wholeheartedly endorsed Sumpitan when he was alive.

The deaths of Sumpitan and Siamae Sanji and the concomitant interpretations arising in opposition to these two men demonstrated not only that alternative, fragmentary explanations existed in the local domain (something a postmodernist might say), but that Sumpitan and Siamae Sanji had been, until their deaths, persuasive unifiers. It was they who had convinced people that umputé meant what they said it did.

After their deaths, Siamae Sanji's visionary legacy continued, while Sumpitan's disappeared. Many new people came to me in the lowlands to give me an alternative to Sumpitan's interpretation, but not one of the new interpreters was able to persuade and unify the community, as Sumpitan had, by convincing everyone that their vision was right. Everyone seemed to have their own idiosyncratic take on umputé. The only common theme I could see at the time was that they all critiqued Sumpitan's ideas. Gradually, however, as I listened over and over to more of these critiques, a pattern slowly emerged. Elites, like the wife of the olongian and a man I call the Haji, blurred Sumpitan's sharp distinctions between immigrants and locals, bad umputé spirits and good ones. In general, these elites tended to use umputé as a symbol and as a metaphor. They were more likely to divide its parts into binary categories and relate them to the social world. Commoners tended to focus on the unifying aspects of umputé. Female spirit mediums, like Siinai Alasan, saw umputé as an indivisible gestalt, while male healers, like the self-assured Siamae Balitangan, tended to question whether spirits were really possessing mediums or whether the mediums were faking the possession. Both Siinai Alasan and Siamae Balitangan emphasized that spirits are not like people and should not be characterized as such. To characterize the spirit world as though it is comprised of individual people would be to "get away from the purpose of worship."

Nevertheless, commoners and elites alike tended to interpret umputé in terms of, and in response to, their own perception of what Islam was. In general then, though these people were members of a group with loosely shared common experiences, they were interpreting umputé as individuals, and thus idiosyncratically. It is this individuality, as well as this loosely shared pattern resembling a collective representation, that I am trying to convey in this book. I am also trying to show how particular people, like Siamae Sanji and especially Sumpitan, with their eloquent, collective political visions, can persuade whole generations of people to believe those visions. After they die, that elusive but coherent idea can also die with them.

2

SIBLING RIVALRY
Competing Histories

Before Siamae Sanji and Sumpitan taught me about the spirit world, the world of umputé, each man, without knowledge of the other, began the process of telling me local histories. Their mutual interest in the past was meant to explain present-day Laujé affairs; thus, it was intertwined with their notions of collective Laujé identity. Siamae Sanji's historical narratives about highland Taipaobal and Sumpitan's about Dusunan, depicted a more glorious past, which was now in decline vis-à-vis neighboring communities. Sumpitan's and Siamae Sanji's historical narratives explained the causes for this decline, repeatedly depicting incidents in which people and groups wrongly separated themselves from their communities, creating social decline in the process. By analogy, they referred these historical separators to the illness-causing aspects of umputé.

In Sumpitan's history it was foreigners who split highland from lowland communities and severed the unity of the Islamic olongian's sovereign rule. In Siamae Sanji's history it was women who married outsiders in non-Muslim, bela communities, or in lowland Muslim villages, dividing kin from the Taipaobal homeland. At the heart of each man's historical narrative was a claim about religious affiliation and ethnic identity. In order to make claims about their own moral community, each man used narratives about evil others, Muslims, immigrants (regarded as foreigners) or non-Muslims (bela), who stood outside their respective communities. Both men pointed their accusatory fingers toward lowland culture. Siamae Sanji found the lowlanders in Dusunan reprehensible, while Sumpitan, a Dusunaner himself, found the lowland life of Tinombo reprehensible. On the one hand, lowland life represented all they desired for their own communities, and on the other hand, it represented all that they wished their own communities to avoid.

Since the turn of the twentieth century, Tinombo had embodied the essence of progressive lowland life; its status as an economic and religious center rose and overshadowed Taipaobal's and Dusunan's status as superior communities. Dusunan was once the home of the Laujé divine ruler and the only Laujé Muslims. Mountain Laujé once looked to Dusunan and the olongian for spiritual and religious guidance, paying the olongian tribute. Once the Dutch brought the immigrant raja to the area, the tribute payments were officially banned. Highlanders had to pay tribute to the raja. Highland attention refocused on Tinombo and the raja. The raja, in turn, began to proselytize against animism and syncretism in rites headed by the olongian. The raja taught reform Islam to eager converts like Siamae Sanji, further separating highland Laujé from lowland Laujé.

Divisions not only existed between lowlanders, but between highlanders, too. From the 1930s to the 1970s, Taipaobal was the home of the only mountaineers with knowledge of a world religion, but in the 1970s that changed. Many bela began to convert to Christianity (through missionization once based in Tinombo).[1] Other bela learned Islam from the Tinombo-trained imam who moved to the village above Taipaobal in the late 1970s. Thus Siamae Sanji's community was no longer the only one with a respectable world religion, and Sumpitan's community, Dusunan, was no longer the only one with a religious and political leader.

To counter this change in status, Siamae Sanji and Sumpitan, both eloquent spokespersons, reconstituted history. They accused others of bringing on social decline. Sumpitan accused the immigrants in Tinombo of destroying the olongian, and Siamae Sanji accused the bela and the olongian of neglecting the "true traditions."[2] By claiming to follow the true and enduring Laujé moral "traditions," each man claimed their community was an innocent witness to the moral decay all around them. They did this to explain a decline that, because it resulted from historical mistakes, could be rectified.

Sumpitan's Narratives: The Good Laujé and the Bad Foreigners

On my first visit with Sumpitan, he told me his father had been imprisoned for hitting (slapping) Raja Borman in the 1920s. It took me a while to make sense of that story and the many other stories Sumpitan told me in urgent, subversive tones when I went with Pak Husin to visit him. His chronicles would shift back and forth between the mythological past, the recent personal past, and present-day politics. The narratives are provided below, but rather than presenting them in the jumbled order in which they were given to me, I have rearranged them chronologically from beginning to end, so that the narratives flow rhetorically. On the one hand, I worry that this rearrangement violates the native voice, but on the other hand, as a cultural broker, I am willing to make the sacrifice for the sake of clarity.

In Sumpitan's stories, the Laujé court in Dusunan existed as a sovereign and indigenous polity until the arrival of the Dutch in the early twentieth century. Sumpitan's version of creation claimed that the Laujé were created first and, therefore, were superior to the immigrants, "the foreigners," who were created afterward:

> The earth was once one giant androgynous body. But it was pregnant and needed a "door" through which the fetus could exit. So, Allah cut the male genitals off the androgynous body. That body became a female and developed into earth and fresh water. From the body of this female, the first child in the world, a Laujé child, was born.
>
> Allah took the bloody male organs he had cut off the androgynous body and threw them into the air. This created the sun and the sky. But the sun born from the male genitals could not stay up in the sky all the time, just as a male's penis cannot stay erect all the time. So, the sun was forced to rise and fall every day, sinking to its resting place in the center of the sea.[3] At the center of the sea, at a much later time, after the Laujé were a populous and civilized people born from the mother earth, foreigners were created from the male genitals. First the Bugis and Mandar, then the Chinese, and then all the others [were born]. That is why the sea and foreigners are violent. They are born of blood. Their home is a temporary place and not permanent. The earth, though, is the place of the olongian. It is the female earth from which we were born. It gives us our food, nurturing, and continuity.

In Sumpitan's myth, blood and immigrants, whom he called foreigners, were associated with the sky, the sun, and the sea (where the sun arose). Sumpitan told me that the sea was a bad place, a place of turmoil and death. He categorized all things good—land, superiority, peace, permanence—with things Laujé, while categorizing all things bad—sea, inferiority, violence, temporality—with things foreign:

> Originally all Laujé people lived in the mountains because they were afraid of the evil "foreign" pirates from the center of the sea. All Laujé people, in-

cluding the olongian, lived in Taipaobal where the "Inscribed Stone" (Polu Irandu) was. This stone marked the spot from which the first Laujé humans emerged. Some Laujé who lived in the mountains would occasionally go to the lowland seashore. There they would make salt. But often the people going to make salt were captured by evil foreign pirates—the *pengayo*, or the *pagoraé*. Some of the pirates were the Mandar. Others were the To Belo. They took our people as slaves, or they killed them. Our ancestors were afraid so they lived in the mountains and did not go to shore unless they had no more salt. It wasn't until our olongian converted to Islam that we had the power to fight off the pirates and live on the shore.

According to Sumpitan, the olongian's conversion and move to the lowlands occurred when the bride, who later became an olongian, asked an imam to officiate at her wedding. Sumpitan claims that for their wedding Allah gave them and all the Laujé, people Islam. No human being, no "foreigner" introduced Islam to us, "we were chosen as special people by the prophet."

Sumpitan portrayed the period when the olongian moved to the lowlands and converted to Islam as a time of peace and prosperity for the Laujé, until the Dutch brought foreigners, for example, Bugis and Mandar immigrants, back to Laujé shores. Dusunan, he said, was the court of an independent Laujé kingdom until 1904 (see Figure 2.1). "It was a Muslim kingdom; the imams came from the same family as the olongian." The court was elaborate and hierarchical with the olongian at the pinnacle. In the old days the olongian was assisted by various titled nobles, each with specific duties appropriate to their title. "Foreign traders also lived on Laujé shores, but their compounds were far from Tinombo. They were in Moutong." The Laujé olongian gave them permission to settle in Moutong and they stayed there only at Laujé sufferance.[4] The Dusunaners had little to do with these foreigners.[5]

Soon, however, said Sumpitan, those Bugis Mandar "foreigners" created turmoil in our peaceful environment:[6]

In 1901 there was strife in the Tomini Bay when distant kin of the dying raja of Moutong resisted the Dutch choice for a new raja of Moutong. The Dutch sent in troops to flatten the people who resisted the Dutch choice for raja. Many people from Laujé communities all along the Tomini Bay, including some Laujé here in Dusunan, supported the resisters against the Dutch. [Others supported the Dutch choice for raja]. It turned into a big war. Brother was fighting against brother, cousin against cousin, father against son. It was a catastrophe. Our olongian said we must have peace or

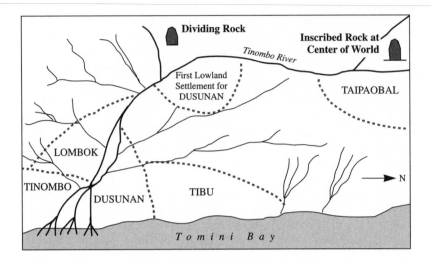

Figure 2.1.   Laujé settlements and points of reference

we would have no descendants left. So she offered her own daughter in marriage to the Dutch choice for raja of Moutong. Then the fighting had to stop.

When I asked Sumpitan the name of the raja, he replied, "he was a Bugis man named Daeng Malino." When I then asked the name of the Laujé woman, the daughter of the olongian who had married Daeng Malino, Sumpitan could not recall it. Neither could the descendants of Daeng Malino recall the name of any Laujé woman who had married the raja. I checked the "ancient" genealogy chart Sumpitan had shown me before and could not find such a marriage listed. This gap in normally well-recalled knowledge leads me to believe Sumpitan fabricated the first raja's marriage to the daughter of an olongian to make a rhetorical point. Sumpitan wished to depict the Laujé as sacrificing themselves and their ethnic purity for the sake of peace. Sumpitan's history blamed the resisters for the brutal Dutch war and the deaths of Laujé soldiers. His history lauded the olongian as a central figure in settling the wars of resistance.

Once Daeng Malino became raja, with the backing of the Dutch, Sumpitan explained the Laujé's adjustment to colonial rule in fairly general terms:

The olongian's daughter married the Bugis man, who became raja. Their "palace" was moved from Moutong to Tinombo.[7] The Dutch began building a modern port—with warehouses, office buildings, and schools. Our Laujé ancestors, being parents-in-law to the raja, had inherited an empire. Soon, though, our ancestors in Dusunan found out how it really was. They could not use their connections. Our noble Laujé ancestors found they had no voice at court. No influence over the Dutch. They couldn't communicate with the Dutch.

See, our ancestors, they were ignorant. They were uneducated. In the early days of colonialism, they did not know any other language than Laujé. The Dutch spoke Malay [now Indonesian].[8] The Bugis, Mandar, and Kaili immigrants knew Malay. They were better able than our Laujé ancestors to tell the Dutch what they wanted. Our ancestors could not say anything. They were quiet. Then, to make things worse, other immigrants— Javanese, Torajans, Ambonese, Arabs, and Chinese—began to move to Tinombo. With all those Malay speakers, no one heard our ancestors speak.

As more Malay speakers swelled the town's population, these people, rather than Laujé, became the backbone of the rajadom. Sumpitan explained that the Laujé waited patiently, hoping their turn would come when the raja's son, a half-Laujé boy, grew up and inherited his father's throne. When Daeng Malino died, however, the Dutch chose the raja's distant relative, a Mandar man named Borman (after a German sea captain entering port during his birth). Raja Borman could speak Malay whereas the Laujé prince could not. Moreover, at least according to Sumpitan, Borman and his relatives bribed the Dutch so that Borman would be selected.[9] Sumpitan said it was at this point, in the 1910s, that the Laujé began to realize they had no access to power, no voice at court.

Sumpitan spoke bitterly about that period of history. He and others regarded the new raja from South Sulawesi, Raja Borman, as a "foreigner," and they vehemently resented this man's power over what they considered their own affairs. Raja Borman, they said, was a usurper who was morally weak and self-indulgent (c.f. Anderson 1972; Geertz 1980):[10]

That raja was such a gambler that he would not only gamble on cards, dominoes and cock-fights, but also on turtle races. He would even bet people as to which lizard could climb a wall fastest. He would bet on little things. Also on big things. He kept horses, in the field where the lower Lombok school is now. He raced them. On Queen Wilhelmina's birthday[11] . . . he would gamble a whole year's salary. The store owners were afraid of him. They let him charge things on credit when he ran out of money. But he went too far.

Once, he was gambling with the head of the Tomini District, one of his underlings. He had run out of money and wanted to keep in the game—it was a game of poker. So, he knew the head of the Tomini District had fancied a beautiful young Laujé girl, the daughter of one of the Dusunan nobles. But, he had been refused her hand in marriage. So, the raja said, "I'll give you the Laujé girl, if I can keep in the game."

Just like that! He made one of our daughters a slave! Well, that raja was not only self-indulgent, he didn't have the power to win a simple card game. He lost that girl to the head of the Tomini District. When he came to get her, we here in Dusunan, poor as we were, had to chip in to pay off the raja's debts so our Laujé daughter wouldn't be forced to marry that "foreign man" from Tomini. All of this because of the raja's decadence.

We got even, though. That raja started to need more and more money. He began to dip into the coffers of the colonial taxes. The Dutch don't tolerate that sort of thing. He went off to prison. His relatives today say that he was put in prison because he was involved in the early Islamic organizations fighting for independence from colonial rule [Sarekat Islam], but we know better. He ended up in jail because he was a cheat and a crook.

With Raja Borman discredited, the Dutch searched for a legitimate heir. But, as Sumpitan explained it, they again passed over the Laujé for another immigrant, Kuti Tombolotutu, who became raja in 1927.[12] Tombolotutu, however, sided with the Japanese during World War II, so when the Dutch returned in 1945, they sought a new raja. This is why Sumpitan and the olongian's family had drawn the genealogy chart I looked at. They wanted to convince the Dutch to reinstate the olongian. Sumpitan believed the only reason Tombolotutu was reinstated as raja in 1945 was because he bribed the Dutch, though, as I said in the endnote on bribing the Dutch for Borman's position, such a scenario was highly unlikely.

After independence, supporters of the olongian, including Sumpitan's father, tried once again to oust the immigrant raja. They sent a letter asking the new president of Indonesia and the "democratic government" to dethrone Kuti because he was "a tyrannical despot." Their letter, dated January 20, 1951, bears the title: "Hadji Kuti Tombolotutu, the raja of the Moutong Kingdom, is no longer suited in the present day circumstances to run the government."[13] The letter received no response. Nor did Jakarta move to dethrone Raja Kuti. Raja

Kuti retained his title and ruled over the Swapraja of Tinombo-Moutong until his death in 1963.

What is interesting to me is that the letter written by Sumpitan's relatives made no mention of the olongian as the paramount Laujé figure of authority. It said: "(1) We ask that the Swapraja be eradicated and joined with the People's Parliament in Jakarta, because we do not have a raja who represents us. He is a Mandar and not one of our traditional leaders (called jogugu or *marsaoleh* as in Gerontalo). . . ." In this 1951 letter, these elites regarded the jogugu or marsaoleh as political leaders, but not the olongian. The focus on the olongian as a sole political power figure and not just a spiritual figure seems to be a rather recent reinterpretation of the past under Sumpitan's historiography. Sumpitan's narratives underlined the political victimization of the olongian at the hands of the evil immigrant rajas, but the local documents did not. Both Sumpitan and the early documents, though, accuse the raja of usurping Laujé power.

Even though Raja Kuti Tombolotutu died in 1963, Sumpitan blamed him for the ban on the Laujé's ritual, the momasoro, which occurred twenty years later. Sumpitan remembered that it was Tombolotutu, in 1951, who had prohibited the giving of first fruit tribute to the olongian.[14] Sumpitan believed it was Raja Kuti's decrees that divided the olongian from the highland Laujé by stopping the main conduit of communication between them—tribute payment. Thus Sumpitan used history to support his claim that it was foreigners' fault, and especially Raja Tombolotutu's fault, that the momasoro was banned.

The View from the Mountains: Siamae Sanji's Narratives

Siamae Sanji's narratives contradict, as well as support, Sumpitan's perception of history. Siamae Sanji believes Raja Kuti Tombolotutu was a laudable leader. The raja was the returned descendant of the first Laujé ancestor. In Siamae Sanji's view Raja Kuti helped the Laujé behave morally and enter into proper reciprocal relations with highlanders, giving them his "new" religion, Islam. By contrast, Siamae Sanji believed the olongian was a failed leader because she or he neglected moral "traditions."

When Siamae Sanji talked about the coastal peoples, he never distinguished foreigners from Laujé, nor Laujé villages from the "immigrant town." Instead, the coast was a single community that he called "the place of the stores." When Siamae Sanji spoke of government in the lowlands, he spoke about a longstanding interdependence between the female olongian and the male *puangé*. Puangé meant non-Laujé Lord.[15] It referred to warriors (tadulako) in the olongian's court or to immigrant rajas who sometimes married the female olongian. In Siamae Sanji's parlance, Raja Tombolotutu, Raja Borman, and Daeng Malino were all puangé and they were respected figures who fulfilled their duties toward highlanders more than the olongian did.

According to Siamae Sanji, a puangé had always been a figure of power and respect in Laujé life. Laujé had always been subordinate to puangé and when they tried to be otherwise, they suffered. Siamae Sanji's story, which he claimed to have learned word by word from his grandfather, depicts such a misguided attempt.

> Long ago, when the sea still lapped at the edges of Taipaobal, the To Belo came to collect cinnamon for the puangé of Ternate. But the puangé discovered that Taipaobal had grown another bush of their own. The fruits were glass beads, iron, and brass trays. The puangé was angry and sent To Belo men to cut down the bush. They burned it to ashes. When the To Belo left, they took the sea with them, leaving Taipaobal high up in the mountains and far from shore. It was a long time before the puangé came again.
>
> Later, when the olongian had already moved to Dusunan, the Laujé had another puangé. A Mandar boat would arrive each year from Cendrana [Cenrana in South Sulawesi] to collect tribute for the Mandar puangé. The tribute had to be paid every year—two fishing nets for every village *(boya)*. After many years the tribute was paid to the Mandar puangé in Moutong. Twenty Taipaobalers were asked by the olongian to go pay labor tribute in Moutong. Panning gold for the puangé who lived in Moutong was their work.

The "words" Siamae Sanji claimed to have memorized and merely repeated have uncanny echoes in Dutch sources.[16] Siamae Sanji's stories indicate that the Laujé "kingdom" was never an isolated and indigenous power. Instead, the Laujé polity had been a vassal to other rajadoms in Sulawesi and the Spice Islands.

Siamae Sanji explained by way of an origin story the reason the Laujé were so willing to serve the non-Laujé Lords. In this story all puangé were the descendants of a Laujé known as the Voracious Child. This is the Voracious Child's story as Siamae Sanji told it:[17]

An old couple prayed that they give birth to a son. Their prayer was granted, but the son was a burden. He ate so much that they could not keep him fed. He also was incredibly strong. He was able to clear seven mountainsides with his machete. Yet it was the boy's appetite that disturbed his parents.

The boy was huge, and while still a child he could eat seven bundles of rice in a day. His father decided to kill the boy. One time he rolled a boulder on the boy, but the boy returned carrying the boulder. Another time he chopped down a tree to fall on the boy, but the boy returned carrying the tree.

The boy realized his parents did not want him and resolved to leave home. His mother prepared traveling food for him and gave him the sacred sword which had come from the Inscribed Rock.

The boy walked for seven days. On the seventh night he came to an empty village. He found a girl hiding inside a drum. He asked her to cook him some rice. She answered she couldn't because the sound of rice pounding would attract the giant bird that had killed her entire village.

The Voracious Boy promised that he would protect her. When the bird came, the Boy used his magic sword from the Inscribed Rock to bring all the souls of the villagers back to life.

The Voracious Boy married the girl. Their children became the people from across the sea—the Chinese, the Bugis, and the Mandar. One of their sons became the first puangé who later returned to the Laujé to marry a daughter of the olongian.

When Siamae Sanji told this story, he told me that I too was descended from the Voracious Boy. "You and we Laujé are all of one trunk," he said. For Siamae Sanji, everyone was one clan. Puangé, olongian, those from the sea, and those remaining in the mountains, were all complements within a single world. Siamae Sanji's story blurred the boundaries that Sumpitan had so adamantly emphasized.

In blurring boundaries, in bringing everyone into his history, Siamae Sanji created one big family. Such inclusiveness seems refreshing in light of Sumpitan's rather vituperative distinctions, but Siamae Sanji's big family was not necessarily a happy one. The moral of the Voracious Boy tale was that the original Laujé parents had cast out their firstborn child and given him their source of power (in the magic sword). Today Siamae Sanji's descendants were compensating for the original sin by paying allegiance to the Voracious Boy's descendants. "Older sibling" is the term Siamae Sanji used to refer to these descendants, who were also the puangé and lowland immigrants from "foreign" lands. They were spawned from the first child, the Voracious

Boy, and thus were "older than the ancestor who sired the Laujé." Siamae Sanji said the people who remained, the Laujé descendants, were
born from the greedy parents who had neglected to feed their own
child. As a result, the children who remained became "junior siblings"
to the puangé. Siamae Sanji said that the past sins of Laujé ancestors
meant that present-day Laujé as younger siblings were obligated to
work or feed the puangé by giving tribute to him. In turn, the puangé,
or older sibling, gave foreign trade items to the Laujé and protected
them with his magic sword.

When Siamae Sanji talked about the sibling relationship, he used
the phrase *vuntuh pusé*, "those who are connected by one navel." He
said it was the most stable familial relationship that existed, because
parents often died before their children matured, but siblings matured
together. Moreover, older siblings often nurtured the younger ones.
Later in life, siblings often built houses near each other. The older sibling usually helped the younger find a spouse, while the younger
showed respect by providing labor and food. It was this bond and
debt which created the closeness between siblings.

When Siamae Sanji characterized Taipaobalers as younger siblings,
and puangé as older siblings, it explained the deference Taipaobalers
felt toward the lowland descendants of the raja. But, according to Siamae Sanji, the Taipaobalers did not always see themselves as the inferior, deferential, younger siblings. In other stories, Siamae Sanji explained that there were subsequent siblings, branches off of the
original trunk, who were younger than the Taipaobal "younger siblings." Siamae Sanji said, for instance, that the lowland Laujé in
Dusunan, descendants of the olongian, were later born younger siblings (thus of lesser rank), while the bela in the distant rain forest were
the youngest siblings of all (and thus of lowest rank). Moreover, both
the olongian's and the bela's younger sibling status was in a state of
decay, said Siamae Sanji, because they had neglected their end of reciprocal gift exchanges and had neglected to show respect to their older
siblings in Taipaobal.

In his narrative about the third sibling, the lowland olongian, Siamae Sanji called her a "younger sibling who failed to return a gift to
the older brother." Siamae Sanji said that during the old days, olongian were all male. They lived in the highlands near present-day Taipaobal. But then a woman named Maulintina, the younger sister of

the Taipaobal olongian, married a Kaili man and converted to Islam. After the wedding they planned to move to the lowlands where immigrant traders lived. At the wedding ceremony, a Kaili imam prayed over the sacred regalia of the olongian. When this happened, the bride told her brother that the office of olongian was now an office for Muslims, not pagans like him. The bride's older brother, the Taipaobal olongian, was shamed into ceding to the lowlanders the office of olongian and the sacred regalia that went with that office. His younger sister promised that in seven generations she would return the regalia and the office of the olongian to the highlands.

Siamae Sanji, along with most of the Laujé patriarchs in the mountains, took the myth's phrase, "seven generations," literally. Thus when the seventh female olongian died in 1955, Siamae Sanji and several of his friends went to the lowlands in a formal delegation to declare that the "seven generations were finished; it was time for the lowlanders to return the sacred regalia." When the highland delegation explained its mission, however, the lowland aristocrats refused to relinquish their claim on the regalia. This was when, said Siamae Sanji, subsequent olongian became less effective in their roles as priest-rulers. The lowland olongian no longer kept their promise to return what their relatives in the mountains had given them.

Siamae Sanji said that the highlanders had "fed" the olongian by providing unhusked rice for seven generations. Highlanders, said Siamae Sanji, had been the "good older siblings" who had sacrificed themselves for the "younger sibling," the olongian. The lowlanders, he said, had neglected the highlanders by not returning the regalia that the myth said was the highlanders' due. The lowland olongian, a female, had refused to return food to the highlanders in harvest rites for them, thus neglecting her younger sibling obligations. The puangé were the only lowlanders who treated the highlanders as they should be treated, but they were older siblings, not younger.

In Siamae Sanji's narratives the moral obligations between puangé and olongian, older sibling and younger sibling, male and female, were clearly delineated. The olongian, as a female younger sibling, was depicted as inferior, while puangé, as a male older sibling, was depicted as morally superior.

The manner in which Siamae Sanji obeyed the puangé or raja illustrated his fealty to the moral point of the myths. In 1927, at Raja

Tombolotutu's request, Siamae Sanji convinced the last of the recalcitrant bela to "come down" from the mountains and swear allegiance to the government. As a token of his appreciation, the raja provided Siamae Sanji with a livelihood. The raja paid Siamae Sanji to lead ebony and rattan expeditions in the mountains. Upon return with the produce, the raja invited Siamae Sanji to dinner, to sleep on his veranda, and to share stories. The raja also discussed Islam with Siamae Sanji. In the 1950s Siamae Sanji sent his oldest son to the raja's veranda to learn to recite the Qur'an. Thus the raja acted as Siamae Sanji's patron. He fed him, provided him with economic opportunity, and opened the door to powerful religious secrets, as was expected of a puangé.

Siamae Sanji's praise for the raja was in sharp contrast to the disparaging remarks he made about recent olongian. Siamae Sanji blamed Taipaobal's decline in rice production on the olongian. The "tradition," according to Siamae Sanji, stipulated that the olongian should not sell food products, because the soul of foodstuffs would leave, never to return. Crops would then fail. He said:

> In the old days, we all gave the olongian the first sheaf of rice *(boké)* from the harvest. She offered it to the spirit of the rice. The rice filled her granary. These seeds were given to those who had none. The olongian fed us when we went to the lowlands to bring our tribute.
>
> But the mother of Isumbi [the present olongian] broke with tradition. She sold food right from her front yard! Before this, Taipaobalers could sell corn. But the smallpox epidemic [of the 1950s] came because the olongian was selling food. So we stopped selling corn for cash.

According to Siamae Sanji, Taipaobal was forced to take on the moral burdens that should have been "carried" by the olongian. Taipaobalers now cannot sell corn for cash because the olongian does so, even though Taipaobalers also provide rice tribute for the olongian's lowland rituals. In Siamae Sanji's narrative, Taipaobal retained the moral superiority which the olongian had sacrificed. Taipaobalers had continued to fulfill their duty of feeding the lowlanders and observing taboos, but the olongian selfishly enriched herself and neglected her own duties. By contrast, Siamae Sanji believed the puangé or raja was the lowlander who behaved as the highlanders expected an older sibling should. The raja's descendants, now living in or around the palace, were to be trusted, while the olongian and relatives were to be regarded with suspicion.

We Give Food to Our Bela: Siamae Sanji and the Female Neighbors

Just as Siamae Sanji believed the olongian and Laujé lowlanders were morally destitute, so he believed the bela were. I learned about Siamae Sanji's prejudice against the bela very early on through his children and my visit to the bela community of Sinalutan. It was this experience and the contagious prejudice against bela that determined I would work in Taipaobal, not in a bela community.

Siamae Sanji believed the tragic split between the bela and Taipaobalers began when he was a young man. Soon after the Dutch conquered the Tomini Bay, they ordered that the Laujé of the highlands move to the coast where they could be more closely monitored. All of the villages to the west ignored the order, and a few Taipaobal families refused to obey as well. According to Siamae Sanji, they "ran away" into the highlands where they formed bela communities like Sinalutan. Most of the families in Taipaobal and the foothill villages obeyed the Dutch command to move to the coast, even though they were reluctant. Siamae Sanji called his own community's move down to the lowlands the "carrying down" *(inalugan)*, a phrase used when a corpse is "carried down." The "carrying down" was a tragedy. The Taipaobalers had to leave their natal village and the bela families who had run into the mountains.

When Siamae Sanji and other Taipaobalers moved to Lombok for the next three years, Siamae Sanji said they were forced to build houses and to work on roads and bridges for the burgeoning Dutch infrastructure:

> Each person was also forced to plant twenty-five coconut trees in their houseyard to pay taxes. We worked so hard there was no food grown. Many people became ill. Most died. After three years we Laujé were allowed to return to our mountain homes. When we Laujé returned to Taipaobal, we found the land overgrown and many fertile fields in which to farm. The fields were five or six times as large as they are now.

Though Taipaobalers' acquiescence to Dutch rule had initially been a tragedy, it had resulted in good fortune, fertile fields. The real tragedy of the "coming of the Dutch," said Siamae Sanji, had to do with those who had fled—the bela. The bela were forced to live a seminomadic existence in the forests because they feared they would be detected and captured by the Dutch. These bela could not plant crops because they were "fearful" they would be discovered. According to Siamae Sanji, it was only when the Taipaobalers returned to the highlands after the Dutch released them from the forced migration that bela were able to survive comfortably. It was at this time that the Taipaobalers began to "give" some of their rice produce to the bela. The bela then brought products which they "gave" to the Taipaobalers.[18] Thus a system of symbiotic exchange was instituted.

Siamae Sanji asserted that the only reason the bela survived during this period was because Taipaobalers fed them rice. "The other food they ate, the taro and ferns, that wasn't real food. We fed them rice and that was food. That was how they lived. The bela did give us return products of taro and rattan mats and bark-cloth, but these were lesser products. These products were not food. We were the ones who fed them with rice and corn." Thus for Siamae Sanji, the Taipaobalers were superior to the bela because Taipaobalers fed the bela as an older sibling feeds a younger.

Siamae Sanji said that the bela relationship should be one of respect and mutual affection. One's bela is like one's spouse or lover—or at least that is the ideal. In the old days people used to marry bela partners' daughters, he said. During the early days of the diaspora, Taipaobal men had many bela to choose from as trade partners and wives. At that time, the bela women moved to Taipaobal to live after marriage. This was because, according to Siamae Sanji:

> In those days, the bela did not have the magical spells to open land to plant. They had no fields. We Taipaobalers knew the spells because we had a planting specialist, the *pasobo* [appointed by the olongian]. We had many rice fields. When a groom married, he didn't move away. He needed to stay in Taipaobal and work in the fields. So, after marriage the grooms stayed in Taipaobal to plant rice. They planted an entire field just for their in-laws.

According to Siamae Sanji, however, a shift in the pattern of brideservice and postmarital residence began to occur in the 1960s. Productivity in Taipaobal began its steep decline when some bela communities "opened their fields for planting without the proper magic spells." These communities began to plant more corn than they needed for subsistence. The bela began to trade corn, even sell it to lowlanders. Siamae Sanji says that to sell corn or rice is taboo. "The ancestors gave us these plants. . . . To sell plants is to sell the ancestors' souls."[19]

Most important, though, the bela began to require that Taipaobal men work in brideservice in distant bela villages. This was acceptable in villages that were close to Taipaobal, but not in geographically remote villages. Not only would such a move make it difficult to visit family members, but it would be a move down in economic status. Taipaobal was one of the few communities that received contracts for work expeditions sponsored by lowlanders. Far away from the lowlands, these Taipaobal men married to bela women could not hope to participate in such expeditions. Siamae Sanji noted this shift when he talked about his own family:

> When I married the first and second time, I didn't live with my in-laws. They were bela from Babong. They didn't have rice fields there. I cut down trees and planted a field here in Taipaobal. I took rice and corn over to my family to feed them. I also worked in expeditions which the puangé asked me to lead. I brought my bela in-laws cloths and machetes.
>
> Nowadays those people in Babong want our children to move there to work when they marry. One of my sons [Sanji] lives there now. His in-laws have a field there and he works for them there. That is wrong. He should not move away and live with them. He should plant fields here. He is too far away to participate in rattan expeditions. He often comes to visit the day the rest of my sons have left on an expedition. My other son, Zhairudden, he married right. We saved money and paid it [bridewealth] to the girl's family in Lalado. They're happy and so are we. Zhairudden and his wife and my grandchild live here with me. They work in the fields here in Taipaobal and take food to the in-laws. That is as it should be. The "older sibling" should feed the "younger" [bela in-laws]. The "younger sibling" should not try to separate families. That is bad.

In the story of his own and his son's marriages, Siamae Sanji gave a clear view of the shifts over time in the Taipaobalers' relations with the bela. What he did not mention in this narrative, though, was that his oldest son, Sanji, married a bela woman in Mambu. Sanji eventually settled in the bela community permanently. Sanji, an old man himself, was not able to visit his father often. As Siamae Sanji's other son said: "The oldest child should take care of the parents when they are old, and then the next sibling will take care of the older sibling. My older brother does not do this. He has neglected us. When my father dies, we will be like chicks wandering about the yard without a parent or older sibling to protect us." By marrying a bela woman, working brideservice, and moving far away, Sanji had severed the connections with his father's family. As land became unproductive in Taipaobal, and as more bela communities opened forest land near their communities, it became more enticing for Taipaobalers like Sanji to marry and move to bela communities. The only way Siamae Sanji could prevent similar "disaffections" by his younger children was by bringing eligible women to Taipaobal for them to marry. In the case of one son, Zhairudden, Siamae Sanji attracted a wife for him by paying bridewealth just as lowlanders did. But, Siamae Sanji had impoverished the whole family in the process (paying over three hundred U.S. dollars). None of the other children, all in their late teens and late twenties, were yet able to think about marriage through bridewealth. As the years went by, they were growing dangerously close to becoming permanent bachelors because their father would not let them marry bela in distant villages.

Siamae Sanji's stories about the relationship with the bela highlighted the danger of marriage to a bela woman. Moreover, when he spoke about brideservice and its drawbacks, he spoke as though it was the bela bride's mother who was enticing the young groom away from her family. One revealing incident occurred with Siamae Sanji's grandnephew through his brother. The young man's mother, Siamae Sanji's brother's daughter, spoke about the incident by using the same themes Siamae Sanji had used. Her story, however, was much more graphic than Siamae Sanji's:

> My son is no good to us around the house here anymore because he is sleeping with a bela girl. He's like a cat. He screws all night and sleeps all day. He won't do his chores. He never fetches water and he let his garlic crop die. He worked on a rattan expedition, made lots of money—(thirty U.S. dollars)—but that girl's mother got him to buy her things. She said they needed some sugar and lamp oil and a new cloth from the store. That bela family is getting my son to do all their work, and he comes home and steals our dried fish. I know the girl's mother put him up to it. Those bela women, they are lazy. They won't work for themselves, but they get others to. Our young boys get hooked by them. They go to the all-night dances [modero], their girls do it with our boys right there. That's why Siamae Sanji wouldn't let his children go to those dances. They would have been enticed by the bela. Bela lie and cheat. Well, my son is not going to marry her. He can screw her as much as he wants, but I'm not giving permission, not me. My son isn't going to marry a bela.

Because a woman oversees the food production within a household, it is often the mother who lures young men to sleep with her daughters so the man will be available to work in the fields. The boy is often treated better there than in his own household. He will frequently move in with such a family and gladly perform their chores. This happens in bela communities and in Taipaobal. The boundaries between them, like those between highlands and lowlands is blurred.

Taipaobalers, however, constantly want to underline the difference between themselves and the bela. Siamae Sanji's son, Zhairudden, told me that "bela don't have marriage ceremonies, they just live with each other." Though this comment was false—women he calls bela do in fact have marriage ceremonies—it is true that marrying such a bela woman is a relatively simple process compared with the more elaborate customs some Taipaobalers use, customs they have copied from lowlanders. A man merely has to give a so-called bela woman's family an antique coin. Due to the ease with which "bela" marriages are conducted, Taipaobal men can more readily marry bela than Taipaobal females. In Taipaobal, the stricter Islamic rules keep the women closer to home and make it more likely the parents will guard against sexual promiscuity. The fact that Taipaobalers like to copy lowlanders' inflated bridewealth exchanges even further constrains Taipaobalers and causes resentment toward the "easier" lifestyle of the bela.

Siamae Sanji blamed the bela for creating separations in the community. He said that "the relatives who carry the same navel should never live far apart. A man and his sons should build houses close together. When Taipaobal men are required to live with bela in brideservice, the family is separated." What was behind his claim about keeping the family together was Siamae Sanji's own desire to distinguish himself and his family from the bela. Through his adoption of bridewealth payments, his association with the raja, and his refusal to let his younger children marry into non-Islamic communities (because of the mistake he had made with his oldest child, Sanji), Siamae Sanji claimed his own superiority to the bela. Siamae Sanji's lament that the bela women lured the men from Taipaobal into marriage, displaced his real agenda—to keep himself and his own family in positions of power and status. He was separating from the bela, not the reverse.

Summary

The focus of this chapter has been on the ways Sumpitan and Siamae Sanji talked about the past to explain the present. Siamae Sanji em-

phasized that females had been the individuals who had only temporary bonds to the community. Females, like the olongian and the bela,
had failed to uphold moral obligations to respect their "older siblings," or had departed the natal village. Only males such as the raja
or puangé had maintained contact with their siblings and nurtured
them through food gifts and hospitality. Siamae Sanji blurred the
boundaries between highland Laujé and lowland immigrants, but de-
marcated the line created by relatives marrying bela women and lowland Laujé women. By contrast, Sumpitan emphasized the boundaries
between all Laujé and the immigrants or foreigners in Tinombo. He
claimed that foreigners had been the individuals who were associated
with violence. Foreigners had cheated the Laujé and divided the once-
unified Laujé nation. In Sumpitan's scenario, the olongian sought to
heal the rifts created by the foreigners but to no avail.

It is worth noting that the themes highlighted by each man, though
particular to them, are nevertheless themes emphasized in other communities throughout the Indonesian archipelago and beyond. For instance, the notion of a prodigal son unwanted by the family, who travels and eventually returns, is common in the I La Galigo saga of South
Sulawesi commonly known as the Sawerigading myth (see Nourse
1998). Also, the story of the earth mother, whose body parts either literally or symbolically become the celestial heavens exists among the
Mambai of East Timor (Traube 1980; 1986), the Bunaq of Central
Timor (Friedberg 1980), Atoni of Timor (van Wouden 1935), and the
Makassae of East Timor (Forman 1980). Moreover, the notion of a
stranger-king hated, but sacred, has been noted by a series of scholars
(Hocart 1927; van Wouden 1935; Dumezil 1970; Sahlins 1981; de
Heusch 1982; Hicks 1978; Francillon 1980; Tambiah 1976) as a
worldwide phenomenon, not unlike the raja/olongian scenario among
the Laujé. Closer to home, the separation between younger sibling and
older is apparent among the Mandar and Bugis of South Sulawesi
(George 1996; Acciaioli 1989).[20] Thus, even though Siamae Sanji and
Sumpitan have obviously constructed their histories to fit personal
agendas, both men frame their political messages within structurally
opposed formats, formats they share with others in Indonesia and beyond. On the one hand, this reveals that underlying their idiosyncratic
constructions are common themes shared by people throughout the
area, but, on the other hand, it reveals the difference between those

other areas and the Laujé. What distinguishes the Laujé case here is the distinctive way in which gender plays into the categories of bela, puangé, and olongian put forth by Siamae Sanji and the way in which that discourse is transformed by Sumpitan into a discussion about indigenous and foreign identity.

Two

CONCEIVING SEX, BIRTH, AND ILLNESS

3

GIFTS TO THE OLDER SIBLING
Siamae Sanji on Umputé

When I first began fieldwork, I had not planned to collect the oral histories Siamae Sanji and Sumpitan were so eager to provide. And just as I had not planned to collect oral histories, neither had I originally planned to collect information about birth spirits. Siamae Sanji began telling me about birth spirits the moment I said I wanted to learn about the Laujé. With Siamae Sanji as my guide, I began to understand how basic birth spirits were to highland cosmology. It was not until three months later, when Sumpitan invited me down to the lowlands to watch the momasoro, that I realized birth spirits were also fundamental to lowland worldviews. Sumpitan began to tell me not only about the birth spirits blessed in the momasoro, but also about the birth spirits addressed in small, individual offerings that resembled, to a certain degree, the rites Siamae Sanji was teaching me. Once I realized there was a common thread connecting highland belief to lowland, I began to rethink the circumscribed notions I had about mountain versus lowland culture. Both men talked in similar terms about umputé. For them it was an "older sibling." And just as younger siblings in the past and the present honor and neglect their older siblings, human beings neglect and honor umputé spirits.

The birth spirits called umputé form a set of concepts that, though seemingly simple, can be played with or "used" (to borrow from de Certeau) in myriad ways. All Laujé with whom I spoke, highlander and lowlander, said umputé nurtured and carried the fetus from the womb into the world. At birth, umputé "died" so that the child could be born. For this reason, human beings owe a perpetual debt to umputé. Without the death/sacrifice of the umputé spirit, there would be no human life. Siamae Sanji and others in Taipaobal told me repeatedly that after a child was born, the umputé spirits could make the child ill just as easily as it could protect the child from illness. It was this paradoxical or contradictory quality inherent in humans' relationship to these spirits that made umputé so compelling. It was also this paradoxical quality that led individual Laujé to disagree as to how umputé should be defined and treated.

Most curers, including Siamae Sanji and Sumpitan, insisted that in the process of birth, humans inadvertently ignored one manifestation of umputé, the birth fluids, while they selected another, the placenta, for special treatment. This neglect happened during the ritualized treatment of the placenta, a practice in which all Laujé participated. Inadvertently, some birth fluids were neglected when they were perfunctorily washed away. The neglected umputé caused illness. To prevent illness or to acknowledge a spirit after illness has been cured, most Laujé make offerings to umputé.

The diversity of approaches to understanding umputé are manifested in the variety of forms that offerings to umputé take. In simple terms, offerings to umputé fall into two categories. One category of offerings signals that a connection has occurred and should be severed to make things proper again. Rites associated with curing highlight this. If umputé "feeds" too long on a body, then a curer can be called to beseech umputé to separate from the human being. The offerings that are made in association with these cures signal the necessity for separation. The second category of offerings are those emphasizing joining or even that an improper separation has occurred that must be rectified. In the more elaborate Laujé rituals—especially the momasoro—offerings of both kinds are given. As a result, a question of priority arises. Is the elaborate ritual to be considered a rite of separation or of joining? This ambiguity allows for considerable interpretative maneuvering among the protagonists in such rituals. In their exegeses about the purpose of such rituals, both Siamae Sanji and Sumpitan emphasized that the parts "should separate" for humans to be healthy. Other healers emphasized that the parts "should join" for humans to be healthy. Still others avoided making any distinctions between the parts or aspects and thus avoided valuing one aspect of the paradox over another.

Birth and Spirits as Taught by Siamae Sanji

As mentioned, Siamae Sanji was known throughout the lowlands and the mountains as a curer or sando.[1] By passing along his knowledge to his sons and close nephews in Taipaobal, the beliefs of Siamae Sanji predominated among sando in and near Taipaobal. Most of Siamae Sanji's knowledge was conveyed through the act of midwifery. He had been a renowned midwife and taught the art of midwifery to his sons, grandsons, and nephews. Most of his midwifery students practiced their art when birthing their own children and grandchildren, but occasionally they were called to assist neighbors giving birth. It was particularly important that a male midwife trained by Siamae Sanji deliver the firstborn child in the family. Afterward, the father could learn the prayers and perform them without a "specialized" sando assisting.

The male midwives who performed the firstborn rites were proud of their expertise. They boasted that it was through their skills that Taipaobal mothers were less weakened by childbirth labor than were women from the lowlands or distant bela communities. It was a particular mark of pride, continually reiterated by both male and female informants, that Taipaobal women were unique—they managed to leave the house a few hours after birth to fetch a load of firewood or bring back water from the stream. Several Taipaobal women said in so many words, "we never lounge in the birth chamber as 'other' women [such as the bela or the lowlanders] do."

Since men praise Taipaobal women's physical stamina, it would seem that they respect the women or at least their role in birth, but women's role in birth is overshadowed (at least in men's conversations) by men's discussion of their own roles (see Nourse 1997). Siamae Sanji and those he trained as sando gave credit for the women's strength to the superior medical and healing powers of the Taipaobal midwives he trained. He, and other men in the community, said that only Taipaobal sando knew the correct procedure for dealing with the umputé spirits. This is why, they asserted, Taipaobal babies usually lived, whereas babies from the lowlands or from bela communities often died.[2] Taipaobal midwives and others in the community regarded the midwives' spiritual knowledge about birth as more valuable than any food or care given by a mother. The mother's contributions—carrying the child during pregnancy, delivery, and nursing the child—were important, but not as important as spiritual knowledge.

Siamae Sanji taught his midwives that the birth spirits were gendered; male umputé spirits were more important spirits than the female umputé. Siamae Sanji claimed that during birth the father must coax the spirits from the womb by coaxing out fluids that are the material manifestation or "bodies" of umputé spirits. One of these "bodies," he said, "is the black blood of pregnancy. The umputé spirit which resides in this body is female. . . . The other umputé 'body' is the placenta, and its spirit is male." According to Siamae Sanji, the "black" blood and its female spirit are first made manifest at birth. This black blood is not the blood that flows in the veins, nor is it menstrual blood.[3] Black blood is the fluid that slowly dribbles out of the mother's womb during the whole birth process. It is the blood that makes the newborn's first stool "tarry black." In Siamae Sanji's scheme, black blood is "dirty," "bad," and "dangerous." Black blood and its umputé spirit are associated with decay, that which is temporary, or that which has caused a separation or interruption in the enduring bond that should be maintained between human souls and the pool of ancestral souls that are waiting to be reincarnated. Because Siamae Sanji characterized the black-blood spirit as female, and because he regarded females in general as social separators, he also implied that the black umputé spirit works to separate the human souls from ancestral souls. In exegeses and in ritual acts at birth, Siamae Sanji and his students characterized the black-blood spirit and the female gender in the most pejorative manner possible.

According to Siamae Sanji, the birth process is especially significant because it is in this context that the umputé spirit of black blood is inevitably ignored and left to decay by the mother-to-be. During birth, the mother-to-be lets the black-blood spirit drop through the floorboards onto the ground.[4] The mother-to-be does nothing to acknowledge the poor neglected spirit, which is left to lie fallow in the filth and refuse under the house. According to Siamae Sanji, this space is particularly dirty because it is

> where decayed objects are thrown, where children urinate and defecate, where crazy people, or retarded people are tied. It is where bela women cook, where the droppings of chickens, goats, and dogs are left to rot. Where witches enter the house. To let a spirit fall through the floorboards into that filth and decay is to neglect and mistreat that spirit. . . . The blame for this neglect is the woman's. The mother-to-be lets the black blood spirit fall through the 'catching cloth' onto the ground.

Because the spirit has been neglected by women, it can return "in anger" to plague humans through sickness and death.

By contrast, Siamae Sanji treats the "white" placental spirit, or "white umputé" much differently. Not only do males taught by Siamae Sanji treat the placenta as though it is like the newborn child, but they also associate the white placental spirit with masculine things. For instance, after the child is born, the midwife or the newborn's father must clean the placenta and thus nurture the placenta's white umputé spirit. Cleaning, however, must be done inside the house—a place of respect because it is high above the ground and because it has been made from the labor of the male's agnatic kin. The father must wash the white placenta in the same fluid as the child, a fluid they call "sperm of the coconut," further emphasizing its symbolic associations with males. Then they carefully wrap the placenta in a bundle and give it to the father, who must hang the bundle in a tall fruit-bearing tree. According to Siamae Sanji, the placental spirit is very important to the child, because

> if treated properly this spirit will wait for the child's soul when it dies and leaves its body. The white umputé spirit waits for the human soul on the bridge between life and death where it meets that soul and escorts it to heaven. If the white umputé spirit were not there to meet the soul, the soul would be doomed to wander forever in the netherworld between life and death. . . . A soul gone to heaven is not separated from his living descendants. That soul is able to find its way home down the path across the bridge between life and death. When it returns to the world of the living, the soul possesses a family member if that family member is a sando. The soul and the sando then can heal others.

These healing spirits usually possess the body of a male sando and not a female.[5] According to Siamae Sanji's son Sair, the white healing spirit may help relatives fight battles against enemies, especially sorcerers, and it can call on more powerful spirits in heaven to assist the sando in healing the afflicted. Thus, even though the white umputé is separated from the child by death, the connections among this spirit, the living, and the ancestors endure through the sando who reproduces and heals.

The role of the sando trained by Siamae Sanji is to maintain the bond between the two realms of life and death. By treating the umputé spirit at birth as a spirit in suspended animation, the continual bond between life and death is sustained. For Siamae Sanji and his acolytes, the white umputé spirit connotes enduring bonds, nurturance, productivity, heaven, and masculinity, while the black umputé connotes females, separation, neglect, death, and decay.

In general, then, acolytes of Siamae Sanji, as well as other Taipao-balers, believe they are indebted to all umputé spirits for nurturing them in the womb as an "older sibling" nurtures its "younger sibling." Because the spirits opened the path for the humans to be born, humans are to honor and acknowledge that debt by nurturing the spirits and the material manifestation of those spirits at birth. Inevitably, though, Taipaobalers believe they neglect to pay their debt to all umputé spirits, especially the black umputé spirit, and this creates a dangerous state of affairs. The blame for this neglect is the mother's and the female gender's. The male midwives, the sando, and males in general, are lauded as the spiritual caretakers of the community because they maintain connections to the white umputé spirit who protects and guides humans on their route to heaven. They also perform rites to rectify the problems that result because the females have neglected the black spirit.

The Teachings of Siamae Sanji: Midwives' Actions during Labor

During birth, the mother-to-be squats in the center of her house and leans against the "living centerpost" or against her husband, the male midwife, who leans against the centerpost. Siamae Sanji said that "the centerpost for all houses must be brought from the last house which a couple built together. Or the centerpost must be brought from one of the houses the husband's own family built." Though Siamae Sanji did not talk about the symbolic importance of the centerpost, it is clear to me that in Taipaobal both the male and this centerpost symbolize continuity and ties with the ancestors. To lean against the husband is structurally and symbolically equivalent to leaning against the centerpost, and against the first tree of life, because all are mythically related. The centerpost signifies the husband's labor, his family, his ancestors, and the first mythic tree of life. Midwives trained by Siamae Sanji ensure that the birth is associated with continuity and fatherhood.

To prepare the mother-to-be for delivery, the male midwife trained by Siamae Sanji, or the woman's husband (they can be one and the same person), loosely wraps several cloth sarongs around the woman's lower torso in a tentlike fashion so that her genitals are not exposed. When the woman spreads her legs, a wide open space is left underneath her through which the fluids fall. The midwives place a cloth underneath her to "catch" the fluids, the spirits, and the child when they are born. Inevitably, however, the cloths become too soaked to absorb the constant flow of secretions from the womb. Thus, some fluids, and the spirits residing in them, fall through the floorboards onto the ground.

When the Taipaobal woman is bleeding and experiencing contractions, the midwife or the father-to-be gives her a bundle of wrapped wood to hold in her hand. The bundle consists of small twigs, no longer than a finger, that the man takes from four different trees in the forest.[6] He knows that these trees are the original four trees of the world, and each is blond or "white wood." The midwife shaves each twig until it is clear of bark and is "smooth" and "slick." After he has collected four different twigs, he wraps them together with the leaves of the "first grass born from earth." He stores this bundle until the birthing day to give to the mother-to-be as a magic talisman to protect her. Siamae Sanji said these pieces of wood "connect" the holder, the mother-to-be, to the forces of the universe and of creation. The wood "make[s] the path of birth [the birth canal] smooth like the woods [*sic*] themselves."

Thus, by giving the mother the "bundle of wood" and by ensuring that she lean against her husband or against the living centerpost as she holds the bundle, the father or male midwife ensures that the child will be "connected" to the following: (1) the founding ancestors who have created the world, (2) the family members through the father's line who have provided the living centerpost, and (3) the family members who have passed down the "medical expertise" for making the birth an easy one. The bundle marks the child's dependence on these patrilateral relatives for a safe delivery into the world.

Siamae Sanji claimed that the midwife's birth medicine induces the fluids to flow out of the womb. This "turns the child around in the womb" so that it exits the birth canal "head first," not "feet first." The midwife ties a black cloth around the top of the mother's abdomen to push the child around, and to start the process of separating child from mother. In Siamae Sanji's scheme, "black blood" heralds birth and carries the child from womb to world. The black cloth signifies that the child will be separated from the womb and mother. This is a good separation, said Siamae Sanji, because it gives life to the child and "leads" the child out of the birth canal head first. Without the midwife to massage and push the child out of the womb, it would not be properly born. In this and other statements, Siamae Sanji claimed the midwife was more spiritually concerned for the child. Thus, males were morally superior to females.

The Teachings of Siamae Sanji: Midwives' Actions after Labor

As soon as it is born, the infant usually makes its first sound, "Oaaa, Oaaa, Oaaa." Taipaobalers said this is the universal cry of all newborns. Siamae Sanji's sons asserted that the cry is a signal that the newborn's soul *(nyaa)*, or its breath (also known as *nyaa*), has started to enter it from the placenta (which may or may not have exited the womb at this point). The cry signals that the breath or soul is traveling through the umbilical cord to reach the child and make it cry.

The soul that enters a child, as well as the souls of its umputé, come from a finite pool of ancestral souls waiting to be reincarnated. Most of these souls are those of remembered ancestors who have died in the not-too-distant past. Some souls are "old souls" of male ancestors who are venerated as men of great spiritual power. The souls tend to be reincarnated from the father's father's family. Thus, just as the actions associated with the birth of the soul and the umputé spirits have a patrilineal bias, so do the origins of the soul and the spirits in the womb have a patrilineal bias.

Additionally, Siamae Sanji's trained midwives act as if the actions of the father, once the child is born, are more important than those of the mother. For instance, while waiting for the placenta "to be born," the father often gives the mother some betel nut to chew. The new father gathers the betel nut and encourages his wife to chew so that the blood will flow through the umbilical cord to the newborn. During this time, the father places the child on a cloth and gently massages its upper abdomen, soothing and rocking it so it will not cry. According to Siamae Sanji, the infant stops crying immediately because the gentle massage rocks the infant's body in a rhythm it finds soothing and comforting.

Once the placenta is born, and before the umbilical cord has been cut, the father treats the placenta as he does the child. He places a clean cloth underneath the placenta and gently massages it until the remaining blood inside the placenta flows through the umbilical cord to the body of the newborn infant. Some fathers place the placenta in its own cradle—a hollowed-out coconut shell that has been cut in half.

They said the placenta is more comfortable "wrapped in a cradle like the father has made for the child."

Next the father or male midwife prepares to cut the umbilical cord and permanently divide the breaths or souls of the child and placenta. In preparation, he must search for a yellow betel nut that has fallen "naturally" from a tree onto the ground. Additionally, the father must pluck some fresh leaves from a *didil* tree.[7] This tree is one of the first mythical trees of the world and it plays a supporting role in all highland rituals concerned with reforging links with ancestors.

Once he finds these, the father returns to the house to prepare the "bamboo knife" for cutting the cord. From the rafters of the bamboo roof, he takes down a sliver of split bamboo to sharpen into a "knife." He places the yellow betel nut on the floor, the green didil leaf on top of the yellow seed, and the umbilicus on top of this. Then he cuts the umbilicus with the sharpened bamboo knife.[8]

All midwives trained by Siamae Sanji insisted that the cord must be sliced with bamboo and not with a metal blade because the metal would "harden or stop the connection" between the placental spirit and the child. In other words, the placenta and child would be permanently separated. Thus the father must avoid cutting the umbilical cord with metal, to avoid acting in ways that connote separation. Siamae Usman, a nephew of Siamae Sanji said:

> A hardened connection means a child, or any human, cannot call on umputé spirits or ancestor spirits to help them in times of drought, floods, or illness. To cut with a metal knife could cause the child to be all alone. Abandoned. That child could die. Very quickly. To cut the umbilicus with a knife would make hard or rigid the connection between placental spirit and child's spirit. The child's soul could be doomed to wander in the in-between world of the footbridge separating life from death.

The iron from the metal knife is said to be a "male" entity. Because males here do not want to separate, it is imperative they avoid using the iron to cut the umbilical cord separating the umputé spirit from the child's soul. Instead, they use bamboo, which, Siamae Sanji says, "belongs to two realms, the sky and the earth." Symbolically it does not separate, but connects two realms. Everything associated with the placenta comes from the sky or high above the ground in a tree or a house. These "high-up" places are significant as symbolic markers of continuity. The sky represents a place of continuing links with spirits, the trees connect the earth with the sky in the origin myths, and the house is a place of shelter and protection continually built by a man for his family. All of these markers of things "high-up," which connote connection, are opposed to the black blood and its umputé spirit. They are all allowed to fall to the ground, a place of filth, decay, and danger, a place where corpses are buried, a place from which Siamae Sanji's descendants in Taipaobal wish to be distinguished or separated. By connecting these two realms, the bamboo symbolically counteracts the negative associations of the ground. Bamboo transcends two symbolic categories, earth and sky, male and female. Thus in cutting the umbilical cord with bamboo, the father works to maintain spiritual connections, even in actions that physically separate entities. Thus, whatever their explanations about why they use a bamboo knife and not a metal knife, the point is that a midwife must make sure he does not close off possibilities in the newborn's future life by cutting the cord with a metal blade.[9]

After the umbilicus is severed, the father/midwife places the placenta and umbilical stub in a coconut shell bowl. Then he takes the yellow betel seed, dips it into the blood of the severed cord still attached to the placenta, and touches the blood-soaked nut to three spots on the infant's face. When he is finished, the child has three little dots, one on each cheek, and one in the center of the forehead.[10] This marks the child's continuous and enduring bond with the placenta, even though their souls (or spirits) and their "bodies" are now separated.

During this period, the child's "soul has not yet come to accept the separation from umputé." It has not come to "rest comfortably in the body of the newborn." Siamae Sanji and other Taipaobalers said: "The sign that the child's soul is uncertain is the soft spot [fontanel] on the top of the head. It quivers as though the soul is coming and going, not able to decide whether it should stay in the infant's body or go through the umbilicus to rejoin the placental soul." To ensure that the soul stays in the newborn's body, the father or midwife gently blows on the soft spot, then places his right palm over the spot. He repeats this gesture three times.[11] Then the mother turns her sarong cloth upside down, the father takes his off and shakes it out three times. Though no informant I asked could tell me why they did this, I think this is to ensure that the soul not flow back into the mother's womb and that it flow from the father's cloth and his ancestral pool of souls

who are waiting to be reincarnated. Afterward, he blesses the child
and then whispers a secret prayer[12] to the umputé spirit. This "answers" the child's "Oaaa, Oaaa" crying. The blessing is as follows:[13]

> Don't walk away
> We ask that you live long,
> Don't cry,
> We ask that you stand upright *(meloon)*,[14]
> Don't be ill,
> We ask for hardiness *(metedes)*.

The prayer is secretly uttered as follows:

> The laws, the laws
> The years of the universe
> You say, Oaaa.

Because the father has uttered these blessings and prayers, the child's
soul will stay in its body, at least for the time being. The father may
now leave the house to wash the childbirth cloths and fetch water for
washing the child and the placenta. Siamae Sanji insisted that the dirty
cloths must not be washed inside the house high above the ground. By
contrast the placenta must not be washed "on the ground," but in the
house high on stilts. "To reverse this order," said Siamae Sanji, "is
taboo *(pepali)*." It would bring almost certain death to the child and
perhaps to the mother as well. Moreover, according to informants
trained by Siamae Sanji, the ground is considered dangerous and polluting. Thus the mother, who is presumed vulnerable to these spirits,
cannot descend to the ground to wash her own birth cloths in the
stream. She must remain separated from the umputé spirits embedded
in the blood-soaked cloths, lest they attach themselves to her and
cause sickness. The black blood spirits are especially attracted to
women.[15]

When the father takes the cloths to the stream to be washed, he is
not in any way polluted by the contact with "black blood." Nor is he
responsible for "neglecting" the blood. No prayers are said to the
black umputé spirit as he disrespectfully kicks the spirit's "body," in
the form of coagulated blood, downstream. According to Siamae
Sanji, it is the mother who "neglects" the black blood spirit when the
child is born. The father has nothing to do with this neglect even
though it is he who kicks the spirit's body downstream.

When the father returns home, the midwife teaches him how ritually to cleanse the child and the placenta. A fresh coconut (often bought at market) has been set aside for the event.[16] It is cleanly sliced open so the shell forms two neat bowls. The placenta is placed inside of it. Then the mother leans against the "living centerpost" of the house once more. She spreads both legs straight out in front of her and places the infant's head at her feet.[17] This head-first position is how the child exited the womb. Near the mother's feet, the father squats with the coconut shell encasing the bloody placenta, the halved coconut shells, some water, and a piece of wood from a didil tree. He carefully washes off the bits of coagulated blood from the placental sack so that the placenta will be "glistening white." Then he cleans the child, washing all the coagulated blood from the child's skin. He avoids, however, the three blood dots on the child's forehead and cheeks, which must remain until they wear off.

Once he removes all the birth blood, the midwife or father dips some fresh didil leaves in a coconut juice mixture. The juice mixed with coconut "meat" is called the *juu nu niu*, the sperm of the coconut. The father or midwife rubs this cold solution over the baby and then performs the same action on the placenta. Thus the father removes the symbolic female fluid (black umputé) and he replaces it with white coconut "sperm," or symbolic male fluid. By this action, the father signals his enduring bond to the child and the white placental umputé spirit. His efforts to bond himself with the child supersede the mother-child bond because the father's bonds include those to the umputé spirit.

Once he finishes cleaning and anointing the placenta and the child, the male midwife shows the father how to wrap the child in a clean cloth, swaddle it tightly, and place it in a cradle he has prepared from split bamboo. The cradle or the "nest" hangs from the rafters of the house. The father ties a string from the cradle to his toe so he can gently rock the newborn while his hands are free for other tasks. While rocking the child, he lines the coconut shells with didil leaves. He places the clean placenta in one half of the shell and swaddles the placenta in the leaves, just as he swaddled the child in cloth. Taking the top half of the divided shell he covers the bottom half, wraps it in more leaves, and ties the whole bundle with a bamboo cord like the one tying the child's cradle to the rafters. The father carries the bundle as he descends to the ground. Walking to a fruit-bearing tree, he hangs the cradlelike bundle on a limb. He then returns home, and the midwife, if not a close relative, prepares to leave.

Before leaving, though, the midwife reminds the father that he has three more tasks, which may extend over a weeklong period. One chore is to bury in the courtyard of the house the betel seed that was used to cut the umbilical cord. This act shows that even though the umbilical cord has been cut and the infant is separated physically from the placenta, the link between them is enduring and productive: The betel nut seed linking the child's blood and the placental blood matures into an areca palm.

After the birth, the father is also responsible for "caring for" the umbilical stump still connected to the child. After a few days, the umbilicus begins to wither. The father must watch the child's navel carefully so he can "catch" the dried cord *(popolu pusé)* when it falls off of its own accord. He must not let the dried umbilicus fall onto the ground, for this would "insult" the cord. The father must gently wrap the cord in a dark cloth and store this packet somewhere in the living area of the house.[18]

The father's third chore is considered the most important and significant for the child's continuing health. It involves procuring food for the newborn so that the mother's milk will start to flow.[19] Siamae Sanji asserted that the mother's milk does not have enough "substance" in it to induce the breast to lactate. Consequently, the father must buy sugar and "hot water" (coffee or tea) at the market to feed to the mother and "start" her milk flowing. In addition, the father must buy the "child's first food." Several of our neighbors came to ask us to sell them the sweets for this purpose, but they could not ask other Laujé in the community for the same sweets. The father had to bring something from an outsider to feed the newborn child and the mother. Usually the "food" is a small package of store-bought cookies or a sweetened rice cake purchased at the market.

In the case of the sweets brought from outside the village for the infant, the father will chew the cookies first, until they are soft enough for the baby to swallow. He will then feed the child in one of two ways. Either he will use his finger to scoop out the masticated food from his own mouth (in the majority of cases), or he will extend his lower lip, until it forms an ersatz nipple, which the infant can suckle. It is important to note that the verb *momaang,* or *pinopa'angomé,* describing the act of feeding the child for the first time, is the same verb used to describe food offerings to the spirit owners of the Land and Water, the global umputé spirits of the momasoro rite.

Once the father has "nursed" the newborn and given sweet tea to the mother so that her "milk will flow," the child is given to the mother so it can be nursed on her nipple. The father may continue to supplement mother's milk with the lower-lip-as-nipple procedure. In this way, Taipaobal fathers trained by Siamae Sanji proudly mark themselves as the nurturers.

In summary, among the Siamae Sanji family, it is the male who marks himself as the first food giver. He maintains a connection with the child's protecting spirits, who are gendered as male. He is concerned with the child's health and safety, and he maintains the child's spiritual links to patrilineal ancestors (even though kinship is reckoned cognatically). These patrilineal ancestors who began the universe and reside in heaven thus have priority over all others. By association with the important patrilineal ancestors, the child gains status. By emphasizing the positive aspects of the male's role, these midwives imply that females neglect connections with people, spirits, and living beings. The mother "neglects" to nurse the child and separates herself from the child and its umputé spirits. This neglect can be dangerous for living and future generations, who may suffer the consequences of the wrath of forgotten or neglected spirits. Thus, females' dealings with spirits and humans are negatively marked. Moreover, the spirits who symbolize neglect or separation are said to be female.

In sum, then, in Siamae Sanji's description of the birth context, males' work is more valued than females'. This promotes health and safety for the child. It maintains the connection to all spirits, though the black ones are connected to humans more tenuously than the white ones.

Repaying the Spirits' Labor: "Feeding Umputé with Our Bodies"

Both black and white spirits are called "older siblings" because they were born first. To call the umputé spirits "older sibling" (with no gender designation) is to acknowledge an unquestionable and immutable relationship between humans and spirits, a relationship of debt and obligation. All Laujé with whom I spoke say the umputé spirits give them life and nurture them in the womb, just as an older sibling does in the family. An older sibling is superior because it was born first, leading the way for the younger. At the early stage of the life cycle, the older sibling offers its own food to the younger, bathes her, plays with her, and protects her from taunts by neighbor children. The younger sibling is forever indebted to the older for these nurturing acts, which can never be "repaid." Siamae Sanji's sister-in-law answered my question about this debt with her own question, "How do you give a gift or offering that is worthy enough to acknowledge the spirit who gave you life?" Her rhetorical question needs no response. There is no gift that can cancel a debt to the older sibling. As Siamae Sanji's son Sair puts it, this does not obviate the need to give gifts through which "humans acknowledge or repay the debt we owe with our own bodies. When we are ill, we are paying tribute *(nokasiviani)* to the umputé spirits. We let the umputé into our body for three days. That is its due. Then we can use 'medicine' to ask it to leave. When it leaves, then we recover." Thus, sickness is a physical form of repayment or offering to the umputé spirit. Humans' bodies are the gift from the spirits. Only through death and return of the bodies to the spirit can humans completely cancel their debts.

Diagnosis and Initial Treatment of Black and White Illness in Taipaobal

The "White" Illness

Ironically, umputé is not generally responsible for serious illness. The mild colds and fevers it brings are tolerated. Death, at its proper time, is expected. But occasionally umputé is thought to overstay its welcome, to inhabit its human sibling's body longer than is healthy or proper. It is in such instances that a sando such as Siamae Sanji is called upon to send the offending spirit home. The curer must diagnose which umputé spirit is afflicting the person. The white umputé causes less severe illness, while the black causes illness that can lead to death. If the afflicted seems weak, listless, and chilled, as one does in malaria, the curer will whisper a prayer to the white umputé spirit over a glass of water. He will respectfully ask the spirit to return to heaven and wait there for its "younger sibling," the human. A sample prayer from Siamae Sanji is given below. It is simple yet polite, and the spirit is named, like a remembered ancestor.

We respectfully ask you the Spirit Rabakah
Who brings the chills, who brings the fever
No more!
Take pity on us, you who live
At the House of Spirits, at the Source of the Waters
Oh Rabakah!

The prayer is whispered over a glass of water.[20] The prayer to the white umputé spirit uses the spirit's personal name, Rabakah, whereas the prayer to the black umputé spirit uses only a generic spirit name, black umputé. The names or locations of these spirit places are not important to the curer in terms of their meaning, but in terms of their efficacy. Siamae Sanji's sons say that the white umputé prayer is more efficacious because they know the spirit's name. They are "close to the spirit." The spirit, they say, is like "a remembered ancestor whose name we invoke when we go to their grave and ask for rain." To know the name of the spirit is to ask the spirit's aid in curing.

After inaudibly murmuring the specific name of the spirit, a sando like Siamae Sanji gives the afflicted person the "medicine," the "blown-on" water to drink. Within a short time the person should be well. If not, then more drastic methods are necessary—a spirit familiar must be called in to possess the sando. When the sando is possessed, he is called a *boliang* (at least, that is, here in the mountains). If the cure works, though, the person who was treated must acknowledge the umputé spirit by giving an offering of thanks. This offering also repays the debt the cured has to the boliang and/or sando. Until the offering is made, the sando/boliang is responsible to the spirit who has left the ill person's body.

White umputé spirits called *pontianak* (in Indonesian and Laujé) must be called in for a cure. They have caused the illness by getting too close to the human. They represent, says Siamae Sanji, "too much connection." A pontianak is generally known throughout Indonesia as a spirit of a woman who has died in childbirth. According to Siamae Sanji, though, the white umputé spirit is a pontianak who died while giving birth to twins. Thus the souls of the twin children, the placental spirit and the mother, are still united, thereby underlining the tragic consequences of too much connection. The twins are little boys who are told by their mother to gather firewood or fetch water. One spirit fetches water and is cold, the other gathers firewood and is hot. When they connect with human bodies, they afflict humans with the hot and cold illness, malaria. For a cure, Siamae Sanji calls on the boys' father's spirit, a white spirit who resides in the sky. The father asks the boys to stop "playing with the human's body" and instead separate from it. If a cure results, an offering must be given.

Siamae Sanji's White Umputé Offering

Though the afflicted may wait as long as a year to save enough money and rice for the white offering, Siamae Sanji says they should repay the spirit and the sando as soon as possible.[21] If they do not, they and the sando could suffer a much harsher illness than the first. The offering for the white umputé spirit is called the "white chicken" rite.

The recovered should have gathered the supplies for Siamae Sanji—rice, a young white cock, eggs from a white hen, golden bamboo, betel nut, and tobacco. Siamae Sanji usually arrives midmorning and works slowly but methodically into early afternoon when the offering is made and all present share a special meal of thanksgiving together.[22]

Throughout the day, the household women usually remain in the kitchen preparing the rice, the chicken with coconut sauce, and the cookies. Some of this food will be offered on a tray for the spirit, some will be used for the festive meal. The household men, guests, and children sit in the "parlor" smoking homemade cigarettes and watching Siamae Sanji make the bamboo offering tray called a *selasa*.[23] Usually these rites serve as a forum for other men to learn the "offering medicine." Often a novice prepares the tray under the careful guidance of Siamae Sanji.

Siamae Sanji teaches how to carefully and artfully weave the bamboo tray in the same basket-weave manner as the walls of a house or the body of a cradle.[24] The tray is flat and approximately six-tenths of a meter (or two feet) square. An acolyte carefully cuts leaves from a *bagis* tree and hangs them around the edges, gathering and tying them like a baby's cradle. Then the novice hangs five bamboo cylinders underneath the tray, filling the cylinders with water "for the white umputé spirit to drink."

When the food is finally ready, the household women set the various kinds of rice—regular white rice, regular yellow rice, sticky white rice, sticky yellow rice—and cooked meat from a white chicken next to Siamae Sanji and the hanging bamboo offering tray. Siamae Sanji places a layer of fresh green didil leaves (about twenty-five of them)

over the top of the hanging tray so that none of the rice will fall
through the open weave of the bamboo tray. He scoops up a fist full of
plain white rice, carefully shaping it into a round mound about three
inches in diameter on the tray. Then he encircles this with a ring of
white sticky rice; then a ring of glutinous yellow rice, carefully washing his hands between "colors." Then, from this central clump or
circle, he shapes four branches or arms of rice from the center to the
tray's edges. The portions of the long arms closest to the center are
made of white sticky rice; then at the end of each branch, he adds
yellow sticky rice.

While waiting for the food to be cooked, Siamae Sanji rolls seven
homemade cigarettes with bagis leaf "papers" "like the ancestors used
to use." He ties the cigarettes in the center with a thin strip of the
strong bagis stem. Once the cigarettes are rolled, he momentarily lights
them, allows them to burn a short time, then he extinguishes the fire
and sets the bundle aside. A small banana-leaf origami boat is used
here to store the tobacco offering before it is placed on the offering
tray with the cooked rice and meat. The cigarettes will be placed on
top of the rice, and on top of all this Siamae Sanji will place an antique
coin called "hard money" *(doi mooas)*, a white hen's egg, boiled and
peeled, and betel nut.

Because Siamae Sanji was unable to walk unassisted, he asked the
apprentice and any other males who wished, to slowly carry the cradle
offering to a tree in the houseyard (see Figure 3.1). There they hang
the offering on a branch of a fruit tree. They place a small white cock
on top of the tray, petting and encouraging the chick to nibble at the
food on the tray. The apprentice utters a prayer inviting the spirits to
take the offering, to eat its essence. The name of the spirit is mentioned
quietly (secretly), but the name of its home is said aloud. The blessing
is polite and serves as an acknowledgment of humans' continuing in-
debtedness to the spirit:

> Respected Spirit named Rabakah
> There at the Source of Water
> At the House of Spirits
> These words we speak, please[25]
> With these words you must take
> All that we are offering and
> Listen to us well
> And do what is good for us all.

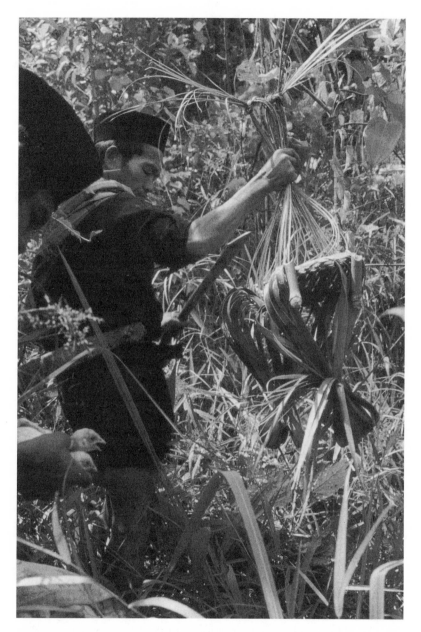

Figure 3.1. Apprentice carrying offering to white umputé spirit

The apprentice deposits the feathers of the slaughtered chickens and the slivers of the bamboo tray further away in the bush. The apprentice unties the young white cock and takes it to Siamae Sanji who will raise it at home. In some cases, the father of the afflicted will keep the cock to raise. Later, the grown cock can be slaughtered for another ceremony provided that it is replaced by a living immature bird.[26]

The participants return to the house to share a festive meal of rice, leftover chicken meat cooked in coconut juice (juu), and, if the family can afford it, another chicken. Betel nut, cigarettes, coffee, and sago cookies are served if possible. Such festive feasts are in sharp contrast to the typical Taipaobal meal of plain rice, dried fish or taro, and crushed pepper with salt.[27] Before Siamae Sanji returns home, he is given traveling food—rice bundles, cooked in little woven squares, triangles, and ovals, called *ampini* (*ketupat* in Indonesian).

According to Siamae Sanji and other Taipaobal informants, these offerings represent not only the world in which humans live, but also the mythological creation of spirits. Siamae Sanji says that the center or navel of the tray is the center of the world. He says the egg is the "shaded or covered place" and it harkens back to the world before earth and sky divided. The center is also the seat of the olongian. He calls this the "essence." It is to this specific spot that the words of the prayer are directed.

Because the offering is made for a spirit to whom he wishes to be close, Siamae Sanji uses a mound of plain white rice, surrounded by a concentric circle of sticky rice, and then another circle of yellow sticky rice to represent the essence of this spirit. This reveals that the offering is for a "pure spirit," the "highest," the "olongian spirit." The rice branches are for the underling spirits, the "servants" of the olongian. Because the central mound representing the ruler is connected to the four corners by long "arms" representing the "servants," servants and ruler are said to remain in a close, patron/client, relationship.

The corner areas, says Siamae Sanji, represent the cured or the sacrificer. "The long arms stretch to the remote corners showing how spirit and human are connected." The corners represent the "four corners of the world, [the] place where the spirits live at the edge of the world." "Humans have a connection with the white umputé spirit" to whom this tray is being offered because "the arms reach out." Though he never explicitly said so, the "connected arms" imply that Siamae

Sanji is reconstituting the social world as it should be; the olongian and her underlings remain in close contact.

The other offered items have significance as well. They mark the rite as one in which distinctions between mythic time, present time, and the time of a proper childbirth are connected and collapsed. The tray's leaves are the same as those used for the placental "cradle." The cigarette bundle resembles the four sticks of wood held by the mother during childbirth. Its tan leaves are from the bagis tree, the tree planted by the first ancestors. The cigarette bundle thus connects the first ancestors to fathers of children who gather the "wooden bundle." It also connects the sando and the patient to the white umputé spirit who is to receive this "cigarette bundle." The fact that tobacco, an exchange item, is used in this offering, may show that some kind of bridge between two worlds is signified, as George (1996) and Hoskins (1997) have shown elsewhere with other exchange items. Tobacco, like resin *(damag)*, was famous as the cash crop in the Laujé mountains from as far back as the days of the Dutch East India Company (VOC, in Dutch, which dissolved in 1798) (Colonial Records of 1820). As bush products, these items acted as mediators between the outside world of Dutch capitalism and the inside world of exchange between humans and spirits. Thus, these cigarettes seem a perfect icon by which the Laujé may also refer to exchanges taking place between themselves and the outside or nonhuman world of the spirits. Normally, Laujé men and women prefer clove cigarettes, which are a sign of status, but the kind of cigarette smoked here must connect the smoker with the past, with the time of the ancestors; clove cigarettes are prohibited, for they are a recent introduction to the area.

The little origami boat the cigarettes are stored in also emphasizes connections between realms. Just the fact that a boat is used here, deep in the mountains, suggests connections of sea and land. Additionally, since some curers, when they are possessed by spirits, are called vessels *(payangan)*, which carry the spirits, the boat may refer to spirits in another realm. Boats are used by outsiders, those from far away, to sail to the Laujé land. Once the traditional ancestors' cigarette bundle is burnt, it signifies a transference of substance across realms and a continuing tie or bond between the realm of spirits, who may or may not be ancestors, and that of humans, who are seeking aid from them. In

general, then, the cigarettes and the boat symbolically suggest continuity rather than separation.

The antique coin, usually a silver *kupang* from the eighteenth-
century Dutch East India Company (VOC), is also significant as an
icon of connection with the ancestors. Because the coin is so old, it
represents links and bonds with the ancestor who saved the coin, passing it down to this generation. The metal substance of the coin, silver,
is also important because, in origin myths, many Laujé say humans
were first separated from the world of the souls, from God's world,
when a silver wall divided the living from the spiritual world. Being
made of the same substance as the dividing wall, the silver coin carries
the message of division, but also of links to the past. As a double-
edged icon, it is used on the one hand to signify separation, distance,
and the cutting of bonds between two mythic realms. On the other
hand, it is used to signify continuity with the recently dead ancestors
who provided it. Thus, using the coin in the offering helps to meld the
distinctions between mythic past, remembered past, and the present.

The peeled white egg signifies that the offering for the spirit of
mythic beginnings when the world was like an egg. It also refers to the
souls of white umputé spirits, the pontianak, which were undifferentiated as fetus, mother, and placenta when they died together. The
peeled egg refers to the pool of souls, the general mass of remembered
ancestors and their particular umputé spirits. All these souls will eventually reincarnate into future bodies. The egg is thus the icon representing the beginning of life, the end of life, and the future bond connecting these souls.

The betel nut signifies an exchange between two disparate realms.[28]
It is given along with the pieces of white chicken meat, the best pieces,
says Siamae Sanji, which are put in the central mound. The word for
the juice or coconut milk in which the meat is cooked, *juu,* is the same
word used for the sperm and vaginal fluids that create a child. It is also
the word used for the placental waters that nurture the child in the
womb. By eating the juice in the present, the participants reconnect
with the umputé spirits with whom they were in the womb.

Time is also collapsed when "old" chicken meat from the white
cock brought by Siamae Sanji is prepared for offering and a young
chick is placed on the tray with the sacrificed "old meat." The young
chick is called the "plaything" of the umputé spirit, just as a younger
sibling is called a "plaything" of the older sibling. Siamae Sanji be-

comes the chick's caretaker and nurturer, but the soul of the chick is the property of the spirit, just as the soul of a child is the property of its umputé.

The rite creates a proper relationship between human and spirit by substituting the chicken's soul for the ill human's soul. It also effects a separation between the spirits who are suspended in time between birth and death. The spirits of the mother who died in childbirth with her twin children did not make the proper separation at birth, and now they are suspended in the in-between world. When the offering is hung in the yard like a placental cradle and the young chick is taken back to the house to raise to maturity, the offering makes the separation and distinction between generational souls that should have been made at birth. By redefining the time period in which it takes a younger sibling to mature, die, and rejoin the older sibling, the rite stops sickness. Specifically it is the male spirit, the father, who ultimately stops the other spirits from causing illness.

From Siamae Sanji's perspective, the whole rite signifies connection, mythic beginnings, fertility, childbirth, ancestors, masculinity, and nurturance. It is a rite that honors the white umputé spirit. It marks the connection humans have to that spirit at the same time that it states that a more hierarchical relationship should exist so that the spirits and humans are separated from one another. The white illness is structurally opposed to the black, as is its cure. While the white illness comes from the placenta and is associated with ancestors and males, the black illness comes from black blood and is associated with females and severed connections.

Black Umputé Offerings: Separating from the Female Spirit

Siamae Sanji says the illness caused by black umputé spirits creates "black" symptoms. An ill person's skin is "black like a monkey's," "black like theirs (bela)," and "black like a woman's skin before marriage."[29] If the afflicted has dark-colored skin, sunken eyes, or a burning hot fever, then Siamae Sanji, or another sando trained by him, will utter a prayer to the black umputé spirit, asking it in less than respectful terms to go home. Though both men and women are afflicted with the black umputé disease (which causes pain when urinating), they call a lingering version of it "the woman's disease." In this way, Siamae Sanji and most Taipaobalers equate the female spirit and black umputé with feminized outsiders, the bela. In other words, Siamae Sanji and Taipaobalers make their own ethnic distinctions through gender differentiation.

And just as they neglect the black umputé spirit in the birth scenario, in curing they invoke the spirit in a rough and cursory manner. The prayer to this spirit is short and rude:

> Go on, go home, you black umputé spirit
> Leave this sick person alone.
> Go home to the Wall of Stone[30]

Siamae Sanji says the spirit is a black pontianak. It can be either the child or the mother who died in childbirth. The black spirit, though, has departed in evil circumstances. It was aborted by the mother. To avenge its own "murder," the spirit waited for its mother's spirit in the blood pond just under the narrow bridge separating life and death. When the mother's soul crossed over the bridge heading to the land of the dead, the spirit (soul) of the aborted child pulled her down into the murky depths of the blood pond.

The fluid in the pond is made from the "blood" and the souls of all persons who died for some egregious sin "before their alloted time." The pond holds the souls of people who have died violently and people who neglected to give food to or responsibly care for their family. Some were masturbators who "wasted sperm" instead of producing a child. Even women who have miscarriages are there because they "neglected their unborn child." Siamae Sanji says most souls in the blood pond were bela women because they most frequently abort their children.[31]

From this bloody liminal netherworld, all these black umputé spirits afflict the living with diseases. Thus, the spirit who hears the black umputé prayer is a spirit who has neglected to nurture her ties to family and has separated herself from connections with others. It is not inappropriate, then, that the offerings to this spirit are those that signify separation, femininity, and neglect.

As was the case with the white chicken rite, the black chicken rite is the means by which the patient repays a sando like Siamae Sanji for getting rid of the black sickness. The sando, in turn, repays the spirit. In contrast to the white offering, though, the black rite is simple and unembellished. The selasa, or offering tray, for black umputé is more hastily constructed. The tray is made outside on the ground rather than inside the house. No one wants to linger at the offering site, much less go to much effort to make the offering aesthetically pleasing.

A sando such as Siamae Sanji hastily plaits the small tray and haphazardly slashes the grass away so he can set the tray down in a little clearing. Then, he casually throws a banana leaf on top. Not bothering to clean his hand before he dips it into the pot of plain "black" rice, Siamae Sanji swiftly scoops up rice and flings it onto the center of the tray. Too hurried to shape the rice into a neat circle, he reaches into another pot of black sticky rice and flings another scoop into the tray's corner. Repeating this pattern four times, Siamae Sanji fills each corner with its own mound of rice, solitary and detached from the central mound. He forcefully stabs four bamboo tubes, about six inches tall, into the ground near the corners, filling each tube with water. Taking an egg that has been cooked in the black sticky rice until its skin is mottled and purple, Siamae Sanji peels the egg. Then he severs the egg in half with an antique coin. One half of the egg is put in the central mound; the other half is cut into four more pieces and placed at each of the four corners.

Lastly, Siamae Sanji reaches for the meat to place on the offering. Rather than selecting the choicest pieces of meat to bestow, as he did in the white chicken rite, Siamae Sanji selects the "worst meat"—the "organs," the "internal parts." He places this meat in the four corners. Finally, he takes the wing feathers from the slaughtered black hen and places them on top of the offering. Siamae Sanji mumbles a quick prayer, without mentioning the name of the spirit, just its home, the Wall of Stone:

> Scram, Scat, Go Home!
> Go Home to the Wall of Stone

No one who has followed Siamae Sanji to the edge of the bush lingers to eat the leftovers. Participants simply grab the pots and trot back to the house. They quickly smoke a cigarette rolled with store-bought paper. Inside, a "festive" thanksgiving meal is served with black rice and steamed chicken cooked in gravy, not in coconut milk. Though the meal is more elaborate than Taipaobaler's daily fare, it pales in comparison to the multiple course meal served during the white chicken rite.

In many ways, the black chicken rite is the inverse of the white chicken rite. Not only are the colors of the rites opposed, but the black rite is "on the ground" and "outside," while the white chicken rite—

by being made inside and hung in a tree outside—effects a connection between "sky" and "house." Instead of the bagis-leaf lining signifying connection to the ancestors, banana leaves are used. Bananas are not plants that are indigenous to the area. In myths about bananas, the banana plant refused to feed its sibling. Banana leaves signify neglect and severed familial connections. The "hard coin" serves as a divider in this rite, symbolically reiterating the rite's theme of disjunction and separation. The coin analogically stops the connection between the human world and that of the umputé spirit, when it is used to divide the egg. It is symbolically opposed to the white umputé's antique coin.[32]

Also, the cigarette rolled from store-bought paper is unlike those ancestorlike cigarettes rolled from bagis leaves in the white umputé ceremony. The cigarette smoked upon entering the house before eating the leftovers is reminiscent of "smoking one's body with a burning log" upon returning from a burial. This act marks a connection to, yet ultimate separation from, the domain of death. By association, the black umputé offering is linked with death. While the black rite uses a grown hen that has hatched several litters of chicks, the white rite uses a young chick. The black hen is at the end of her life cycle, ready to separate from life. The white cock is at the beginning of his life ready to be nurtured.

The foods placed on the offering tray duplicate this theme of death and separation. The rice in the center is not connected by rice "arms" or "legs" to the four corners, as in the white rite. Internal organs and scraps, rather than the choicest meat, are proffered in the black rite. The feathers of the slaughtered hen, which are tossed into the bush in the white umputé rite, here, in the black, are placed on top of the offering. The black spirit's name is "forgotten," and only a generic name is given in the short black rite, whereas in the white rite a proper spirit name is used and a long respectful prayer is uttered. The oppositions between the two rites are as follows:

Black Umputé	White Umputé
Separation	Connection (and some separation)
Severed egg	Whole egg
Dead hen (female)	Young cock (male)
Outside	Inside (and outside)
Inedible meat	Delicious meat

Imperfection/incompletion	Perfection/completion
Earth (female)	Sky (male)
Ground	Hanging

Under Siamae Sanji's tutelage, the black chicken "medicine" relays the same message communicated in the birth process: The black blood umputé spirit is neglected and thus dangerous. The black spirit is associated with females. It is treated with a minimum of respect. A radical separation between it and the space of human habitation is effected. As such, the rite reiterates the birth scenario, but in an exaggerated form. In the birth scenario, "black blood" is inadvertently ignored. Here "black blood" is put in its place—on the ground, away from humans.

Though all Taipaobalers with whom I spoke say one should be respectful to all spirits, repay them for the "sweat" of their labor—which carried humans into the world—this black umputé spirit is mistreated even when it is ostensibly honored. This marks the ambivalence Siamae Sanji's family has toward these spirits. All Taipaobalers acknowledge that they "should not ignore any umputé spirits" because of their debt to the spirits. At the same time, however, Taipaobalers who respect Siamae Sanji distinguish between umputé spirits, honoring the white spirit more than the black.

In some respects, the category including white umputé does not simply contrast with the black umputé category, but also encompasses it. Just as the placenta encompasses the fetus, the white umputé encompasses black. Thus rather than a straight binary opposition in which the two halves are equal, here, there is a hierarchical opposition in which the encompassing category is superior. Such a hierarchy is predicted in the structuralist writings of Dumont (1970), Maybury-Lewis (1989), and Traube who say that all oppositions, if researched sufficiently, logically progress and evolve into encompassing hierarchies.[33] In the Laujé case, white umputé is the encompassing category because it is associated with both outside and inside, rather than simply inside, and because it deals with both connection and separation, rather than simply connection. The important thing to note is that white umputé, especially as it is embodied in the placenta, is discussed in positive terms. It is always associated with nurturance and referred to as the "older sibling." Moreover, Siamae Sanji associates it with the positive aspects of males, ancestors, and the olongian. In sum, then, the white umputé is superior and more encompassing than the black because it is more valued and more inclusive.[34]

Other Manifestations of Umputé Spirits in Taipaobal

Siamae Sanji teaches that umputé spirits originate from the birth fluids and the placenta, but they may manifest themselves in many forms, including that of humans. Because the body of the white umputé, the placenta, is nurtured and hung in a tree, it is less likely to leave its body and take human form. Black umputé whose "body" is carelessly allowed to fall onto the ground is most likely "to leave the ground" and appear in human bodies.

Usually, when the neglected black umputé spirit manifests itself in human form, it is more a harbinger of illness. Siamae Sanji and his trainees say the black umputé spirits can appear as lowland traders or animist bela. In whatever form they appear, though, they are always "unknown strangers." Usually the black umputé spirits are dressed in black clothing, the clothing of outsiders.[35] Because any stranger may be a black umputé spirit in disguise, these Taipaobalers say one must never refuse a stranger's request. To do so would ignore the debt one has to the umputé spirit and thus could cause one to become ill and "die before one's time." Taipaobalers must be careful not to anger the spirits lest they cause an epidemic.

The black spirits, however, are not completely pestilent. Siamae Sanji's son Larsen says the black umputé spirits possess great wealth. They live in "stone houses," and being intermittently invisible, they can walk into the stores of Tinombo and steal money. They have the power to create wealth objects not produced in the Taipaobal highlands. If one acknowledges these umputé spirits' superiority by giving them food or drink, they may, in turn, bestow riches on one. Thus, says Larsen, all Laujé should treat everyone, stranger or family member, equally.

Of course, this description is an idealized model that is not necessarily followed in everyday life in Taipaobal. Most Taipaobalers try as best as they can to avoid acknowledging any debts they have to strangers who might be disguised spirits, unless they see that they may gain something in return. My fieldnotes reveal how the Taipaobalers first regarded me as a black umputé spirit:

When Eric, Pak Husin (my language teacher), and I arrived in Taipaobal for the first time, all the doors to houses we approached were shut. No one would answer our questions as to where we could find water. We knew people were in the houses—we could see their eyes peering out—but no one was brave enough to speak to us. It was only after Siamae Sanji recognized Pak Husin as a former colonial officer, that someone acknowledged our presence. Siamae Sanji warmly took us in as guests.

But a month or so after we settled in Taipaobal, we were invited to spend the night at the house of one of the people who had ignored us on that first day. Siinai Usman, the woman of the house, explained she had been at her in-law's when we asked for water and no one answered. "My in-laws were deathly afraid of foreigners," she said. "Though I knew you would not harm us, I could say nothing as a guest in my in-law's house."

Now in her own home, she wanted to pay back the "neglect" by inviting us for a chicken dinner—a very special treat. She slaughtered a black chicken, shared "foreign" clove cigarettes with us, and made homemade cookies with sugar she bought from the market in Tinombo. She seemed warm and friendly.

Later in the evening after long conversations, the woman finally blurted out a question as though she had been waiting to ask it all night long. "So, I want to know the secret now, tell me the place to find your money machine, your *rupiah* machine." She thought that foreigners like myself had "the secret" of making money, and she wanted the knowledge too. Rather ineptly I tried to persuade her that I did not have a money machine. The woman, however, did not believe me. Hurt that I would reject such a request, her wellspring of hospitality dried up. I soon found out from Larsen that the woman and her husband had thought we were black umputé spirits who when fed in an honorific manner as we were, were supposed to respond with a gift from "our land." The woman truly thought we were spirits. After this incident, she kept her distance from us, often giving us suspicious looks. At her expense, I learned about the black spirits.

Black umputé spirits can manifest themselves as foreigners such as myself. The spirits are often women. These spirits have access to externally produced, non-Laujé products—sugar, cookies, clove cigarettes, and paper money. They visit for a short period of time and may bring sickness. A sando like Siamae Sanji wants to separate himself from such spirits and identifies them as foreign or other (in his case as female spirits).

By contrast, Siamae Sanji characterizes the white umputé spirits in ways that are identical to his role as a sando, a curer, or a boliang. *Boliang* also refers to the spirit familiar that possesses the medium to cure an illness when simple white umputé prayers have not worked. The boliang spirit exhibits many characteristics of the white umputé spirit, though it is slightly different. Its home is the sky, near where the white placental spirit lives. The boliang and the white umputé spirits can be called to leave their "home" and come cure humans. The spirit will travel from the sky to earth so it can possess curers' bodies.[36]

Siamae Sanji "calls" the boliang spirit by playing a sequence of notes over and over again on a lute. The notes are those that the "first ancestors played." The spirit "floats in on a white cloud" and possesses Siamae Sanji. This enables him to "see things human beings cannot see" and thereby effect a cure.[37] Though boliang spirits are not the same as the white umputé spirit, both are characterized as nurturing, healing spirits connected with the ancestors, the sky, and, for the most part, with men.

In sum, Siamae Sanji characterizes curing rites for the white and the black umputé spirits in structurally opposed terms just as he characterizes them as opposites in the birth scenario. The white spirit is categorically superior to the black because it represents positive values like nurturance and because it encompasses, literally as a placenta and figuratively as a separator and connector. The key scenario of birth, one which everyone experiences, sets up these relationships. During the birth scenario, the importance of the woman's nurturing is minimized, while the father's nurturing is accented.

Though a pure postmodernist may find my analysis of umputé too totalizing, reading too much into the "native point of view," this is Siamae Sanji's analysis. His exegesis demonstrates the depth and detail of a particular "native's" structural worldview. The postmodern way to make sense of his structural/symbolic perspective, is to assume that this is his and not everyone else's way of seeing the world. My point, layered on top of the postmodern perspective, is that his symbolic and structural understanding of the world is not created in a vacuum. Structural and symbolic perspectives like his abound throughout Indonesia and beyond.[38]

Additionally, Siamae Sanji's emphasis on umputé is not an isolated case. The literature on birth siblings in Indonesia alone is extensive. On Sulawesi there are several examples. Kennedy's survey of ethnographic work for the Celebes and Sunda notes that the Balantak have a religion based on the placental amniotic fluids (1953). The Balantak also have a six-day festival in which a boat is cast off to sea with offerings of rice, etc. Acciaioli briefly mentions the notion of spirit siblings among Bugis immigrants in Central Sulawesi (1990:207–35), while also discussing how foreign migrants may try to usurp rituals oriented to local spirits. More discussion of placental siblings among the Bugis can be seen in Gibson's (1995) work. On another island, Bali, placental spirits, called *kanda mpat rare,* are well documented; Anthony Forge (1980), Hooykaas (1974), and Linda Connor (1986) have written about placental siblings as have local authors like K. Tonjaya (1981). On Java, Ossenbruggen (1977) and Headley (1987) discuss the *monca-pat.* In Sumatra, John Bowen writes about the significance of placental spirits among the Gayo (1993:118) and Steedly (1988) among the Karo Batak. Josselin de Jong (1965) mentions placental siblings throughout the Indonesian archipelago.

The cluster of ideas that the Laujé call umputé are probably Austronesian in origin, since they exist beyond Indonesia into the Malayo-Polynesian, or Austronesian-speaking world. For instance, in Malaysia, Laderman (1991; 1983) discusses the widespread beliefs in birth siblings among Malays in her extensive research on midwifery and spirit possession. R. McKinley (1981) also notes Malay beliefs, while Signe Howell mentions birth spirits among the Orang Asli in Malaysia (1984; 1985). Hart (1965) discusses the birth siblings in a Bisayan Filipino village, Coughlin (1965) in a Vietnamese village, and Rajadhon in a Siamese village (1961). Such far-flung and well-substantiated cases leave little doubt that birth siblings are an Austronesian phenomenon.

Taipaobalers who agree with Siamae Sanji, then, draw upon general Austronesian themes and interpret them in ways that specifically relate to their everyday lives. Umputé becomes the idiom through which their symbolic categories of male and female, inside and outside, and nurture and neglect are expressed. It is through the shape and substance of offerings taught to them by Siamae Sanji in his own idiosyncratic way that these Taipaobalers make the distinctions among umputé spirits tangible. Such oppositions and ideas articulated by Siamae Sanji would not resonate with other peoples' ideas, however, if they were not shared by a number of people. Thus, it is through discourse about the characters of these spirits, and their propensity to cause illness or cure, that the "tangible" distinctions of umputé reiterate and reinforce broadly shared, more or less collective representations, of social distinctions in the Laujé community.

4

FATAL ATTRACTIONS
Sumpitan on Umputé

L ike Siamae Sanji's, Sumpitan's characterization of umputé spirits associates spirits with colors. But rather than monochromatic themes,[1]
Sumpitan draws from a more colorful palette. Sumpitan's four-color
symbolism for the umputé spirits—white, yellow, red, black—is shared
widely throughout the Indonesian archipelago (Geertz 1960; Fox
1980; Forman 1980). Both Acciaioli (1989) and Pelras (1996) even
mention the necessity of similar sticky rice offerings of all four colors
in Bugis rituals. Also found in other parts of Indonesia are the spirit
pairs that Sumpitan invokes in blessings for the colored rice offerings
(Fox 1980; 1988; Kuipers 1990; Metcalf 1989; 1993; Traube 1986).[2]
Thus, Siamae Sanji and Sumpitan are not alone in the way they present umputé. What makes them both unique, however, is that they introduce a new moralistic twist to color patterns and umputé categories
found elsewhere in eastern Indonesia. Thus, even though Siamae
Sanji's scheme is quite different from Sumpitan's in the particular references he makes to birth and sexual fluids, the general patterns, the
structurally opposed categories dividing nurturing and connection
from neglect and separation are very similar.

Elite Laujé Worldview: The Teachings of Sumpitan

Just as Siamae Sanji divided umputé spirits into two categories—one
nurturing, the other neglected—so did Sumpitan. Like Siamae Sanji's,
Sumpitan's umputé spirits had the same personalities as his historical
characters. For Sumpitan the placental spirit was analogous to the
olongian who nurtured the Laujé people and connected them to the
mythic beginning of time. Sumpitan's red blood spirits were analogous
to the foreign raja who "separated" the community and ignored his
responsibility to his subjects.

Sumpitan's teachings about the umputé spirits, however, were more female-friendly than Siamae Sanji's because they did not characterize the evil other as feminine (although they still did not give the female a central role). When Sumpitan talked about umputé, he combined spirits into couples and then divided them into good and evil pairs. The white spirit, he said, was "married to yellow. They are good. Black is married to red. Both are bad." In effect, Sumpitan associated the white and yellow spirits (the light-colored ones) with sexual foreplay between Laujé men and women, the red and black spirits (the dark ones) with coercive sex, foreign men raping native women.

According to Sumpitan, it is when the white umputé spirits, the spirits residing in vaginal fluid and sperm, meet and mix together that yellow umputé appears. He said only a man who is a Laujé aristocrat knows how to call forth these spirits in sexual fluids and thus only a Laujé nobleman can sexually satisfy a woman. Sumpitan said:

> The white umputé spirit responds to our prayers which only elite Laujé know. When we Laujé people say secret prayers, we call forth the white umputé spirits. We call forth the clear liquid secreted by women and men during intercourse. We recite a secret prayer . . . and then we entice the white umputé spirit to flow into the womb, and then we ask the white spirit to guard against the red spirit. We Laujé elites know how to do this by reciting a prayer called *pombirih salah* on the wedding night. The others, the foreigners and the commoners, they don't know this. Only we Laujé.

Sumpitan also said:

> Without this liquid, the penis of a male will not enter a female. Just as this clear [liquid] if present will let any size penis enter a woman if it is present—try putting your fingers in your nostril, even the thumb will fit, right? [He pauses and sticks his finger up his nose, encouraging me to do the same.] You can do this because there is a clear substance there. This clear [substance] is what wraps the baby while it is still in the womb. . . . It is the white umputé.

Sumpitan claimed that no child would be born from any sexual union unless the two sexual fluids, the white umputé fluids, from the woman and the man are joined together "like two index fingers touching. If the substances are unequal, they will not touch, but pass by to the right or left. If the substances touch equally, then the two white fluids turn yellow, swirling together in a whirlpool." This yellow substance "congeals into the first thing formed in the womb, the eyeball." Sumpitan said that a golden knot is tied around the four "characteristics" from the mother and four from the father combining to make the eye of the child (see Bowen 1987). He said the dark center or cornea of the eye is the part inherited from the child's father. The white matter encircling the iris is the part inherited from the mother.[3] Only the "pure" Laujé umputé spirits can create this eye or egg.

The "foreign" umputé spirits cannot create life. They symbolize the "absence of life." When the red umputé spirit appears in the form of red blood it appears without the white umputé spirit.

> Without the white spirit present, a male cannot easily enter the female—she would bleed. Does a Laujé man come to the house and push his way into the door? This is what the foreign barbarian does—the red-turbaned one [the red umputé spirit]. No. The Laujé man arrives gently with his palms outstretched [like a good Muslim asking forgiveness]. Then the door will be open.

The door is a common euphemism for the woman's vagina. The "red turbaned one," said Sumpitan is "the red umputé," the "foreign warrior," or "the red umputé spirit who is like the raja and resides in red blood." Laujé women's "doors" are closed to foreigners, but open to Laujé men because the latter summon the white umputé spirit so that it secretes the sexual fluids.

The white "native" spirits are calm, nurturant, and fertile. The red "foreign" spirits are wild, barbaric, and bring death or uncreated life. These red "foreign" spirits refer to the spirits of menstrual blood—the spirits that herald another unfertilized egg. Red umputé spirits also reside in the red blood from "foreigners." "Red blood" and the volatile "red umputé spirit" of the foreign raja appear because a foreign male does not know how to summon the white umputé spirit of the vaginal fluids. Sumpitan said: "When this red umputé spirit appears, it is a sign that no child will be born, just as menstrual blood is a sign that no child will be born. The umputé spirit of the red blood is not a good spirit. . . . The red umputé spirit is wild and untamable, like a violent storm at sea . . . and it means infertility and violence." Sumpitan said elites believe that the white umputé spirit guards the door of the womb to keep the spirit and the food for the infant from flowing out. If a Laujé woman marries a foreign man who does not know these prayers, "the white umputé spirit does not guard the womb" and thus "all the forty-four kinds of sickness brought by the red umputé spirit are allowed to enter the woman's womb." The more she has sex with the man who does not know how to call the spirit of white umputé and "make her fluids flow," the thinner she will become.

Pregnancy Taboos from Sumpitan's Perspective

The pregnancy taboos mentioned by Sumpitan also distinguished foreigner from native. For instance, Sumpitan said:

> During pregnancy, the woman must guard against eating foreign food. Both the mother-to-be and the father-to-be cannot eat at foreigners' houses, because if they do, then something that is dirty might attach itself to the placenta, making childbirth difficult. But the couple must be especially generous in sharing food with Laujé relatives. All the couples' relatives should visit each other while a family member is pregnant.

During pregnancy if the mother-to-be goes out of the house, she should always wear a machete or at least be armed with a knife. She should carry it as a man does, on the hip. The man must avoid wearing pants, he must wear a sarong, as his wife does, and he must cook for his wife while she is experiencing labor pains. The man must weed and harvest the household garden where the woman normally works. Sumpitan said that an elite Laujé woman who is pregnant is brave, just like a tadulako warrior. She is "hard," and her skin cannot be pierced by "foreign objects."

> She is like a person of spiritual power. She must fight all the forty-four kinds of sickness that come to her through the barbarian red umputé spirit. The evil foreign spirit, the red umputé spirit may try to enter her womb at any time during her pregnancy and the mother-to-be must resist. The father-to-be must remain more sequestered during his wife's pregnancy. He must resist contact with foreigners, lest his actions harm the child. He must refrain from joking or flirting with women who are not family members. Otherwise, the child born will be thin and easily covered with sores.

Curing Rites for the Red and White Umputé Spirits in Dusunan

In Sumpitan's curing rites there is a very clear division made between offerings to the red spirit and offerings to the white. Though both spirits cause illness, Sumpitan says the "white illness" is less severe. If a person is feverish or chilled with malaria, or if they are listless and depressed for a long period of time, then it is because the white umputé spirit has been "visiting" them. The white spirit is the spirit of sexual fluid. She appears in dreams as a beautiful woman. "She hugs you, (male or female), you get excited or frightened and wake up weak or sick." She is a calm spirit, the spirit of sexual longing. To cure someone of the white illness Sumpitan skewers a clove of garlic with a small knife, usually a special one with a carved wooden handle, and immerses the knife in a glass of water. He blows on this water and quietly mutters the following prayer:

> Our Mother
> Our Father
> Bring down the fever, the chills

The prayer to the white umputé, says Sumpitan, is to "our mother, our father," rather than to a specifically named spirit, because the spirit represents "the lost possibility" of maternity and paternity through spent sexual fluids in nocturnal dreams. There is no specific child created, so there is no specific mother and father named. The terms for mother and father, however, are idiomatic Laujé and thus they reflect the identity of this spirit as Laujé. Sumpitan says, "this white spirit is Laujé." She comes from the "top of the mountain near the center of the earth by the Inscribed Rock." She is "one of the original Laujé ancestors. The prayer to her signifies connection to Laujé ancestors at the same time that it blames the white illness on the transgression of the spent sexual fluid that separates one from the ancestors.

The white umputé offering continues the theme of sexual longing and the deep bonds of commitment between Laujé lovers, even if they are separated from each other. These bonds can become so deep that they lead to incest between a father and a daughter. Sumpitan says the offering to the white umputé spirit is to Laujé spirits who have become too close:

> A Laujé man who was the father of a baby girl decided to go to Mecca on the pilgrimage. He did so during the days when the pilgrimage took many years to complete. So the man told his wife that he would be gone a long time. He said she might not recognize him when he returned. So he reminded her of the bald spot on his head which he always covered. His bald spot was in the shape of a cross. His wife said she would not forget.
>
> Many years later, when the wife was on her deathbed and her husband had not returned she told her daughter, "Wait until your father returns to

marry. If your father returns you will know him by the cross on his head." The girl remembered this. Many suitors came to woo the girl, but she wanted no one, until one day a suitor came with a white hat on his head. She fell in love with him. When he came to ask for her hand in marriage, she accepted. Excited, he took off his hat to bow down to her. She saw the cross on his head and realized that he was her father. She told him her story and he acknowledged that he must indeed be her father.

But both were already in love. They decided to keep their relationship a secret and marry according to traditional (non-Islamic) custom. During the wedding ceremony, however, an imam asked the father to remove his hat.[4] When he did, the imam realized who this stranger was.

The imam decreed that the man and wife were father and daughter and must be punished for the sin of incest. They must be tied to a rock and thrown in the sea. When the couple was thrown into the water, two white chickens, a female and a male, floated up. These white chickens were the first chickens in the world. Ever since they replaced the father and daughter, the Laujé have offered chickens in sacrifices rather than killing those who sin.[5]

Though this couple was punished for their sin, the story is one of love and nurturance to the point that categories—generational, religious, and temporal—normally separated are collapsed. The young girl married her father, thus dissolving generational and familial distance. She married a Muslim according to animist vows, thus uniting disparate religious categories. The couple's early relationship of too much distance merged into a relationship of too much closeness. The not-so-distant past when the Laujé went on the long pilgrimages was fused with mythical time when humans' corpses turned into chickens. The message of the story was that sickness comes from those who collapse hierarchical categories that should remain distinct.

If Sumpitan cures a person from the white illness, they must give an offering called the "white chicken rite" to the spirit via Sumpitan. For the rite, Sumpitan places yellow and white rice on a plate. On top of this plate, he adds a *whole* roasted chicken with head, beak, and feet still intact. The body is dry and brown.[6] The chicken's breast is split and the body splayed so it will lie flat on the rice. This plate is placed on a *flat* antique tray near the living centerpost of the house (where mothers give birth to children).

Sumpitan carefully skewers a whole, boiled, shelled egg onto a stick, adding to its top and bottom two flat Laujé cookies made from sago and red palm sugar, and two antique coins with holes in the center. On "top" Sumpitan carefully pierces a blossom from the red *ja-jambo* flower. The skewered egg with cookies, coins, and a flower flanking it is then poked into the middle of the chicken's back. Beneath the chicken's beak, a cup of water is placed so that the chicken might "drink it." The chicken faces the sea (in the east), where it arose in the incest myth. Toward the west, other plates of yellow and white rice topped with a whole egg, tobacco, locally rolled cigarettes, and betel nut are offered. In addition, a plate of puffed rice and some sprigs of the "first four woods of the earth" are set out.

When the food is arranged, Sumpitan calls both the father's and the daughter's spirits. He quietly whispers their names into his cupped hand, in which he holds two antique silver coins. He sits behind the feet of the chicken, facing the sea, "just as a woman giving birth would sit." Sumpitan sets down the coin for the male spirit on the right, the coin for the female spirit on the left. Each time he sets down a coin, he burns fragrant "wood of the ancestors" to call up the spirits. Then he presses his palm down on the plate with the puffed rice kernels and blesses the offering:

> The Radiance
> He/She, The Radiance or Light
> The ??? *(Bada)* Radiance
> Let this be received
> This we send to you
> To ask forgiveness
> To arrive for the Laujé ancestors
> Allah, give us long years
> Ancestors, give us long years
> Stop don't arrive again
> We Pray to our Grandparent
> To make long the Unwi[7]
> We place our palms upward in submission

He then grabs a small handful of the puffed rice and passes it around to the people in the room who quietly pray with their palms skyward. Sumpitan chants:

> We pray to the Ancestors and Allah to make us safe
> While we are here in the world
> Until we arrive in heaven
> [These three lines are repeated three times.]
> It is true the world is one
> And misfortune is far away.

When all finish praying, everyone turns their palms down *(tabanamé)*, spilling the puffed kernels onto the floor. Sumpitan tips over his left hand, but takes the rice in his right hand and throws it out the front door and into the bedroom. With this part of the ceremony finished, each participant eats some chicken and rice.

The prayers and substances used in this offering emphasize connection to Laujé ancestors. The prayer also invokes Allah. Thus, animism and religion are collapsed. Likewise, rice conveys a sense of fused time. Sumpitan says the white and yellow rice are equally "pure" because both came from the beginning of the universe. The white rice signifies male and female sexual fluids, the prelife state. The yellow signifies fertilized fluids, the beginning of life. Puffed rice is the "original" form of rice mentioned in the creation myth. It also signifies pregnancy of present day humans. Cooked rice and puffed rice signify mythic time as well as the time of procreation.

Similarly, Sumpitan says the skewered egg repeats the pattern in which the world began. In the mythic past, the earth and the sky were merely separated by an egg. The sky was a brass tray and the earth was a brass tray. The coins and the brown cookies that surround the egg on the skewer iconically repeat this fertile beginning in the mythic past. Concomitantly the skewered egg represents the fertility of a new bride, the white spirit who married her father. Sumpitan says the delicate red flower, jajambo, immediately falls off its vine when it is touched. In a similar way, a virgin's hymen "falls off" when it is touched. Thus, the image of the red flower, sweet cookies, and whole egg collapse the mythic and historical past. Moreover, the single undivided chicken represents the Laujé father and daughter who have neglected to separate as they should.

Sumpitan's message in this rite is that sickness occurs because categories that should remain distinct were collapsed. The rite offers a substitute "body" to the spirits so that humans do not repeat their mistakes, do not nurture so much that they collapse the hierarchies and categories that make the world what it is.

I Dreamt I Saw the Soldiers: The Red Umputé Spirit and Its Offering

The red umputé illness is much more severe. Its spirit, red umputé, connotes violence. Sumpitan invokes the red umputé prayer[8] when a person is afflicted with a fever, bleeding excessively in childbirth, or vomiting or passing blood. Before the prayer is uttered, Sumpitan prepares a glass of water. With a small knife, he stabs a red shallot clove and immerses the impaled shallot into the water. Sumpitan blows three times on the water and whispers the prayer:

> The King of Horns
> And She-Goddess Unasara
> Bring down the fever

This prayer, as well as the offering given after the prayer works, was introduced by a famous sando, Siamae Arbou, who arrived in Dusunan sometime in the 1910s. At that time, there was a dysentery epidemic. The cure for this disease came to Siamae Arbou in a dream he had about a raja who had sided with the Dutch against the local people. This raja, a "foreigner" from South Sulawesi, was a despot who required his subjects to work in forced labor at high noon during the Islamic fasting month. Angered at such cruel treatment and finding their pleas to rest ignored, the people turned on the raja.[9] They murdered him, the Dutch officer in charge (the *kontrolleur*), the colonial chief of police (KPN), and the Javanese soldiers who guarded the raja. Siamae Arbou said that it was the spirits of these "foreigners," the raja's red spirit and his underlings, the black spirits, who came to locals in the form of a severely debilitating dysentery.

In his dream Siamae Arbou's spirit-other, a boliang, gave him the cure for the illness in the form of a name and a prayer for the raja's spirit.[10] The prayer invokes not only the raja himself, Raja Tandu, but also his wife, Siti Unasara, who was a local woman. She was physically diminutive, but because she was "of the earth" (a Laujé), she is invoked in the prayer to restrain her husband, the raja, from causing severe illness. This offering served as a sacrificial substitute for the Laujé who became ill. It also acknowledged the high status of the raja, something the murderers had neglected to do.[11]

Today, Sumpitan's family still uses the "red medicine" that was given by Siamae Arbou's white spirit in a dream. If the prayer directed at the raja's spirit cures the patient, then the patient must make an offering to the red umputé spirit. The family also offers the red medicine annually as a preventive measure to ensure that the "red and black spirits" do not bring illness to the Laujé.[12]

In the offering for the vicious red umputé spirit, social rank is emphasized. To acknowledge the status of the raja's spirit, the offerings to the lesser officers and Javanese guards are segregated into two sections, the "big red" and the "little red," with a third "black" offering for the Javanese coolies.

Rank in offerings is signified in two ways: (1) by location of the trays either inside (high rank), or outside (low rank), and (2) by use of pedestal (high rank) or flat (low rank) brass trays.[13] The "big red" offering is for the two murdered officials, the raja and the Dutch kontrolleur, who were of the highest rank. For them, Sumpitan places plates of cookies, rice, scrambled egg, roasted chicken, tea, coffee, and cigarettes on brass pedestal trays *(dulang dadangki)* inside the house. Each item has its own plate or cup. One glass of water has three Dutch coins immersed in it. The "red" rice is mixed with the blood from the red chicken that had been slaughtered. A scrambled egg is placed on top of this in the center of the high pedestal tray. Other plates surround this central plate.

The "little red" offering is for the chief of police (KPN), who was a local man in colonial service. For it, Sumpitan places individual plates of rice mixed with blood, meat, cigarettes, and cookies on flat trays *(dula jepang)* in the house near the door. To signify the police officer's Laujé status, a whole egg is given instead of a scrambled one, and coffee instead of tea.

At the threshold, an offering to the highest Javanese guards is given. It consists of two coconuts, said to represent the soldiers' heads, each of which is pierced with two long sticks impaled with clove cigarettes (see George 1996). The cigarettes are taken from the chief of police's offering plate because the police officers "always gave their guards cigarettes." In each of the offerings, an Islamic prayer, an *aruwa*, or funeral dirge, is chanted. The prayers ask that the raja, the kontrolleur, the chief of police, and the guards leave the Laujé people alone and take what is offered, rather than the bodies of the Laujé.

Most of the items used in the offering are not locally produced. "Foreigners," usually Mandar and Bugis, introduced these items to the Laujé region. The plates and trays, as well as the coffee, tinned biscuits, sweet tea, and rolled cigarettes signify externally produced items owned or traded by people of high status and wealth. These items contrast sharply with the less hierarchical Laujé products.

This "lesser" offering to the foot soldiers who wore black is placed on the ground outside the house. The "black" offering is reminiscent of Siamae Sanji's black chicken offering. First, the items are carried to the edge of the houseyard. There, tall weeds are quickly slashed away. Blood from a slaughtered red chicken is poured over white rice and the chicken's heart, which rest on a sago leaf.[14] This bundle is wrapped up and the bloody red chicken heart is placed on top of the bundle. One boiled egg is divided into four parts and placed around the edge of the wrapped bundles; four homemade cigarettes are wrapped in black palm fiber and momentarily burnt; four betel nuts, gambier, and lime are wrapped in black cloth; and all are placed on the ground. Then the Islamic blessing (aruwa) is chanted, asking the spirit of the soldiers to leave the villagers alone.

Sumpitan says this offering signifies hierarchy and respect, as well as separation and impermanence. Each item offered is placed on individual plates rather than "connected" on one tray. Dark meat, the internal meat that decays the quickest, is used rather than "good" white meat, which is eaten by everyone. Chicken blood, which is thrown away in other offerings, here is mixed with the rice. Some informants sympathetic to Sumpitan say this resembles the blood and sperm that are mixed in an unfertilized womb, or the bone, blood, and skin that "mix together" when someone dies a violent death. In many respects, this offering signifies life and all the internal substances of life that a human body has, but also the transitory nature of those substances, the chaos and violence of "mixed" categories.

The egg offering in the "big red" for the raja's spirit, is the only one of all the Laujé offerings in which the egg is scrambled and then fried (like an omelette).[15] The scrambled egg, together with the bloody rice, symbolizes an abortion or rape. Sumpitan says that fierce foreign men often rape Laujé women or make them bleed on their wedding night. I could never discern whether or not rape is a reality or Sumpitan's metaphor for the political rape of the Laujé by "foreigners." Whatever the case, this offering to the red umputé spirit signifies that "foreigners," especially rajas, are spiritually inept and dangerous because they do not protect the human body, the egg. The rite effects a separation from the foreigner and thus, it neutralizes foreigners' effect on the Laujé.

The red umputé offering is not about nurturance, sexual longing, and deep bonds of commitment between Laujé lovers; it is about foreigners, violence, murder, and rape. The red umputé rite remarks that too much hierarchy has been effected. Its Islamic prayer is a funeral dirge for recently dead souls who have not yet found heaven. The message this rite conveys is that foreigners never reach heaven; they are too hierarchical and violent.

When comparing the two rites and the egg offerings in them, the divisions between foreigner and Laujé become more clear. The egg of the white offering is left intact because the spirits receiving the offering were both Laujé. The egg in the red umputé was broken and bloody because the spirits were foreign men of high status. The two umputé rites differ in this way:

Red Umputé	White Umputé
Foreign raja spirit	Local man and woman
Murder	Incest
Ranked offerings	Flat offerings
Hierarchy	Merging of hierarchy
Scrambled eggs	Whole egg
Chicken parts	Whole chicken
Separate plates	One central plate
Foreign food	Local food
Arabic prayer	Local prayer

Through Sumpitan's interpretations, these rites enact the limits of hierarchy and divisions. The foreigners take the divisions to extremes and separate themselves from their subjects, while some Laujé avoid hierarchy and distinctions to the point of committing incest. Sumpitan's message is a multilayered one: (1) to stay healthy, humans should make proper distinctions in the social and the spiritual world; (2) nurturance, love, even incest, are better than murder, rape, and separation; and (3) to be too close to fellow Laujé is dangerous, but to be too close to foreigners is fatal.

Birth in Dusunan: Complications in Sumpitan's View

Sumpitan's outline of spirits made perfect sense to me as long as he used it to analyze sexual matters. It became more convoluted, however, once I carried his ideas to the realm of birth. Sumpitan loved to talk about sex and the umputé spirits, but he never initiated any conversations with me about birth. Nevertheless I was interested in the topic since Siamae Sanji had emphasized birth so much in his outline of spirits and I wanted to compare highland birth to the lowlands. Thus, after I had been studying for several months with Siamae Sanji, and had come down the mountains to visit Sumpitan, I asked him about lowland birth rites. Rather than the long, detailed answers I normally received, Sumpitan rather stiffly told me "in the lowlands, a person of any gender can act as a midwife. But they have to know the right Laujé rituals." Sumpitan told me that if the father-to-be is from another ethnic group, and thus unfamiliar with Laujé customs, "he and his family would not be asked to assist in the birth." Sumpitan concluded, "the birth customs of the Laujé must prevail [because] men from other ethnic groups are not concerned with nurturing."[16] Sumpitan's response to my questions, on the one hand, made logical sense; he tried to carry the same oppositions—that Laujé are nurturing connectors while foreigners are violent separators—from the sexual to the birth scenario. On the other hand, his lack of enthusiasm and failure to provide specific details about birth puzzled me.

I talked to other Laujé aristocrats about how the umputé spirits were involved in birth. The neat divisions and structural oppositions Sumpitan had so carefully outlined did not readily appear in their depictions. I recorded their information, but regarded the discrepancies as failure on their part to understand the collective representations as Sumpitan did. It was only later, in writing up my material, that I began to reassess how the lowland birth rites seemed to contradict Sumpitan's neat scheme. The main thing these aristocrats revealed, contrary to Sumpitan, was that Laujé fathers engage in separating activities associated with death when they care for the newborn and the placenta. When the lowland Laujé father cuts the cord, he ties black thread around the umbilicus in two spots. He then uses a *metal* knife to cut the cord between these threads. The "black thread" said one elite lowlander, "signifies separation." The father's use of a metal knife is associated with a final act of separating the placenta from the child.

When a Laujé father cleans the placenta, he treats it as though it is a human corpse. The father is forbidden to speak while cleaning the placenta, just as Sufi Muslims are told to avoid speaking while cleaning a corpse. The father cannot allow the blood on the placenta to touch his hands. He must let the water rinse the placenta clean. This action is the same as when a corpse's fluids are "rinsed" away. The father then cuts a coconut in half—to place the placenta inside it—and inserts a fish bone, a wad of cotton, and several raw, husked rice kernels. The fish bone represents something dead from the land of the souls, the sea. The cotton represents a trade item introduced by foreigners from "across the sea" in the "land of the dead," and it is an item used to "stuff the corpse's orifices" in an Islamic funeral. The husked, raw, white rice represents rice that can no longer grow. It is hard and stiff like a corpse. When the lowland father fills the "coconut nest," he wraps it in didil leaves and ties it with a rattan cord. In the lowlands, the didil leaves are used to line the grave of an olongian, to "make the grave clean." Thus lowland fathers treat the placenta as though it is dead and they separate it from the living child.

The separating acts become even more evident once the nest is filled. The lowland Laujé father prepares to walk outside the house to put the placental nest in its "resting place." The female midwife places a white cloth over his head, the same cloth worn by mourning females when they attend funeral services at the mosque. With his white head covering and his cloth sarong (the father cannot wear trousers), he looks like a female carrying an offering to a funeral. He is dressed this way to "trick" the placental spirit into thinking it will be nurtured by a female and not sent away to the land of the dead by the father.

The female midwife accompanies the father while she holds a lantern of clay, lit with *pa'an* oil, the oil that is burned at a funeral. The midwife leads the father to a hole that has been dug in the ground near the river's edge, or near the family burial plot. The father places a hard coin in the ground, one that has been used in the prayer to "harden the soft spot" of the newborn child. He places the wrapped placental "nest" on top of this. Elites said that to keep the child's soul stationary, the flow of its soul back into the ground must be stopped. Hence, the hard coin is used because it blocks the path of things, and solidifies, rather than liquifies, the connections.[17]

After the placenta has been placed in its grave, the father covers the grave with dirt, but again he cannot use his hands, only his forearms. Sumpitan's nephew said the father must use only his forearms because this will make the child grow as strong and as big as the father is.[18] To mark this as the place of decay, as well as rejuvenation, a green coconut fruit collected by the maternal grandmother of the newborn is placed on top of this buried bundle. The "grave" is completely covered with dirt. Then the clay lamp (something made from the earth) is placed on top of the placental grave, and every evening (for seven days if one is closely related to the olongian, for three days if one is distantly related), the maternal grandmother returns to relight the clay lamp and "water" the grave. This is the same procedure as that followed when a family member has died. Soon thereafter, the place of decay becomes a place of rejuvenation, for the coconut grows from this spot. The child who once shared the placenta is said to be as strong and productive as the coconut. This strength is due to the maternal grandmother who "watered" the "grave" and to the mother who is associated with things from the earth that provide the sustenance to reproduce and live. Moreover, once the placental nest is buried and watered, it is said to have returned to the source of all fluid, mother earth. Once it has "given what it has gotten," then the mother of the child will give fluid—her milk will start to flow. Several days after this, the father clips the umbilical stump from the infant's navel. It is wrapped in white cloth (*gandisé* or funeral cloth) and stored by the mother. This act marks the final separation from the forces of creation. In general, then, one could say that the lowland elite father behaves toward the white placental umputé spirit in ways that associate his actions with death and separation, while the mother or females behave toward the white placental umputé spirit in ways that associate their actions with nurturance and rejuvenation.

The question is, Why did Sumpitan neglect to discuss this information with me? It could be that Sumpitan avoided discussing the separating role elite Laujé men play in dealing with the umputé of birth because these actions would have negated his rather simplistic contention that all Laujé, no matter what gender, are nurturing, while all foreigners, especially men, are violent separators. To say Laujé men engage in separating activities would contradict or obviate his simple scheme of binary oppositions. He wanted very much to prove his good-versus-evil point for my book on the Laujé. Ironically enough, his avoidance tactics defeated his goals. If, in burying the white placenta and therefore the white umputé, Sumpitan had admitted that Laujé males were associated with separation and death, it would have meant that their symbolic category, the white and the yellow, would have been more complete, more encompassing than the black and the red. The white and the yellow would have been associated with life-giving properties as well as the lack of life. Because more of everything would be associated with the white, which he in turn associated with

Laujé identity, Laujé identity would have encompassed and therefore superseded the foreign, black and red, categories. Such completeness reinforces the same point made about white umputé in Siamae Sanji's scheme. White umputé are not just contrasted to the other colors of umputé but are more complete, therefore superior to and encompassing all others.

Sumpitan, however, could not have known the subtleties of symbolic analysis, so he may indeed have neglected to tell me about the role of Laujé men in burying placentas, because it contradicted his logical scheme of a simple binary opposition. Then again, Sumpitan was a crafty analyst with an almost lawyerlike skill in manipulating ethnographic facts. He could have argued, had he wanted to, that when the father buries the placenta he is a nurturer. After all, the effort and care given to burying the placenta and giving it an elaborate funeral connotes nurturance, not neglect and division. Why did Sumpitan not argue that Laujé fathers follow funerary rituals that nurture the placenta on its way to heaven? Why did he avoid talking about birth in the lowlands?

I can only speculate here, but with some well-founded assumptions. One likely answer is that Sumpitan had heard highlanders denigrate lowland treatment of the placenta and did not want to give me information that contradicted too strongly the information he knew I was getting from Siamae Sanji. I say this because whenever I visited him after studying with Siamae Sanji, Sumpitan acted less sure of himself. He would repeatedly ask me, "What do they say up there in the mountains? . . . You've heard the same thing from the original Laujé up there in the mountains, haven't you?" Sumpitan wanted me to write about a unified Laujé culture that was distinct from foreign ethnic groups. To differ too greatly from Siamae Sanji's scheme would undermine his own goal of presenting the Laujé as one united ethnic group. This explains, I believe, Sumpitan's reticence about discussing birth, and his tendency to make simplistic divisions between Laujé and foreigners. But, as I will show below, Sumpitan was not always consistent.

Comparing Siamae Sanji's and Sumpitan's Worldviews

Though Sumpitan and Siamae Sanji exhibited similar reactions to the social "other" and expressed their ambivalences through the umputé concepts, the significant feature differentiating the two men's concepts of umputé spirits and the world was that Sumpitan used ethnicity to convey messages about otherness, while Siamae Sanji used gender.[19] Yet, Sumpitan could just as easily have used gender, that is, maleness, to convey otherness in his scheme. Instead he consistently said the despised umputé spirits were "the foreigners." The spirits were not just males, but foreign females too.

Similarly, Siamae Sanji could have designated the black umputé spirit as "foreign" since the concept of "bela" with which it was associated implied foreignness. But instead of calling the bela or the umputé spirit "foreign," Siamae Sanji preferred to designate the despised black umputé spirit as female. Why were the significant others for Sumpitan and Siamae Sanji designated in terms of gender or ethnicity and not vice versa? To understand this, we have to understand how Sumpitan and Siamae Sanji conceptualized who they were. Then we can understand how they conceptualized who they were not.

As mentioned above, Siamae Sanji continually remarked that the most important means for determining how the community of Taipaobal was comprised was through determining agnatic bonds of kinship, bonds through the male line. "All kin, *vuntuh pusé,* (literally "kin connected by the navel"), should stay together," said Siamae Sanji. But it was "most important for brothers to stay together." When he traced the genealogical connections of heads of households in Taipaobal, he always traced their relationships through agnatic lines, rather than through in-marrying or out-marrying women. Though he did include female kin of his own generation and those of his descendants, when tracing backward, Siamae Sanji reckoned as "kin" only the male ancestors who had remained in Taipaboal.

His reckoning was significant, for as mentioned in Chapter 2, Siamae Sanji believed that the kin who had remained in Taipaobal were descendants of males, while the lowlanders and the bela were descendants of females who had moved away. Because he believed these bela and lowlanders were not to be trusted, he also characterized distant kin, related through uterine links (i.e., links through the female line), and women, in general, as untrustworthy. Thus, the way in which Siamae Sanji characterized otherness depended upon how he perceived his own community's "sameness." Others were the opposite of his community; others were female, his own community was male.

Similarly, Sumpitan's way of characterizing otherness depended upon how he perceived his own community's "sameness." Sumpitan was an aristocrat and identified himself and those in Dusunan with the olongian. Though the olongian had been female until recently, for the last twenty-five years, the olongian had been male. Thus gender designation and unilateral kin reckoning were not criteria for distinguishing who was a member of Sumpitan's elite community comprised of descendants of the olongian. Affinity to the olongian was the main criterion for distinguishing elites from commoners.

But this "order" began to change for Sumpitan at an early age. When Sumpitan was still a young man, his father had been mayor of Dusunan. Sumpitan went with his father to visit the raja and the colonial offices. He told me he saw, even as a young man, that "the raja, just a mile over the river in Tinombo, helped people of his own kind, from the Mandar ethnic group, enrich themselves. . . . They got the meat [of the coconut] while we Laujé were left with empty husks." Few Laujé had as clear a view of otherness as Sumpitan had. When he reached young adulthood, Sumpitan was drafted into the Japanese army, and later into the Dutch KNIL army. He continued several years after independence (until 1957) to serve in Java with the first Indonesian armed service. Though Sumpitan describes those years as times of hardship, emotionally trying (because he was forced on occasion to fight his fellow Indonesians), and physically draining (with little or no food), he nevertheless found them intellectually rewarding. He told me: "I saw how those other people, the Batak, the Javanese, the Bugis, how they got things. They united themselves against the others. They stuck together and helped each other. I was the only Laujé man there was. I didn't have anyone to stick together with. But I watched and learned how to ask superiors for things." When Sumpitan returned to Sulawesi, he soon became the mayor of Dusunan. The wife of the olongian told me: "Sumpitan was young, but he knew how to talk to the others. He had been abroad and he came back to help us." Sumpitan's experiences made him acutely aware of the Laujé as an ethnic unit.

This was important because the newly independent Indonesian state began to deal with their constituency on the basic of ethnic identity (see Henley 1996). Locally, though Sumpitan hated the Mandar as an ethnic group, in Tinombo where the raja was Mandar, others of Mandar ethnicity assumed positions of status and marked Laujé of all social groups as inferior. Thus, as Sumpitan began his political career, the means for determining status in the region shifted from an internal aristocratic/commoner distinction to one in which affiliation to one's land of origin, one's *suku,* or ethnic group, became primary. Some of the reason for this shift had to do with the way in which the newly independent Indonesian government treated the olongian. As mentioned in Chapter 2, in the early fifties, prior to independence, Sumpitan and other elites had unsuccessfully tried to reinstate the olongian as ruler over the Laujé commoners in the lowlands and the highlands. They had lost to the "foreign" raja and now they were "paying" for it by lack of opportunity. The only way these elite Laujé could hope to claim more right than the raja to rule over Laujé commoners was by emphasizing that the olongian's family was Laujé, just like the commoners. In other words, the elites like Sumpitan began to emphasize their identities as Laujé—their similarity to and affinity with the commoners—in contradistinction to their identities as foreigners like those in power. This was Sumpitan's aim in revealing the information about foreigners and Laujé for my book. He hoped to reinstate the olongian as an autochthonous ruler by outlining the distinctions between his own community of Laujé and that of the foreigners in Tinombo.

This is not to say that Sumpitan was completely consistent about the unity of the Laujé as an ethnic group. Whenever I talked to him for a long period of time, his neat, logical "us" versus "them" distinctions dissolved into internal hierarchies. Basically his narratives switched to another "us versus them": Whatever highlanders did, lowlanders did the opposite. When I asked Sumpitan, for instance, why the people in Taipaobal suspended the placenta from a tree branch while aristocratic families in Dusunan buried it, he explained that it was because the kin of the olongian were superior and "of the earth," while highlanders were inferior to the olongian and not "of the earth." Sumpitan said that the highlanders could not bury their placentas in the earth, because this would have been an act of arrogance, an act claiming that highlanders were just like lowlanders. To Sumpitan (and other aristocrats), the difference between their customs and highlanders' reflected a hierarchical relationship between the two communities. Lowland elites performed their birth rituals as they did to signify incontrovertibly that "we are elites and thus our rituals are more elaborate and distinct from highlanders' rites."

In turn, Siamae Sanji's relatives claimed that their rites nurtured the umputé spirits, while lowlanders' rites "killed" the white umputé by treating the spirit like it was dead. For Siamae Sanji's relatives, their umputé rites were superior to the lowlanders' because their rites emphasized nurturance and continuous bonds to the placental spirits while lowlanders "severed connections" when they wrapped the placenta in white funeral cloth and buried it. Though Siamae Sanji's relatives used the rites to claim that males were associated with nurturing spirits and therefore were superior to females, they also used the rites to claim that Taipaobalers' were superior to the so-called elites in the lowlands. And though Sumpitan used his rites to claim ethnic identity for the Laujé, he also used his rites to claim that elite Laujé were superior to commoner Laujé. Consequently, Sumpitan's and Siamae Sanji's rites not only delineated who was in the defined group and who was considered "other," but it also distinguished levels of social status.

Though it should be obvious that the symbolic distinctions Sumpitan and Siamae Sanji made between umputé spirits were reflections of the social context in which those distinctions were expressed, it must be remembered that these are distinctions primarily made by Sumpitan and Siamae Sanji and not by other leaders in their community. The way Sumpitan or Siamae Sanji described the events of birth by selecting certain colors or characteristics of umputé to emphasize and dichotomize revealed the particular issues each man saw as important. Thus, while highlanders may have hung a placenta and lowlanders may have buried a placenta, only Siamae Sanji equated the placental spirit with males and only Sumpitan equated the placental spirit with the Laujé olongian. It was each man's perception of hierarchies in the social world that allowed him to refer those distinctions and hierarchies to the spirit world.

In their rituals, Siamae Sanji and Sumpitan exaggerated the positive qualities of the white umputé spirit as they exaggerated, in their historical narratives, the positive qualities of "our category of people," the olongian or men. In their narratives, they also exaggerated the negative qualities of the social "other" by symbolically marking the "other" as dangerous and inferior. By differentiating and exaggerating similarly negative qualities of the umputé spirits, these men linked the social domain to the spiritual domain and implemented "models for" an ideal world.

It would be tempting to take the views of Siamae Sanji and Sumpitan as representative of Laujé "culture," since the rituals taught by these men were highly regarded in their respective communities and since their perspectives fit with symbolic anthropology's assumptions about the relationship between ritual and social structure. Nevertheless, their interpretations cannot be taken as the collective voice representing the total philosophical rubric of umputé. Yet they are not idiosyncratic either. Siamae Sanji's and Sumpitan's interpretations of umputé did reflect their own views of social decline and their own attempts to restructure that decline through ritual action, but they also tapped into the same themes others throughout Indonesia employed.

The following two chapters reiterate this same point by focusing on Sumpitan's portrayal of social and spiritual hierarchy through the momasoro curing rite. The oppositions he draws in these smaller curing rites are restatements on a grander scale for the momasoro. In the momasoro, Sumpitan was able to exaggerate the distinctions between umputé spirits in such a way as to make explicit his critique of foreign domination implied in the story of the murdered raja. Later, after Sumpitan's death, other interpreters chose to submerge his interpretation in favor of one that stressed the connection to and the unquestionable superiority of the red umputé spirits and the foreign rajas. Though we will return later to a discussion of how these interpretations resonate with structural distinctions people make throughout the Austronesian world, for now it is important to remember that Sumpitan's (and Siamae Sanji's) heavy symbolic interpretations are dependent upon divisions and separations they believe exist in the social *and* spiritual world. Their divisions are then tied to more enduring and pervasive notions of illness and health.

Three

CONCEIVING THE MOMASORO

5

CASTING OUT
THE FOREIGNERS
Sumpitan's Momasoro

It is not surprising that Sumpitan explained the momasoro as a curing rite writ large. He carried into this communitywide rite the same oppositions and messages he had underlined in his individual curing rites: Foreigners are making the Laujé ill. Sumpitan's view of the momasoro was not only convincing to me but seemed to be accepted by everyone in the community who was tired of the ills, figurative and literal, brought by immigrants or foreigners. Sumpitan said the rite's name, *momasoro*, meant "to stop." The community had been plagued by "foreign" presence and this illness would only be stopped if the ritual redefined and reinvigorated the community. Participants would redraw the boundaries of the Laujé kingdom, while casting out the foreign illness and the metaphoric foreigners in a boat. This, he said, would "seal," if temporarily, the boundaries of the Laujé community, making it a discrete and autonomous entity. Thus, as Sumpitan explained it, this curing rite was a profoundly political act in which a reinvigorated and purified people would emerge.

Sumpitan said the rite propitiated the umputé spirits involved in the procreation and birth of individual humans and in the birth of the world. In the creation myths, which the momasoro enacted, all umputé spirits were once joined in the "womb of the world" near the Inscribed Rock at the "center of the earth." When the world began, the sea separated from the land and its rivers to form two complementary halves—the sea and the land. The land and its rivers remained the nurturing and healing part of the world. This was where the first people, the Laujé and their umputé spirits, arose. Later, the sea formed the pestilent, diseased part of the world. This was where the foreigners and foreign umputé spirits arose.

Sumpitan said that the sequence of offering rites for the momasoro reenacts the way the world was created. The first rites in the moma-

soro begin near the mountains and the navel of the world, the Inscribed Rock. They serve as blessings to the Laujé umputé and the
original Laujé ancestors. Later, rites for the umputé of the first Laujé
Muslims are held downstream at the spot where they first settled. This
sequence of rituals, said Sumpitan, circumscribes Laujé territory and
"marks the Laujé umputé as the first in the world." At the next stage,
another set of umputé spirits, pestilent sea spirits, are invited in to
shore to meet the nurturing Laujé spirits. "The sea spirits," said
Sumpitan, "represent the later-born foreigners who became a separate
[and therefore] secondary group." Both sets of spirits are feted for
seven nights. At the culmination, a boat carrying offerings to foreign
spirits is cast out to sea, thus separating Laujé spirits from foreign. The
rites, then, recreate the origins of humans and umputé and, according
to Sumpitan, distinguish Laujé health from foreign disease and Laujé
land from foreign sea. When the boats are cast off to sea, they stop the
illness, physical and analogic, brought by foreigners (see Figure 5.1).

Sumpitan was the choreographer for the whole event. He organized
the curers, sando,[1] who, in turn, helped to call in spirits to possess
mediums *(to pensio)*. The to pensio sang blessings to these spirits and,
along with various sando, made offerings to spirits. Sumpitan, a sando
himself, oversaw the other sando offerings and arranged where mediums would sit after they were possessed. His central role allowed him
to orchestrate the rite so that his antiforeign, pro-Laujé message was
especially clear.

The Context in Which the Voice of Sumpitan Prevails

Recall that the momasoro rite had been banned by Muslim officials in
Tinombo for two years prior to its reinstatement in 1985. Sumpitan
and many other lowland Laujé believed this ban was one more attempt by "foreigners" to hammer a nail in the coffin of Laujé custom.
Sumpitan was unaware that such struggles were common throughout
Indonesia (Geertz 1973; Acciaioli 1985; Atkinson 1987; Kipp and
Rodgers 1987). Muslim fundamentalists who wished to purge custom
or *adat* from local rites fought indigenous peoples wanting to hold
onto those rites. While Laujé were Muslim, most practiced a version
of Islam that was coming to be increasingly contested by Islamic
purists or fundamentalists. Laujé custom in general, and the momasoro in particular, were targets of these purification efforts.

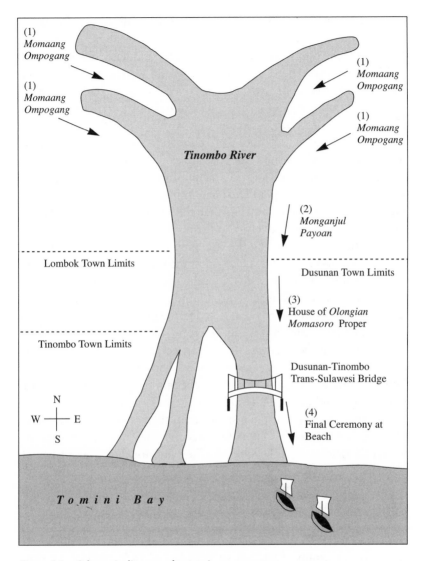

Figure 5.1.   Schematic diagram of events in a momasoro

In the early part of the twentieth century, the Laujé in Dusunan practiced a syncretic Islam, typical of communities throughout the archipelago (Geertz 1960; Bowen 1986, 1987, 1993; Hefner 1985). Newcomers, especially the immigrant rajas, who were better educated in the reform Islam they learned from Arab teachers, disapproved of the Laujé's blend of Islam and animist tradition, but tolerated rites like the momasoro.[2] One Tinombo immigrant, who was born in 1917 of a Laujé mother, recalls being a spectator to the momasoro when he was a child: "We used to go to watch. We would watch the dancing. We would follow the boats down to the river. Everyone had a torch. [It was] beautiful. But later [when I was older] our parents forbade us. They would try to scare us. 'Satan' they would tell us. 'The dancers are Satan!'" Such Laujé practices were abhorrent to the first wave of reform Muslims who would not tolerate syncretism in their own children's beliefs, but would allow Laujé to practice and believe what they wanted. Thus, the Laujé in Dusunan kept their religious practices to their side of the river, knowing that the immigrants disapproved of them, but would not actively stop them.

Over the years, however, the changing politico-religious demography of Tinombo made it less likely that the momasoro would continue to be tolerated in this way. As Tinombo grew during the late colonial period and the early independence period, more fundamentalist Muslim immigrants not directly connected to the government arrived. This "second wave of immigrants" to Tinombo, less wealthy, less educated, and less tolerant, were, more often than not, followers of a more fundamentalist Islamic sect called the Muhammadiyah (see Peacock 1992).[3] Muhammadiyah's imams taught that religious syncretism was wrong and would not be tolerated in others. The Muhammadiyah followers took a more proactive stance than the first-wave reform Muslims. Muhammadiyah sought to eradicate rites like the momasoro, which they believed to be satanic. They did not, however, attack all syncretic rites with equal vigor. They ignored, for example, the Kaili, Bugis, Gorontalese, and Mandar rituals held by Tinombo's elite and concentrated on Laujé "custom" or adat.[4]

Preaching against animist rituals like the momasoro came to a crescendo in 1982. At this time, during one of the seven nights of the momasoro, a group of Muhammadiyah teenagers from Tinombo went to the momasoro to mock the festivities. A fistfight ensued between the Muhammadiyah and Laujé youths. This incident became the excuse the Muslim fundamentalists had been waiting for. Arguing initially that a ban of the momasoro was necessary to keep the peace, fundamentalists who worked in government later asserted that a permanent ban was appropriate on religious grounds. Tinombo's chief of police joined forces with the head of the Religious Affairs Office to declare the rite illegal, justifying their decision in terms of national development policies.[5] They said that the momasoro "wasted food" or "encouraged beliefs in traditional healers rather than western doctors."

Though the reform Muslims of Tinombo initially supported the Muhammadiyah-led ban against the momasoro, their support began to weaken when Sumpitan and others threatened to stop voting in the next election for the bureaucrats' political "group" (GOLKAR).[6] As mentioned, most of the reform Muslims were descendants of colonial-era bureaucrats, and they, too, occupied positions in the local government. Their positions in local government, to a certain extent, depended upon local support of their national group, GOLKAR. If they could not "control" the locals by garnering votes for GOLKAR candidates in the next election, then they too would lose power. Thus the Tinombo establishment, more interested in maintaining their own political positions than in asserting ideological religious dogma, responded to Sumpitan's threat to withhold votes. The "first wave" reformists split with the "second wave" fundamentalists and realigned themselves with the Dusunan elite. The "first wave" Tinombo reformists, many of whom were descendants of Raja Kuti, publicly acknowledged that the momasoro ban was wrong. Officially overriding the fundamentalist Muhammadiyah, these "first wave" elite reformists in positions of power gave permission for the rite to be performed after the harvest in December. This reinstatement, however, took nearly two years. In the interim, much resentment and anger seethed just under the surface of interactions between Tinombo officials and Laujé lowlanders.

When the momasoro was reinstated in 1985, it was an event that dramatized local tensions centering around ethnicity and religion. Most Dusunaners, including Sumpitan, found the religious issue surrounding the momasoro ban and reenactment the most insulting. They resented all Tinombo immigrants, reformists and fundamentalists alike, because it was Muslims from Tinombo who had branded the Laujé elite as heretics. It was Sumpitan, and others like him, who characterized the ban as more than just a religious problem. For Sumpitan the ban was an ethnic affront. Sumpitan argued: "We have been Islamic since the first ancestors moved to Dusunan. Our rites always praise 'the disciples of the Prophet Mohammed under the wind.' How can they say this rite is banned [and not Muslim] but continue their own Bugis and Mandar curing rites?" Sumpitan had a compelling case. After all, it was only Laujé "customs" that were banned as heretical, not the ancestral and equally heretical customs (adat) of the higher status immigrants.

But it was not just these circumstances that led Sumpitan to his position. Sumpitan's own personal history suited him for the role he played as chief protestor against the ban. Sumpitan was, in a sense, a rebel always in search of a cause. And this particular case was exceptionally well suited to him. Sumpitan had a reputation as a leader and a hero. During the Permesta rebellion, he had joined antigovernment (anti-Sukarno) forces to fight as a guerilla. Later, he served as head of the local trade union. Through the 1970s, as mayor of Dusunan, he had fought to find meager government benefits for his "Laujé" people.

Because Sumpitan had considerable standing in Dusunan, he was the man to whom the Tinombo officials wanting peace in Dusunan came. Though Sumpitan resented having to discuss Laujé matters with outsiders, he was anxious to reinstate the momasoro. Thus government officials, along with representatives from Dusunan, began to hold "planning meetings." At one of these meetings a Tinombo official, interested in drawing Dusunaners back into the GOLKAR fold, mentioned the possibility that the *bupati* or regent of the province might come to witness the momasoro. He also suggested that the Tinombo Office of Education and Culture, which he headed, might be able to secure funds from the provincial government to build a "traditional shrine house" for Laujé rituals.

Ironically enough, Sumpitan was thrilled that a "foreigner" like the regent might come to the momasoro, thereby legitimating the Laujé's rite beyond the local arena. Sumpitan was even more thrilled about the promised funding, spreading the news in the Laujé community that if they could capture government funds to build a shrine house, maybe the Laujé could buy costumes for the dancers and reinstate permanent ritual officers in the manner of the precolonial kingdom. Sumpitan began to speak about these possibilities in inspirational, revitalizing terms. In a speech he delivered during a local planning session for the momasoro (to which I, but no Tinomboers were invited), he said:

> For a long time we have been governed by others because we didn't have the knowledge. But the spirit of the land promised that we would once again rule ourselves. Maybe, maybe 1985 is our year—the year it will start again. . . . We already have some of our own [Laujé] in the government and in the universities. . . . Maybe this year the government will recognize us

and give us money to build a really good shrine house, to buy materials for this ceremony, so that things will be right again.

Ethnic pride and optimism about redressing past wounds were the major factors in how the momasoro was perceived by Sumpitan and others. It was these circumstances that made Sumpitan's declaration that the momasoro was a curing rite to "cure" the illness brought by "foreign spirits" a compelling one.

Outline of Momasoro

News arrived from the provincial capital that the regent did plan to attend the momasoro. Funds for a shrine house and costumes were handed over to Sumpitan. He was ecstatic and went into high gear, preparing all for the regent's visit. He arranged for the little shrine house to be constructed behind the main house of the olongian, whose "court" was located "halfway" between mountains and shore. Sumpitan also contacted other communities so they could plan the preliminary rites prior to the momasoro at the house of the olongian. Everyone was involved.

A date had to be selected for the regent's visit that would correspond with plans for the local ceremony. Sumpitan repeatedly traversed the river to the *camat's* (county leader's) office to radio, via shortwave, to the regent's secretary in Palu. When he found a date from the secretary, he would go back to the community ritual specialists in the foothills above Dusunan, asking if the selected date would coincide with expected harvest time. The momasoro was normally performed at the end of the dry rice harvest season. Because of variations in rainfall patterns, though, communities farther inland harvested their rice earlier than the closer-in coastal communities. Thus, foothill communities held the first thanksgiving rites. Now, however, these rites had to be coordinated with the regent's return from a meeting in Jakarta. After much back and forthing, dates were confirmed. The regent was to attend the next-to-the-last and the last day of the momasoro on January 8–9, 1985.

Rites Leading up to the Momasoro

Before the main momasoro, each individual community had to perform its own small thanksgiving offerings. These smaller rites normally signified that the harvest was complete. Neighbors usually gathered at the headwaters of the little springs that flow into the branches of the Tinombo River to give two offerings. One was placed upstream for the spirit of the source water and the other downstream for the spirit of the river water.

After the olongian was notified that each of the participating communities had performed its local offerings, plans were made to gather at a downstream location at the confluence of the headwaters for the "floating," or "casting-adrift-the-outer-covering" rite *(monganjul poyoan)*.[7] This place was called the "trunk," the "tap-root," or the place of origin of Laujé land and rivers. It was also the original home of the first lowland olongian located three kilometers upstream from the river's mouth. It was here that the rite was to be held. Families would bring small packets of rice wrapped in woven coconut-frond "sacks" or "skins" (ampini) and pile them up for the olongian and the umputé spirits to consecrate. At the end of the rite, a sando would bless the rice sacks and then give the nod. Hundreds of children would rush to the piles of rice sacks, grabbing what they could. The sando would toss packets near him to the smaller children on the crowd's periphery. Eventually, after everyone ate the rice packets, the sando would gather the discarded outer coverings and toss them into the Tinombo River to float downstream. Thus, rice grown and cooked at home is redistributed once it has been blessed and the outer covering is "stripped away." Also, during the ceremony, several sando will make two rice-offering trays. One offering will be made near the pile of rice sacks and possessed mediums. It is a large tray mounted on four posts stuck in the ground. A smaller offering tray (similar to that in the white chicken rite from the mountains) will be hung in a tree a few dozen yards downstream.

Sumpitan's Interpretation: Purging the Foreign Illness from Laujé Land

Though the monganjul poyoan is definitely associated with the harvest season and is regarded by many as a thanksgiving ceremony for the spirit owners of land and water, Sumpitan tended to downplay the harvest aspect of the rite, instead emphasizing its curing qualities. I believe his curing emphasis was primarily influenced by the fundamentalists' prior ban on the momasoro. Whenever Sumpitan spoke about this rite, the references to pestilent foreigners were always apparent.

For instance, Sumpitan explained that the current site for the ceremony marked "a border."[8] He explained the border in terms of the tides:

> There are seven tides from the sea that travel like waves up from the sea into the Tinombo River. Even the highest streamlets or offshoots of the Tinombo are populated with crabs which come from the sea. [The crabs eat fish that people would normally eat.] If crabs don't have enough food they can eat people [thus] bringing illness. This rite stops those [crab] spirits of the sea from climbing any further upstream. They are stopped here at the border. Later at the momasoro, they will be invited to enjoy themselves. Then they will be sent back to the sea.

The crabs represent the unwanted foreigners who have traveled to the first border, sometimes called the "parlor of the Laujé house." These pesky crabs need to be feted and entertained so they will not travel any farther across the Laujé border, consume all of the Laujé's food, begin to eat their bodies, and thus cause illness.

To reach this border area where the sending-the-crabs-downstream rite would be performed, Sumpitan, the wife of the olongian, Eric, and I walked approximately two kilometers upstream from the center of Dusunan, where the house of the olongian is located. Sumpitan told me that all Laujé, highlander and lowlander alike, would gather at this upstream location to give offerings or "tribute" to the olongian, but I had always doubted highlanders would attend a lowland ceremony. When we arrived, my suspicions were confirmed. I found only lowlanders with no highlanders in attendance at all.[9] Sumpitan insisted I bring my tape recorder to place in front of mediums who were to be possessed by spirits of the land and river (which Sumpitan called the white and yellow umputé). The wife of the olongian, who was to be possessed, did not seem bothered by the prospect, so rather reluctantly I brought the tape recorder along.

As we approached the crowd, five mediums sat with their backs to the Tinombo River. These mediums were all women from foothills communities.[10] They were all commoners except the wife of the olongian, whose status was achieved through marriage to the olongian, not through birth. Sumpitan told me the mediums were already possessed by spirits, as their bodies were taut. I was a bit disappointed, having arrived too late to see the process of possession. I could not dwell on this for long, though, because Sumpitan grabbed my tape recorder and

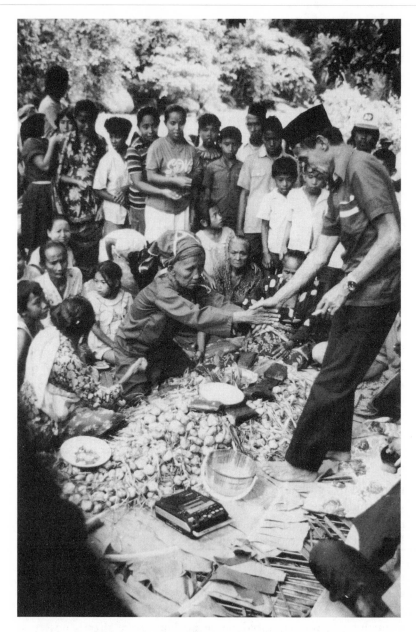

Figure 5.2. Sando shaking hands with spirit medium at monganjul poyoan

boldly placed it in front of the possessed mediums, on top of the piles of cooked rice wrapped in coconut frond packets (ampini) (see Figure 5.2). Sumpitan said the five mediums were possessed either by sea spirits or land spirits. He said the sea spirits came from the sea and entered the mouth of the river to travel upstream. They followed the same path taken by pesky sea crabs and illnesses. Two of the five possessed women were dressed in bright colors—reds, purples, dark blues—and they spoke in a "foreign" language, Kaili. They were possessed by sea spirits. By contrast, three of the women wore white and/or yellow. Their heads were wrapped in the cloths the ancestors used to wear. They were possessed by the spirit of the land and rivers—the spirit of the first Laujé ancestors who are said to reside at the "original rock" or the "navel of the earth" from which all humans sprang (Polu Irandu). When they were possessed by old spirits, these mediums bent over as if they had arthritis. Their heads almost touched the ground as they spoke. One of the mediums, dressed in white and possessed by an ancient Laujé umputé spirit, immediately spied my tape recorder, which Sumpitan had set in front of her (see Figure 5.3). The spirit became furious and spoke in a loud, forceful voice to the tape recorder:

> You humans have neglected to follow ancestral custom (in the past two years) and now you are going against custom by having foreigners here.

Sumpitan humbly asked forgiveness and said:

> The government would not let us perform the ritual. The people wanted to, but the government would not let us. We have brought rice packets, betel nut . . .

The land spirit interrupted (a rarity):

> I am angry because I remember that the custom was not performed right. But, if people promise to do it right, perfect this time, true to form, then I will no longer be angry.

Sumpitan implored:

> Please do not hide from us humans, for our grandchildren must know you and your customs, or else the spirits of the outside will inundate them. They must be overseen by you, the Laujé creator of the Inscribed Rock at the center of the world.

The Spirit answered:

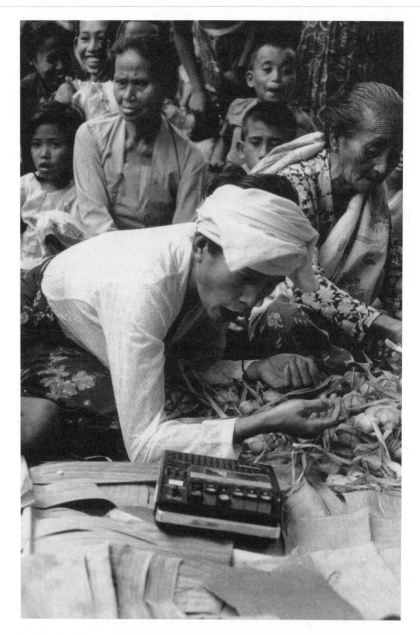

Figure 5.3. Possessed spirit medium talking to a tape recorder at monganjul poyoan

It is I who guard over the treasure of the Inscribed Rock at the Center of the World.

Sumpitan excitedly responded:

That's it, that's what we ask for so that we can hold on to it there and exchange sickness for cure. All ethnic groups blossomed from there. The powerful of the earth first came from you. Whatever you ask we will give; you are the essence, the root. That's why these foreigners and the anthropologists are here. They search for the essence.

The Spirit answered:

After the world opened up, after the sky broke in two, there were humans who came from this navel, this womb. All moved from the original Rock, they moved to the west, to the east . . .

The discussion continued with Sumpitan trying to induce the spirits to make an explicit statement about the relationship between the Laujé as an ethnic group and the foreigners as ethnic groups. The spirits offered answers that were cryptic, giving Sumpitan the opportunity to interpret them later.

After this dialogue, the wife of the olongian, dressed in red warrior clothing, and possessed by a Kaili warrior (tadulako) spirit, began to sing a song in the Kaili language. The song was a chant announcing who the spirit was—the spirit from the middle of the sea. Then the other mediums sang their songs.

Subsequently, spirits dressed in white blessed the giant offering tray for the Laujé spirit of the "womb of the world." The four posts of the tray stuck in the ground were four tree trunks. The tray itself was approximately 2 by 3 meters and it stood 1.5 meters off the ground. Ancestral didil leaves lined the tray's bottom. It was topped with a central concentric circle of white and yellow rice with four arms stretching to the tray's corners. On top of the rice was a whole egg, an antique coin, sweet cakes, tobacco, betel nut, taro, cassava, and cornmeal. All these were locally produced products. Also on the tray were young white chicks that would be blessed by Siamae Asarima, a local sando, and then raised by him.

The blessing invoked at this offering tray followed Sumpitan's guidance. The theme the blessing emphasized was curing:[11]

This is meant we say to come to ask of	Njeine antuonyé peu mai mai pomongi
The spirit of the land and river	Li Togu Petu, Togu Ogo
That is we mean to say	Antuonyé peu mai
Wherever there is hotness [fever]	Liga sanu moonda
Wherever there is coldness [chills]	Liga sanu mojolo
By fever, we mean,	Antuonyé sanu mapalaé
That which flows in	Sanu moonto
That is certainly is what is to be	Njeiné tetap
Carried back down river	Moanjuli
This is to be floated down river	Molondong patuiné
To be swept down river	Molondong patuiné
To be cast adrift, those outer skins	Noanjuli lemaonyé poyoané

The blessing not only enlisted the spirit's aid in casting off illness, but asked for strength, health, and fertility from the "spirits of the surrounding mountains." The blessing then returned to the subject of illness, using the image of "chills and fever" to admit that some illnesses still might cross the "border" from the sea. But it requested that the spirits only send humans "the warm breeze" or "the cool breeze." This meant minor illnesses, not death:

That means that for you humans	Antuonyé emé manusia
There will be equal measure	Notindana
Equal measure from the breeze	Notindana li sanu moonto
Of the spirits of the	Li sanu mahalus
Surrounding mountain sides	Li vuyul molintaba
So that all will be steadfast (everlasting)	Bai sanu moloon
Be sturdy, be fruitful	Sanu metedes
Be fresh,	Sanu moloba
Be pure	Sanu mamanta
Only the warm breeze	Bui moonto sanu moonda
Only the cool breeze	Bui moonto sanu mojolo
Will come to us bringing	Bia moduaé
That which is bitter	Sanu mepeit
That which is spicy	Sanu mananas
This we ask	Pomangité
In the name of Grandparents	Li topé Siopu
who are Muslim	Ata Allah
That we humans are only given	Amé manusia bui njané
What keeps us steadfast, sturdy, everlasting	Naagaad sanu metedes, moloon

The tray for the umputé of the sea was filled with the same shape, a central mound with four arms reaching to the corner. This tray, however, was about half the size of the other tray and was hung on a tree. Its rice was divided into two halves. No chick was placed on it; nor was an egg, a coin, or local foods. Only bananas; red, black, white, and yellow rice; sweets; shrimp; and sea crabs—all foods from foreigners. The blessing to this sea spirit was intelligible, though quiet and short. In this prayer the umputé spirit was acknowledged more explicitly with the euphemism "sibling":

This is for the "sibling"
Who is washed up with the tides
This is meant for those spirits
Who float up to here
We mean that if you come and happen upon us humans here
We mean do not come to us humans
Don't come with crudeness
Don't come with difficulties
If you must come, bring the simple hot and cold
  [the minor illnesses]
Come with goodness, come with proper measure.
[Bring only] the simple [illness] nothing more.

While the sando were reciting the finishing prayers for these trays, the five possessed mediums returned to the huge mat filled with what I estimate to be about 3,000 rice packets (ampini) located near the river.[12] A Laujé imam[13] recited an Arabic chant (tulabala)[14] over the rice offerings. Then the mediums came out of trance and stepped back. Sumpitan announced that the children could ransack the pile of blessed rice packets. Gleeful shouts sprang from the eager children as hordes rushed in to grab ampini, peeling off the outer wrappings, and stuffing as many cooked rice balls in their mouths at once as they possibly could. After an amazingly short period of time, Siamae Asarima gathered the scattered "outer skins" of the ampini and cast them down the Tinombo River while uttering (secretly) a prayer (see Figure 5.4). Then Siamae Asarima bathed the participants in the stream water. Many people asked Siamae Asarima to fill small lengths of bamboo with consecrated water so they could take a healing bath at their own houses. Participants then went home and planned, in two or three weeks, to gather further downstream at the house of the olongian for the momasoro proper.

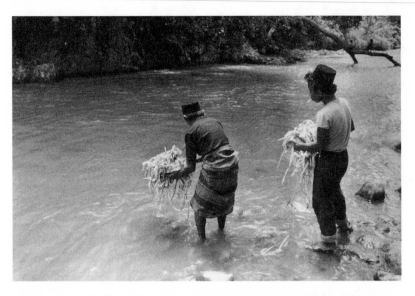

Figure 5.4.   Sando, Siamae Asarima, sending skins downstream at monganjul poyoan

Though local sando like Siamae Asarima, from the commoner villages, made the actual offerings, Sumpitan was able to oversee the
whole operation and make sure it fit with his interpretation of
umputé. For him, the rite's purpose was to propitiate the two kinds of
umputé, the more pure and the less pure, and then separate them. The
offering trays iconically reiterated this theme and the characteristics of
these spirits. Sumpitan insisted that the sea spirit's tray be divided into
two yellow and white halves, rather than concentric circles. "Foreign
substances of procreation cannot easily mix," he said. "They cannot
form a child, because they are not the spirit of creation, but a secondary, less powerful one." Thus no rice colors on the trays were allowed to touch each other. He said this foreign offering was "the opposite of the tray for the land and river spirit because foreign spirits
can't get along with each other." By contrast the "white Laujé" tray he
called a "fortress" (from Indonesian *benting*). Like the Laujé spirit, it
represented strength and sturdiness. Its concentric-circle-shaped rice
offering of white in the center, encircled by yellow, then by white, represented, said Sumpitan, the olongian at the center of the world and all
the Laujé people touched by the olongian. It also represented a fertil-

ized egg in the womb, all parts, male and female, yellow and white intertwined. The four posts of the tray, Sumpitan said, were the "four
pillars which hold up the four corners of the world." Without these
pillars and this spirit, "the world would collapse." The prayers to this
spirit, he said, were uttered to ask the Laujé spirit, the olongian spirit
who anchors the world and keeps earth separate from sea and sky to
continue to do so.

More important, though, Sumpitan said that the rite was to honor
the olongian as the primary healer of the Laujé people. The participants, he said, brought rice packets as a form of tribute for the olongian. After these rice packets were blessed, the olongian redistributed
them to the people. This act, said Sumpitan, purified the rice and made
the people who ate it healthy. When the outer wrappings were removed and the "skins" floated downstream toward the ocean, it was
done under the orders of the olongian to ensure that the people were
disease-free. "Diseases," said Sumpitan, "enter Laujé bodies through
the black hairs of the outer covering of our skin." The rite served "to
strip off" the illnesses that might have entered the community as a
whole and infected the "body" of the land and its rivers.

In Sumpitan's view, this rite propitiated the cruder umputé from the
sea, but it also stripped off the outer layer infected by its crudity so
that the Laujé people could reach the core or essence of all that was
Laujé. The rite, then, was a preparation for the momasoro in which
seven days of prayers and chants from the spirits of the first beings of
the universe rejuvenated the core or essence. They made Laujé bodies
—individual and social—strong enough to withstand illness brought
from the outside.

After the upstream gathering, everyone returned home to wait two
weeks, when the new moon would signal the beginning of the momasoro rite. The momasoro, in contrast to the family-oriented fare of the
monganjul poyoan, will be conducted at night and will attract adults
and only a few children. Its purpose, while still festive, is more serious
than the monganjul poyoan.

Nevertheless, the potential visit of the regent to the momasoro
meant there was extra preparation work. Busy parents could be heard
in the ensuing weeks ordering their children to fetch palm leaves to
make the archway decorations or find wood to cook offerings. In one
way or the other, everyone was involved.

The Momasoro at the House of the Olongian

The momasoro is a seven-night fete at the house of the olongian to which all Laujé are invited. Because of the regent's visit and because of the two-year hiatus, more curiosity seekers from surrounding towns were attracted to the nightly rites. Flickering lanterns owned by cigarette and snack vendors hoping to earn an extra 100 rupiah lit the road to the house of the olongian. Shadows of people slowly navigating the crowds were intermittently illuminated by the occasional flashlight or gas-pressure lantern. The mood was celebratory, but mysterious. Shadows passed by; no one knew if they were spirit or human.

Spirit possession was what the momasoro proper was about. All the spirit manifestations of illnesses and cures were invited to the house of the olongian to possess mediums (to pensio). These embodied spirits spent their time either in the public space of the house (the "parlor" or "big house") or in the ritual hut behind the living quarters of the olongian (the "hearth" or "little house"), which was constructed, ironically enough, with funds from the immigrants in Tinombo.

Sumpitan says the gathering of the spirits of the "little house" who chant the story of the creation of the world is the "core" or "essence" of the rite. Their chanting reinvigorates the power of the olongian. Two kinds of spirits possess mediums, who are dressed in either white or brightly colored clothes. White usually represents Laujé spirits, says Sumpitan, and colored usually represents foreign ones. The "white" spirits tend to calmly and melodiously chant lullabies and blessings that depict the beginning of the earth, the creation of trees, land, and rivers. In 1985 Sumpitan choreographed the rite so that most of the white spirits possessed mediums in the shrine house or little house.

Inside the little house, on each of the seven evenings of the momasoro, the ceremony begins in the same way. The lead medium, the boliang, begins to breathe in the damar incense and chew the betel nut an assistant prepares.[15] The smoke from the incense, and the mild stimulus of betel nut, trigger trances. First the boliang, seated cross-legged on the floor, moans and sways languidly with closed eyes. As she rocks back and forth, the deep moans gradually meld into a chant. Usually she begins with the Budding Tree chant. After the boliang has sung her first song, the other mediums follow the same procedure. The boliang is the first to go to the altar and offer quiet blessings while also singing her psalms to the tune of a lullaby. Others soon follow. Their moans slowly meld into recognizable tunes. Onlookers often comment at this point that "the spirit has come to sit in front of" the medium. At the altar, while chanting, the spirit places kernels of raw white and yellow rice (husked and unhusked) in the offering plate at the altar. When this spirit is finished chanting, another spirit (possessing another medium) approaches the altar.

The altar in the little house serves as the repository for sacred carved objects including the regalia of the olongian and a sliver of the first tree. The regalia, *ginaling*, were wrapped in layers of homemade bark-cloth and machine-loomed white cloth enclosed within a pyramidal shrine about 1.5 meters high.[16] This was called the *vunkeng* (see Figure 5.5). Other objects in addition to the sliver of the "first tree" were covered with cloth inside the shrine. Sumpitan said these objects had been handed down from the first ancestors and marked the Laujé shrine as a center of power. The wrapping, first in bark cloth, then in white, said Sumpitan, represented the "first egg of the beginning of the world."

Here at this altar, spirits chant about the birth of the world, the separation of the healing from the pestilent spirits, and the creation of the first ethnic groups. While the spirits chant, they offer raw, husked rice kernels to the tree shrine. Occasionally, they massage the olongian. Throughout the seven nights of the ritual, the olongian sits in passive silence beside the shrine. This part of the momasoro is carried out in relative seclusion. The small audience is composed of the olongian, some of his immediate family, a few other aristocrats, possessed mediums dressed in white, and the boliang who often carries bark-cloth *(donu)* pom-poms to ward off bad spirits (see Figure 5.6).

More boisterous spirits possess the brightly clothed mediums in the parlor. These possessed mediums dance before a large public audience every night.[17] Their dances are called "play." They dance wildly, fight mock battles among themselves, jump on drums, and wave swords at audience members who scream in feigned fright, sometimes running into the courtyard to escape from the so-called sea spirits. Most of the mediums possessed by these spirits dress in colorful outfits. Some, however, wear the white and blue clothing of Muslim mourning.

Sumpitan told me that in the past, before the momasoro was forbidden, many of the possessed in the big house walked on hot coals or pressed sharp machetes to their chests without letting the machete pierce their skin. Other possessed persons would intentionally cut

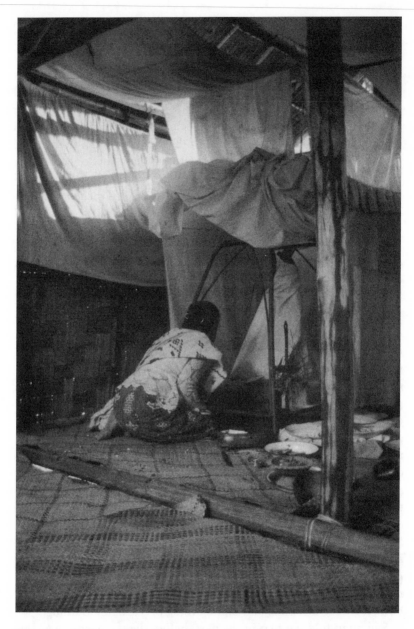

Figure 5.5. Medium placing offering at a Laujé sacred altar (vunkeng)

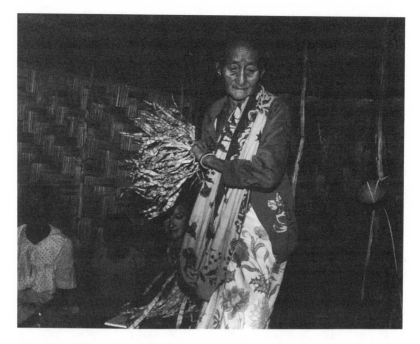

Figure 5.6.   Boliang Siinai Samaliu, at a momasoro

themselves, bleeding profusely, then with one stroke wipe all the blood away, so the wound would disappear. Though such flashy possessions no longer take place, the atmosphere in the big house is still one of frenetic excitement. It contrasts sharply with the quiet solemnity of the little house.

Whether in the shrine house or the big house, possessed mediums speak in a language said to be an "ancient" form of Laujé no longer used in everyday speech. Spirits' speech is often obtuse, oracular. Spirits, if they are to be "authoritative," have to speak in couplets; they use esoteric and convoluted constructions analogous to the King James version of English (see Fox 1988; Metcalf 1989, 1993; Kuipers 1990; J. Errington 1988, 1989, 1998; Zerner and Volkman 1988). Spirits never use the familiar thee or thou, but always the formal and inclusive we (something like a cross between the French vous and the proverbial royal we). Spirits never use the exclusive I, but the inclusive we. Spirit language is punctuated with formal, almost rhetorical phrases, such as "it is said," "it means," "that is to say."[18] Because audience members cannot understand spirits' oracular and antiquated language, they rely on various sando, always male, to translate.

Momasoro Proper: The Little House

Sumpitan explained that every year the Laujé must give offerings to the Laujé shrine in the little house, so that the "invisible" tree continues to stand up straight and tall. If they do not, it will shrink into the spherical, egg-shaped entity it was at the beginning of time, and the world will collapse along with it. According to Sumpitan, the shrine house containing the sacred regalia is "the center," the "true focus" of the momasoro. It is "Laujé." Sumpitan said that all the ritual actions that consecrate this shrine are opposed to the rites that will be held simultaneously in the parlor of the olongian's house. The actions in the other house will involve possession by foreign merchant *(pedagang)* spirits from the sea who represent the lesser-ranked red and black umputé. Those rites will be for the public, for Laujé and foreigner alike. The regent will be given a special seat here. Spirit possession in the "big house," or "foreign trader house," will be "play" and therefore unimportant. By contrast, the rites and chants in the "little house" are "prayer." These rites will help to purify the community and its people, and only pure Laujé and anthropologists who promise to only speak Laujé are allowed here.

After Sumpitan told me about the differences in the two houses, I wondered if, when the regent came, Sumpitan, in a show of deference, would also allow the non-Laujé-speaking regent into the sacred shrine. I had a suspicion he would, but could not be sure. For now, I was glad I had met many of the spirit mediums prior to this rite so they would not be shocked by my tape recorder and camera as they had been at the monganjul poyoan.

The Little Shrine House: The Laujé Spirits of the Land Are Invoked

Even though events in the little house were roughly the same on each of the seven days, the rite created a sense of a slow, but perceptible, accumulation of all things good, vitalizing, and nurturing. On the first morning of the ceremony, the shrine frame and the inner walls of the house were bare. On every subsequent day, however, cloth was added until the seventh day. By then, the yellow bamboo walls and ceiling were covered in white. Sumpitan compared this to the creation of a human being inside the womb. "Each day the fetus grows more and more, until it becomes big enough to be born."

The possessed mediums reiterated this theme every evening. At the altar they would chant about the beginning of the world. As they sang, they would take rice kernels from what Sumpitan called the "male side," and transfer them to the "female side" of the altar. Sumpitan called the vertical trapezoidal part of the shrine "female" because, he said, the triangular shape (from the front) was like a woman's vagina. The three porcelain plates in front of the altar were "like the fertile parts of the womb." One plate had husked, dry rice kernels, another puffed rice kernels, and the third antique coins, tobacco, and betel nut. These were all the "original" substances passed down from Laujé ancestors.

Sumpitan called the other side of the shrine "male." He did not have to explain why. Its shape was decidedly phallic. A long sheathed and intricately carved machete was stretched out between two brass plates. One plate contained puffed rice, betel nut/tobacco, and gambier offerings; the other raw rice. When the mediums transferred raw rice seeds, a few at a time, from the "male side" of the altar to the "female side," Sumpitan said this was like impregnating the female side with fertilized sperm. At the end of the ceremony, accumulated rice kernels would form a symbolic "child."

Most of the mediums who chanted at the altar, including the boliang, were commoner women.[19] All were said to be possessed by the Laujé spirits of the land and rivers. The chant sung by the boliang invites in those spirits of the land and rivers who stay at the "womb of the world" near the Inscribed Rock. After these spirits "enter" or possess her, the boliang invites in the other spirits who will possess all the other mediums. None of the others can be possessed until the boliang chants the following:

Yeli ijatié
Who guards the Inscribed Stone
O Divine Body of Light which is eternal
Conscript of the Muslim God
Descendants of the First Woman
Descendants through the generations
No less, No more
O Divine Body of Light which is eternal

The Muslim God of Gods
The descendants of Manangka Allah
Guarded by the First Tree
At the navel of the world
Came with power *(baraka)*
Came to rule over us
We, the disciples of Mohammad under the Wind
Which shelters the World
The world which has four corners
O Radiance of Allah
O Minangka Allah
Who is the one of power
Who rules over us
We are ruled by you
We are empowered by you
We the disciples of Mohammad
under the winds
Hey, the Efficacious Raja
O, the Raja who rules us
O Healer who has power

Sumpitan pointed out that the first spirit the boliang calls is named "Yelé Ijati'é."[20] "Yelé" is an honorific that refers to a female spirit. "Ijati'é," says Sumpitan, "means genuine, original or pure." "Such a name is ancient" and therefore indigenous. After "Yelé Ijati'é" is called, "Manangka Alla, guardian of the first tree" is invoked. According to Sumpitan, the purpose of mentioning this spirit and others is to reiterate in sequential order how the various guardian spirits who resided at the center and the four corners of the world were created from the original deity at the navel or womb of the world. Sumpitan said that all of these spirits, despite their different names, were merely various forms of umputé. He gave no explanation of the words in the chant that implied that the Laujé were subservient to a Muslim god and to a "Raja who rules over us." He only said, "these are the names of the original Laujé spirits."

With this chant, the boliang asked the spirits who resided at the points of power—at the womb of the world and the center of the sea—to participate in the momasoro so they would recognize they were honored. The hope was that the spirits would leave the humans free from epidemics. The boliang also asked the spirits to carry messages to the ultimate deities at the points of power. Those ultimate deities were the highest spirits, who did not leave their "homes" to possess people and receive the offerings.

Once the boliang had called upon all these spirits in her chant, she announced that all the spirits were gathered together in the shrine house. These spirits of land and rivers then possessed the other women who served as spirit mediums. The women were the "vessels" through which these spirits would speak. Each woman took a turn at the altar. Their chants—sung rather than spoken—echoed melodies typical of Laujé lullabies. A typical chant was the "tree song." In it the tree divides at the river's source and continues to branch and bud to its mouth. Then the tree returns to the source, the "tap-root."

O progeny of the first tree	*O bija nu ayué*
Just a tap-root rooting	*Boi nepamayolé*
Rooting-rooting deeply	*Saba mapamayolonyé*
Gave root to a single root	*Nelali selalié*
And sprouted a single trunk	*Meboto sobobotonyé*
And grew a single skin (bark)	*Neungkulé soungkulungaonyé*
And branched a single branch	*Nendaangi sadaangonyé*
And sprouted a single leaf	*Nolongi sololongonyé*
And sprouted a single bud	*Noloba solobalobanyé*
And sprouted a single flower	*Nebansa sebansabansanyé*
And sprouted a single fruit	*Nevua sovuavuanyé*
Later it budded, it budded	*Bia malobaé molabaé*
From the source of the river	*Lae matanyé*
Until it reached the coast	*Dua dua li bambanyé*
At the coast it budded	*Moloba li bambanyé*
Returning again to the source	*Dua dua li matanyé*
[in the mountains]	

As Sumpitan explained it, the "dividing river" and the "budding tree" chants were both about creation, but from two different, yet complementary, perspectives. The dividing river referred to the creation of "poison and cure." Sumpitan said that the river divided when the foreigners were separated from the Laujé. The foreigners became the "poison" and the Laujé became the "cure." Though the chant did not mention foreigners as opposed to Laujé, Sumpitan said that when it referred to poison it meant foreigners and when it referred to cure it meant Laujé. At the creation of the world, poison went to the center of the sea while cure stayed at the navel or womb of the world.

The "budding tree" song referred to a slightly earlier moment of creation. Its point of reference was the large tree that separated earth from sky. The song told how the tree grew from the first rock of creation and budded from the trunk or source. The limbs of the tree "reached the coastline" and then "they grew and returned again to the source." Sumpitan used the song about the tree to talk about the hierarchical relationships within the Laujé community and outside it. The original trunk, he said, was Laujé, but the further it branched and grew away from the center, the more foreigners or pestilent spirits embodied its branches. The tree eventually had "seven buds and seven branches," seven being the Laujé number of infinity. Seven also was commonly used in everyday speech to signal all the ethnic groups of the world.[21] The whole tree or land became ill, said Sumpitan, when the branches returned to the trunk.

By interpreting these images of trees and rivers as though they were images of ethnicity, Sumpitan married his political message to the esoterica of Laujé ritual. Sumpitan claimed that the momasoro showed that the Laujé were the "first people," the "source of all creation," "the trunk," "the headwater," the "womb of the world." He asserted that the Laujé people were themselves representations of, and represented by, the olongian, who was the most "pure" representation of the umputé of creation. By contrast, he claimed the foreigners were "secondary people," "the branches," the "mixed," the "impure ones," "those who come from the sea," or the "land of death."

Conversations in the Little House: Dialogues between Spirit and Human

Interspersed between the songs by the possessed mediums (to pensio) and the chants at the altar were audience members' requests for sando to interpret spirit chants or to ask spirits to cure them of illness. Thus sando, boliang, and to pensio worked in tandem with each other. Sando like Sumpitan were the most visible participants in the momasoro. Boliang and to pensio speaking in spirit language were the major attractions as far as most audience members were concerned but, they were unintelligible; spirit speech was too oracular for ordinary Laujé to understand. Sando thus acted as translators or intermediaries between audience members and spirits. If someone was ill and wanted a spirit to cure them, they would ask a sando to act as go-between. Sando like Sumpitan could then interpret spirits' esoteric speech in a way that fit their own interpretation of the spirit world.[22] Sometimes, this meant that the sando superseded the spirits and gave their own versions of spirit speech. This is not to say, however, that Sumpitan or other curers, did not respect spirits. Sumpitan listened very intently to what spirits said and told me their words were sacred if the medium was not faking possession. Sumpitan did seem to me, though, to interpret spirits' words contrary to spirits' intent.

The following vignette exemplifies the different ways in which sando and spirit speech is understood by audience members. A spirit possessed the medium named Siinai Alasan, who was a widow of about forty and a descendant of commoners. Siinai Alasan's spirit used her oracular speech to speak for all spirits possessing mediums, defining their position in direct opposition to Sumpitan and sando in general. The vignette begins when a man in his sixties, Pak Lamané, entered the little house seeking Sumpitan's aid in finding a spirit to cure his persistent cough. Pak Lamané was a "half-Laujé" man from Tinombo who had grown up speaking Indonesian and only a creolized Laujé; thus, he needed Sumpitan to act as translator. Ironically, Pak Lamané was the father of one of the fundamentalists in Tinombo's Department of Religious Affairs who had been instrumental in banning the momasoro. Sumpitan relished his role as Pak Lamané's intermediary, telling me after the "curing session" that he, Sumpitan, had shown Pak Lamané "how Muslim our ceremony really is." When Pak Lamané nervously entered, Sumpitan said:

> Come on in. . . . Later when that spirit is finished, that one is the clear one, that one is white. That spirit is from the center, the navel. Later we'll speak with that spirit. That one is strong.

As Pak Lamané entered, the spirit possessing Siinai Alasan begins to lecture Pak Lamané on the interdependence of religion and custom:

> This rite should not be destroyed, it is said. . . . This rite [custom] which is being observed now, it is said . . . is not just a custom, which was just picked up on the streets. This is a ceremony of the ancients. . . . It is the heritage that has been passed down to us humans.

Sumpitan interrupts the spirit:

> We ask forgiveness, O Honored One. This one, the disciple of Prophet Mohammed, has a pain in his chest. O Pure White Spirit, it seems that something has been forgotten. . . . Before the connection [to the spirit] is broken we come to [you] spirit, asking for help. That is how it is.

The spirit entity possessing Siinai Alasan responds:

> This ceremony, this customary rite, this here, this now, that which is seen
> now, that which is before you now, is not to be trifled with, is not to be
> played with. . . . We of the spirit collectivity [umputé] were put before you
> by Allah to speak the words that are the ceremony, to give the words that
> heal, that are the charms.

Sumpitan leans over to Pak Lamané and says:

> The spirit says a little side ceremony, probably a white offering for the
> spirit-who-has-died-while-on-the-*hajj* should be given. It is obvious you
> have forgotten to give an offering to the white spirit of-the-one-who-died-
> while-going-to-Mecca (on the *hajj*).

After speaking directly to Siinai Alasan and identifying her possessing
spirit as "the white one," a euphemism for the purity and high status of
the possessing spirit, Sumpitan turns away from Siinai Alasan and
speaks sotto voce to Pak Lamané, systematically going around the room
naming all the spirits possessing the mediums who are sitting there. In a
loud stage whisper Sumpitan says, "that one, which is from the Center
of the Sea, it sits on a golden throne . . . that spirit helps to cure chills
and aches . . . That spirit there is a quiet one, it is a white spirit, named
The-spirit-of-those-who-have-died-on-the-way-to-Mecca. It is old."

Siinai Alasan's spirit responds to Sumpitan's attempt to identify the
spirits as discrete individuals:

> Generation upon generation, the inheritance from our ancestors is this
> ceremony here. This is the voice that is heard here. What is seen before
> [you] is one. Everything. Just one. We [spirits] are many, but of one view,
> of one body, of one tongue. . . . This ceremony, this chant [uttered by spir-
> its] is what comprises your muscles, the blood in your body, this ceremony
> of custom here. We [you] must bow our heads low, so that all can be heard,
> be seen, this is the chant, the regalia, the words that comprise us [and you],
> punishes with illness and heals from illness. This that we [you] hear is what
> will heal. We submit to it.
>
>   This custom, this inheritance should not disappear. . . . This is the spirit
> collectivity [umputé], that which connects us to our past, our ancestors,
> who gave us knowledge of the spirit collectivity [umputé]. . . . This, here is
> the root. . . . When the root of a tree is pulled up and . . . one looks up into
> the sky and sees that the leaves of that tree have shriveled and died. . . . If
> all one waits for is to pray to Allah [but forgets the root, the customs], then
> the tree will die branch by branch.

Despite the spirit's admonishments, Sumpitan persists in "identifying" or labeling her. He says: "That spirit who speaks is the olongian of all spirits. It says that you will be cured if you follow the white ceremony." In this "curing episode," it is clear that the spirit possessing Siinai Alasan says nothing about performing an additional "white ceremony." The spirit speaks directly to Pak Lamané about the relationship between custom and religion, saying custom is like the root of a tree, and religion is secondary. It is like the branches of a tree. The spirit warns Pak Lamané not to follow Islam exclusively, while forgetting custom.

What is murky here, and cannot really be answered, is whether Sumpitan neglected to translate this portion of the spirit's prayer to Pak Lamané on purpose or if it was an oversight. If he did purposefully neglect to translate, was it because he was trying to avoid embarrassing Pak Lamané (the spirit rudely told this devout Muslim that custom was superior to Islam) or was it because he wanted to direct Pak Lamané's thoughts in another direction, toward seeing the spirit as a white one? Sumpitan tells Pak Lamané that a particular cure is necessary, one that Sumpitan just so happens to know. Sumpitan, like the spirit, leads Pak Lamané toward adat and a curing rite outside the realm of Islamic religion, but does so without explicitly preaching to Pak Lamané as the spirit does. Sumpitan also takes great liberty in translating the old Laujé language and the spirits' intent so it coincides with his own. The result is that Sumpitan does proclaim himself an expert. Whether he is grandstanding or playing the diplomat can never really be answered.

What is significant and clear here, despite the murky qualities of the interaction, is that Sumpitan behaves toward Pak Lamané and toward the mediums (and boliang) in a way that is typical of sando/medium interactions. (More of this will be discussed later, but it is worth noting here). After this fairly typical interaction, the boliang sings a song to send the spirits back to their "resting places." Then she returns to her normal nontrance self. All sit quietly smoking cigarettes or chewing betel nut.

Foreign Umputé's House

Meanwhile, the atmosphere in the big house could not be more different than that in the house with the sacred shrine. Here, the ambience

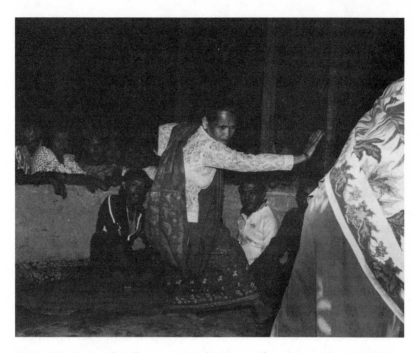

Figure 5.7.   Possessed medium assuming the posture of a male martial arts specialist

is rowdy, boisterous theater verging at times on parody. Female and male mediums are possessed by loud and arrogant male spirits, usually those who speak in "foreign" languages of neighboring ethnic groups, such as the Kaili. The spirits are called trader (pedagang) spirits and are said to come from the sea. They often dance to the rhythm of the two drums with the brass gong constantly playing in the background. Every so often an especially wild spirit will jump on top of the drums, gyrating to the drumbeat and shouts of encouragement from the audience members. Usually, the mediums possessed by these spirits pair off and engage in mock battles with swords and shields. Their dances imitate the movements of martial arts *(kongtau)* combat (see Figure 5.7).

Some of the spirits, wearing the red head-wrap and carrying the spear and shield of the tadulako headhunter, shout and whoop as if they are in a battle with an invisible foe. Some spirits smoke store-bought clove cigarettes. Clove cigarettes represent the outside, foreign world. The spirit mediums smoke those cigarettes with the lighted tip inside their mouths, the unlighted tip turned outside, to show they are spirits "from the other side" (the spirit world). These spirits always shout rather than talk. They scold the audience members for failing to obey the "traditional customs." Other spirits dance and dart around the large concrete floor, threatening the audience members hovering in the corners of the room with words such as, "I'll slit your throat if you don't properly follow the customs (adat)."

The spirits' songs are a mix of Laujé and Kaili languages. They are often muffled by the other spirits who are loud and disrespectful. Many times various spirits sing at the same time as others. Their combined voices become a jumbled cacophony. This contrasts dramatically with the spirits in the little house who always wait until one spirit's song is finished before they start their own. To the audience members in the big house, the general effect of the spirits and their physical and verbal competition with each other is confusing, cacophonous hysteria.

There were a few quiet spirits in the foreign umputé house. They were dressed in white headdresses and blouses, with blue and white sarong wraps—Muslim funeral dress for women. These spirits do not dance. They sing haunting songs that are eerily beautiful, reminiscent of funeral dirges and redolent of a siren's sensuous call.

Sumpitan said that these spirits are the rulers of the spirits from the center of the sea, the white umputé of foreigners, the umputé of sexual fluid that never merged into yellow to create a child. They are from the world of sterility and this is why the spirits wear funeral clothes. Below is a sample of one of the funeral songs sung by a medium named Kaija who was dressed in white. The language is Kaili:

Hey, we come and show our respect for the Creator	*E, no bilangé nosumba Ala'é*
We sit here in the place where the Creator lives	*Ita dunko-dunko Alaé tuvu*
And respect him from the tips of our toes to the tips of our hair	*Nu biisa laé pusé tuvu nu lubaoté.*
Remember us we are from the eye of the sun at the center of the sea	*Tora tora kami Dakori mata eo ri pusé nu dagaté*
We have come to see you the children and to give our voices to you	*Liendemé umama lampé nopoloiloi opu mobolé aivuonyé suaranyé*
So later you can show your respect to us your siblings	*Biapé mogama palé kaitu to siaanga*

An altar for all these spirits was placed in the back corner of the room where the shield and sword of the tadulako were stored. The altar was called the altar of the "red and the black," or the "many-colored." White and yellow rice and seven other (dyed) colors of rice were artfully piled around the circular altar. It was similar to the red umputé offering for the foreign raja.

According to Sumpitan, the seven different colors of rice on the offering represented seven different ethnic groups and seven different sicknesses. The "black umputé illness" occurred when foreigners did not follow Laujé custom. Then, "dead blood" was mixed with "live blood." That was when a foreign male forced a female to have sex before the post-partum forty-four-day taboo had expired. Then, he said, the black blood of birth would pollute the sperm. This would cause the next child to be born with a disease resembling leprosy *(pudung)*.

Most red umputé illnesses manifested as fevers. Sumpitan told a myth about the origin of the first red umputé disease.

> The spirit of red umputé originally lived on top of the mountain, but one day he became so obsessed with making a boat, he came down to the coast to build a boat. The sea rose and the people became sick. He filled the boat with *lipat,* a red vine that grew around the brackish lowland marshes and he put the boat into the sea. The sea fell back, taking the boat and the sickness with it. This was the first momasoro. From then on the red fever mainly came from the sea. We have to give offerings to the red umputé to show it respect.

To represent this fact, a sprig of lipat leaves was placed in a jar of water in front of the altar for the foreign umputé spirits.[23] Every time a spirit possessed one of the female mediums, she went to this altar and placed her right hand on top of the coin plate on the pedestal containing the rice. There she muttered an inaudible prayer.

After the initial blessings and prayers to the altar of the foreign spirits, or "trader spirits," were uttered, the mediums sang about the spirits possessing them. Usually, they were possessed by one of the foreign spirits originating from the outer reaches of the Laujé kingdom.[24] Sumpitan said that the variety of spirit personalities reflected the variety of foreigners who lived in the four corners of the earth. "Just as the world has all kinds of foreigners, this house has all kinds of spirits."

Very few people actually asked serious questions of these spirits, a fact that contrasted markedly with the situation in the smaller sacred house. Some audience members even openly mocked the spirit mediums by commenting "that one's a fake." The audience members had to be careful, though, for the spirits could retaliate if angered. To avoid incidents between audience members and spirits, a male sando acted as the referee. He calmed and soothed inflamed spirits. This sando, dressed in black, often had to separate spirits who tried to verbally or physically attack each other. He was charged with keeping the spirits happy, passing them tobacco, cigarettes, and betel nut when they requested it.

On the next to the last night, excitement was in the air. The caravan of cars bringing the regent, his servant, his secretary, his driver, and other underlings had arrived in Tinombo. The regent was spending the night in the former raja's palace and was expected to arrive via jeep once night fell at the house of the olongian. Preparations were made for the closing ceremonies. The mediums from the Laujé shrine house came into the big house to sit with the "foreign" spirits. The olongian also came into this house for the first time. A possessed medium dressed in white sang a song to the olongian. She held and kissed the hand of the olongian. The olongian sat in a chair, while everyone else sat on mats on the concrete floor.

The black-clad sando officiating in the big foreign house stroked and petted a goat to be sacrificed. The wife of the olongian, still possessed by a tadulako spirit and speaking in Kaili, threw some of the colored rice from the "foreign" altar onto the goat. She and the sando forced the goat to lie before the olongian, who was seated in the chair. The olongian put his right foot on the goat's head. The sando cut the goat's ear, daubing blood on the olongian's forehead while prayers were uttered. This, said Sumpitan, marked the olongian as the ultimate Laujé leader and identified the sacrificed goat with him. The goat's head was offered to the umputé spirit of the land and rivers at a site upstream. The meat from its body was later shared by the participants who remained in the house of the olongian after the boats were cast away. Sumpitan said that the sacrifice of the goat was to ensure that the olongian himself would live long and that the whole Laujé kingdom would be strong as well. Sumpitan had wanted the regent to witness this rite, since it would underline the importance of the olongian in indigenous ritual and culture, but as yet, the regent had not arrived. Sumpitan asked a teenage boy to run across the river and find out when the regent was coming. "Tell him the spirits are being entered" said Sumpitan.

In the big house, the Laujé spirits finally met the foreign spirits and they began battle for the first time. Up until this night, they had remained in their separate houses. The boliang arrived from the Laujé shrine house. The mediums possessed by the Laujé umputé of land and rivers followed her. Laujé spirits bravely waited while the boliang spirit coaxed the foreign umputé onto the "battleground" to "fight" the Laujé spirit from the navel or womb of the world. Many of the mediums were old, in their seventies and eighties, but spirits inside them moved them to dance and threaten others with agile martial arts postures. The battles began in a hierarchical fashion, with the lowliest spirit from the sea, a red umputé warrior, battling the lowliest spirit from the land. They continued until they reached the highest spirit from the sea.

The outcome of these battles was predictable. The Laujé spirit from the womb of the world won every battle. This spirit was the oldest spirit, said Sumpitan, it was the native Laujé spirit from which all others sprang, including the spirits from the sea. Therefore, it was superior. As the evening wore on, each possessed spirit engaged in battle. Whether winner or loser, all possessed spirits concluded by bowing to the olongian and his family.

It was nearing midnight and no regent or teenage messenger appeared. Sumpitan ordered his nephew to go see what was wrong. The exhausted mediums continued to do battle, but finally gave up at two in the morning. The regent and the messengers never returned.

Preparing for the Last Night

The next morning was a late one. Too much betel nut, too many cigarettes, too much battle with possessed spirits. At noon, Sumpitan's nephew returned to a still-groggy crowd sipping coffee on Sumpitan's porch. The nephew's hunched shoulders and hangdog look told most of the story before he opened his mouth. He and the other Laujé messenger had been roped into listening to the Muhammadiyah imam lecture the regent and his entourage about the evils of spirit possession. No one could interrupt or leave the imam, who piously pontificated until the wee hours of the morning. Sumpitan's nephew and the other messenger had fallen asleep on the raja's palace porch (as Siamae Sanji had before). He had come home without ever speaking to the regent or to his staff.

Despite this bad news, Sumpitan was still sanguine. "The regent promised to attend," said Sumpitan. "The government sent money for this rite. They have to come to enjoy the fruits of their gift," said Sumpitan. "It would be bad luck *(ampunan)* to promise and not follow through. The regent will be here." Sumpitan ordered people to prepare for the final night. Slowly those around him began to buzz with activity.

The Last Night

The seventh night of the momasoro was the culmination of all the other nights. It was at once the focus of the whole rite, and paradoxically, the point when so many activities occurred at once that nothing was focused. The most important moment on the seventh night would be when two boats, filled with rice offerings in the courtyard belonging to the olongian, would be carried to the sea in a long procession with lanterns, drums, and festive participants. The boat filled with offerings to the foreign spirits would be cast out to sea at the mouth of the Tinombo River. Following it, an escort Laujé boat would be cast out.

Before taking the boat to the sea, however, a whole series of offerings must be made. The atmosphere was one of chaos and celebration. On the first six nights, public activities began around eight P.M. On the seventh and last night, however, people gathered before sunset (at five) to prepare for and watch the performance of the final rituals. Sumpitan orchestrated the myriad culmination rituals so his ultimate message, that foreigners should not mix with natives, was underlined. Paradoxically, though, he went out of his way to arrange for the regent's visit. At his own expense he had ordered that multicolored flags be made to grace the entrance to the courtyard of the olongian. He arranged their installation so the yellow and white flags, representing the Laujé, were placed slightly higher than the other colored flags. The multicolored flags, he said, each represented a foreign ethnic group and thus a foreign umputé. The flags were appropriate for a regent who governed so many ethnic groups in his province. Sumpitan also arranged for young women to decorate a special raised chair with palm fronds so the honored guest could watch the ceremonies unobstructed. I found Sumpitan's obsequious attitude ironic, given his anti-foreign message.

Sumpitan began the evening by asking a sando to replace the raw, colored rice in the foreign umputé altar with cooked rice. He told me this meant that the foreign spirit could not eat its last meal here. It also meant there was no produce from the foreign rice; it was not fertile. Immediately after that, Sumpitan went to the shrine house for a white chicken offering. Here a whole roasted chicken was given as an offering to the umputé of land and rivers. It looked like the individual umputé offering to the white spirit, but it did not have an egg and a red flower on it (a symbolic hymen). In this offering, the "symbolic hymen" was replaced by a womblike pyramid made of wrapped rice bundles *(baundaké)*. Sumpitan never interpreted this, but following his reasoning, it suggested a child already conceived. During the week of ceremonies in the little house, Sumpitan had arranged for each possessed medium who came to pray at the Laujé altar to transfer puffed rice seeds or kernels from the male side of the altar to the female side of the altar. Sumpitan had told me earlier that these male and female rice kernels represented sexual fluids, and that the tentlike shape of the offering in the white chicken rite was like a fertile womb. Because the two offerings looked just alike, I surmised that this one represented the culmination of the transference of seeds, a fertilized fetus, conceived in the Laujé shrine house. It replaced the white umputé rice kernels, which would be cooked and buried in the ground. It underlined Sumpitan's point that Laujé spirits conceive with each other, not with foreigners.

Sempaang: The "Symbolic Child"

Outside, Sumpitan orchestrated a similar message with the symbolic child offering (sempaang), which iconically reiterated the burial of a Laujé elite child's placenta. First, a square tray was prepared in the shrine house with only white and yellow cooked rice topped by a whole boiled egg placed in its center. The rice used had been consecrated at the Laujé altar. It was cooked and covered by another woven tray. Both were tied together and prepared to be planted in the ground. Sumpitan pointed out that this was also how the placenta was bundled before it was buried. A male sando carried the tray outdoors. He was covered with a white sheet, just as a lowland male father was covered with a white sheet when he buried a placenta [see Figure 5.8]. He placed the tray in a hole in the ground at the edge of the houseyard of the olongian. The sando then covered it with dirt by using his forearms and elbows, just as the father of a newborn does when he buries the placenta.

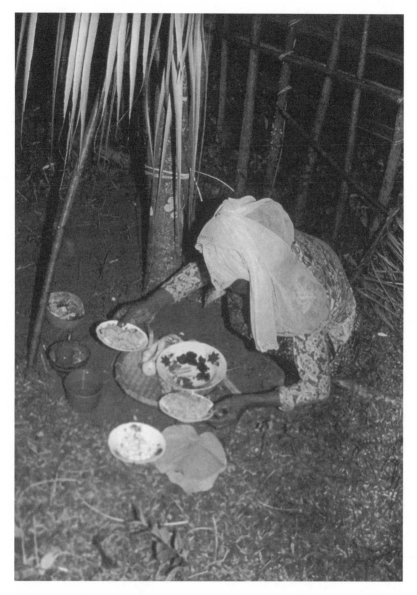

Figure 5.8. Setting up the offering of the symbolic child (sempaang) at the momasoro

According to Sumpitan, the sempaang offering was central to the whole momasoro. A three-sided offering tray with only yellow and white rice and a whole boiled egg and betel nut was hung over the buried tray (much as a tray had been hung at the initial monganjul poyoan rite at the boundary of lowland Laujé territory). Hung underneath this triangular tray was a huge coconut with a hole pierced in the bottom of it. The juice from inside the coconut seed dripped down onto another tray placed over the "grave" of the buried-offering tray.

The sempaang offering in the ground looked like the rite for burying the placenta. But the triangular tray was for a female spirit, said Sumpitan. The coconut beneath her tray was "like the womb." The dripping coconut "sent its fertile juices [translated literally as female sperm] to the male tray on the ground." This substance was what created the fetus and the placenta buried in the ground.

All of these ingredients for the offering had come from the Laujé shrine house and they had been blessed only by Laujé spirits. Sumpitan said the whole offering was a sign to the foreign spirits that Laujé women would create children only with Laujé men. They would not create children with the foreign spirits.

Mantalapu Rite: Preventing Infertility Caused by Foreigners

Other smaller rites were prepared by sando from the big house for the foreign spirits. One, the mantalapu, warned foreign spirits, said Sumpitan, not to bother the Laujé by preventing fertility in the lineage of the olongian.[25] In this rite, the Laujé boliang spirit, armed with a machete, cut down three banana stalks planted in the courtyard. Bananas were said to be "the plants of foreigners." By cutting down the phallic-shaped banana stalks, which represented foreigners or outsiders, the Laujé ensured that no foreign spirit would create Laujé children and no foreign spirit would intervene when Laujé spirits fertilized plants and bodies.

Dabang: Headhunting Rite

Meanwhile, at the threshold of the big house, the wife of the olongian, possessed by a Kaili-speaking warrior spirit, prepared the headhunting rite. Dressed in red, this spirit, though foreign, was a great headhunter who protected the boundaries of the Laujé kingdom by keeping out other foreigners. Two coconuts, representing the heads of two foreigners the spirit had killed, were placed at the threshold with red rice offerings. The spirit asked the Laujé who were inside the big house to place their hands on the hunting spear and the shield. They whooped and chanted along with the spirit as though preparing to hunt heads. They shared a glass of "blood" (coconut milk with red syrup) said to be from the heads of foreigners captured in war. The spirit dipped "four woods" in the "blood" and rubbed it over the participants' faces and feet. This, said Sumpitan, made the participants invincible in war against foreigners who threatened their borders.[26]

Filling the Offering Trays for Umputé of the Land and the Sea

Sumpitan also arranged that the offering trays in the boats and the giant trays to be hung for the umputé of land and rivers symbolically reiterate the differences between foreign umputé and Laujé umputé. The Laujé tray for the umputé of land and rivers sat in front of a boat dressed with a large yellow bark-cloth sail. This tray held the rice and the slaughtered goat's head that the olongian had stepped on the night before. This Laujé tray was taken a few kilometers upstream from the house of the olongian. Sumpitan said this tray strengthened the olongian and the kingdom. It marked the bonds between the umputé spirits of the land and the olongian. Another tray was filled for the same spirit. It was to be placed at the edge of the Laujé kingdom—on the beach. This offering and prayer, said Sumpitan, asked the Laujé umputé of the land and rivers to guard against foreign umputé who entered Laujé shores from the sea.[27]

As soon as he finished telling me about foreigners on Laujé shores, Sumpitan remembered the regent. He had not yet arrived, so Sumpitan dispatched his nephew to return to the foreign raja's palace and find out what the delay was.

Meanwhile, other sando filled two more trays inside each of the two boats propped up in the courtyard. The boat with the white sail, made of funeral cloth (gandisé), was said by Sumpitan to signify foreigners, since foreigners had first brought that cloth to the Laujé. He also said the offering was for the sea spirit, or foreign umputé. Sumpitan made sure that the sando filled this tray with red, black, yellow, and white mounds of rice. According to Sumpitan, each mound represented the umputé of all the foreign spirits who brought illness. Sumpitan claimed that these foreign, or merchant, spirits brought epidemics from Mecca, where such illnesses originated. He said the supreme disease, smallpox, the "golden" disease, the lord of all diseases, sat on the golden throne at Mecca and controlled whether or not epidemics struck people. This image of the golden throne had been used by others as a euphemism combining Mecca with heaven. Sumpitan's comment implied a hierarchical distinction between imported or foreign religion and local religion. Even though Sumpitan considered himself a Muslim, the circumstances of the banning of the rite may have led him to emphasize that the worst of the diseases came from Mecca itself.

As mentioned, the other boat was adorned with a bark-cloth sail "made by Laujé ancestors." "This boat," said Sumpitan, "would escort the 'foreign' boat out to the center of the sea." This boat was "owned by the spirit of the land and rivers." It would sail behind the white-sail boat, making sure the white boat did not return to shore. This boat embodied a messenger spirit for the supreme creator umputé. The messenger was a "pure" Laujé. The sando filled the "Laujé" boat with rice offerings of white encircled by yellow. No other colors were "mixed" with the yellow and white. Sumpitan said the boat also represented the olongian, who was the embodiment of the supreme creator umputé.

After prayers and distribution of rice packets, ampini, the boats were put on oxcarts to be carried to the sea. In years past, the descendants of the warrior tadulako escorted the boats to the seashore, carrying burning torches, waving swords, and beating drums or gongs to ward off any umputé spirits who did not manifest themselves in possession (and who were more dangerous). In 1985, though, many people were embarrassed to be seen at the seashore where more devout Islamic Laujé lived. Thus, only a few people accompanied the boats on the six-kilometer hike to the seashore and back. Those who remained at the big house shared in a communal meal of cooked goat and rice. The goat was given by the olongian. The rice was donated by individuals from Laujé communities along the Tinombo coast. Sumpitan told everyone the regent would be at the shore, but others were beginning to lose hope.

The Beach: Casting the Boats and Foreign Spirits Out to Sea

When they arrived at the beach, no regent appeared. Young people set the boats on the shore and laid out the mats. More wrapped rice packets were piled up for another Arabic blessing and redistributions for the participants living in seaside communities. Small crowds of coastal dwellers surrounded four possessed mediums (all commoners) sitting in front of the rice packets. The sound of the waves crashing against the shore muffled the quiet prayers.

The waves, however, did not muffle the sounds of a large entourage of cars zooming past on the coastal highway, casting long, disturbing shadows over the boats, not even slowing to see what was happening. I knew this had to be the regent's motorcade and felt simultaneously angry and humiliated for Sumpitan's sake. After the thirty or so jeeps sped by and the dust settled, the velvet darkness of the night sky quietly blanketed us on the beach. Everyone knew what the passing cars meant, but no one said anything about the regent. I looked at Sumpitan, but he revealed nothing. After this incident, though, I knew his message would have a more poignant impact. Never trust a foreigner.

Two men took the tray for the Laujé spirit to the mangrove woods at the edge of the beach and hung it on a branch. A sando uttered a prayer asking the Laujé umputé to prevent sea spirits from flowing upstream. Sumpitan said that this tray marked the edge of the kingdom of the Laujé umputé spirit. If it did its job, it would only allow in those sea spirits who brought minor illnesses to the Laujé land. Never would it allow a severe epidemic to enter the Laujé community.

After the offering and the rice packets were blessed, the sando went to the boats to inspect the offerings there. When they cast the boats into the water (see Figure 5.9), youths from neighboring ethnic groups set sail, grabbing the small white chicks that had been placed on the white-sailed boat for the sea spirit. No Laujé could retrieve these chicks, said Sumpitan, for they were now the property of the foreign umputé. Now, said Sumpitan, all major illness would be washed out of the community. Illness would return to "the place it belonged," in the land of the foreigner, the sea.

This marked the end of the momasoro. All Laujé must obey restrictions on work for three or seven days (depending upon their status). They could not work in the fields, chop wood, hunt, fish, or engage in any violent or "separating" activity that might have attracted the

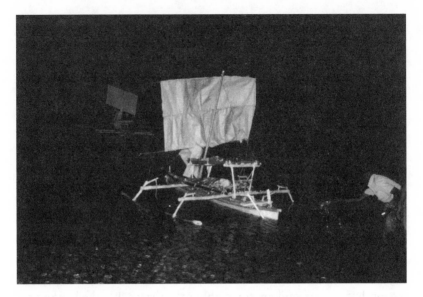

Figure 5.9.   Casting off the boats at a momasoro

umputé spirits back from the sea.[28] To end the period of taboo, the olongian sacrificed a wild chicken.

The next day, the Tinombo official who had originally invited the regent appeared. He told us what we already knew; the Muhammadiyah imam had convinced the regent that the momasoro was a form of devil worship. Scared for his own safety and his political future, the regent had left without gracing the rite with his presence.

Nagging Questions about Sumpitan's Interpretation of the Momasoro

The fact that the regent never appeared was indeed an embarrassment to Sumpitan since he had made the regent such an integral part of the ceremony. This left me with some nagging questions. Why had Sumpitan been so eager to have an immigrant official at the rite when its ultimate purpose was to rid the community of foreigners? When Sumpitan began to explain the "meaning of the boats" from the night before, I began to understand his behavior a little better. The so-called foreign boat was laden with gifts for the spirits from the sea, which are all of lower rank, said Sumpitan. Even though these lower-ranked spirits were invited in as guests and feted for seven nights, they were ultimately asked to leave. The boat laden with food was their going-away gift. It showed the spirits that the Laujé people respected them, but it also made the ultimate point that the spirits were guests and not indigenous Laujé.[29] "Such gifts," said Sumpitan, "showed the difference between the Laujé and the foreigners. One does not have to give gifts to a close relative." By giving food gifts or offerings to umputé of the sea in such an ostentatious manner, Sumpitan said the Laujé marked their distance from, rather than proximity to, the sea spirits as foreigners. His message was clear and, to a certain extent, explained why he had been so solicitous when preparing for the regent's visit. His actions underlined his distance from, rather than servitude to, the foreign official.

Sumpitan also explained that even though at the rite the spirits were only periodically called umputé, the momasoro was still about umputé, but umputé of two kinds. On one level, there were the individual umputé of sexual intercourse and birth. These were the umputé that also caused sickness to individuals throughout the year and could be treated by sando with the rites described in Chapter 4. These umputé could be divided into the nurturing Laujé kind and the pestilent foreign kind. The momasoro was a curing rite writ large because offerings were given here to all the individual umputé of all the Laujé and all the foreigners, in the hope that no individuals would fall ill. On another grander, global level there were umputé of the environment or first creation. These umputé represented places like the center of the earth and the center of the sea. Sumpitan divided these global or environmental umputé so that the nurturing Laujé spirits from the Laujé land and rivers and the womb of the world were separate from the pestilent umputé of the foreign sea. Contained within the simple story of the separation of umputé at birth was, therefore, a whole story of the world's creation and eventual differentiation into hierarchically ranked and color-coded entities. It is this issue of hierarchically ranked entities and the way Sumpitan color-coded them that ultimately poses logical problems.

Recall that Sumpitan treated the global umputé spirits just like the individual umputé. In the momasoro, he said the global umputé of the land and rivers was equivalent to the white and yellow umputé of procreation. As he saw it, when the world was created, the land and rivers were separated from the sea, just as the white/yellow umputé of fertility were separated from the black/red umputé of violent sex. The relationship between sea and land was therefore parallel to the relationship between "red"/"black" umputé and "white"/"yellow" umputé. Yet, he never was consistent about this equation, especially in his comparison of the global umputé of the sea with the red umputé of violent sex or murderous deaths. The red in the individual rites Sumpitan outlined to me (as described in Chapter 4) incorporated a clear ranking of spirits, the highest representing the murdered raja, the next the colonial officers, and on down to the chief of police, and the Javanese coolies. Why was he now denying that the global umputé of the sea was hierarchical, while in every other way he showed how much it was like the red, hierarchically ranked, umputé spirit from the red chicken rite?

I suspect it was because he was trying to force the umputé spirits into logical divisions for which the spirits and their categories were not originally intended. He could not always make the spirits be sterile, pestilent, and without rank. So that Sumpitan could make these inferences, it was necessary that he ignore or gloss over much of the potential significance of the umputé categories and the momasoro rite. For instance, if the evil foreign spirits were related to the evil foreign rajas of history, why was Kaili spoken in the foreign house and not some other language, like Bugis or Mandar, the language of the hated foreign usurpers? Historically, Sumpitan had claimed that it was the Bugis, Mandar, Chinese, and Arabs who had dominated the coconut trade and the bureaucracy, taking from Laujé what was rightfully theirs. Yet the only "foreign" language consistently spoken in the "foreign" house was that of Kaili. In Sumpitan's portrayal of history, the Kaili had had little, if any, role. I suspect he never broached the "Kaili language" question because it would have punctured his depiction of the Laujé as "pure." I later found out that many lowland Laujé, including his own grandmother, had married Kaili cloth traders in the nineteenth century. It is from these traders the Laujé learned the ethic of tadulako warriorhood and it is probably from these ancestors that much of the Kaili adat in the momasoro was learned. Sumpitan wanted to purge all memory of non-Laujé ancestors, but the Kaili language of the mediums revealed that his anti-Mandar/anti-Bugis message was his own invention and not one inherent to the rite itself.

This might explain why Sumpitan chose not to remind me of his earlier statement that the rank of the white sea spirit dressed in Muslim funeral clothes was high, that that spirit was the "sterile ruler of the sea spirits who sat on a golden throne." That spirit always spoke in the Kaili language. To draw attention to the spirit would underline the spirit's ethnic identity, something Sumpitan probably wanted to avoid. Moreover, had I been thinking about the spirit, I might have questioned why the spirit possessing Kaija had no "sterile," or cooked, rice representing it at the foreign altar on the last night. I later found out that, in previous and subsequent years, the Kaili-speaking white/yellow umputé spirit brought rice from his big house altar (Kaija was always possessed by a male spirit) to the little house altar to create the symbolic child for the sempaang. In other words, foreign umputé and Laujé umputé *did* finally have symbolic intercourse, but it was only after Sumpitan was gone or before I was there to question his logical inconsistencies. Sumpitan's scheme emphasized that white and yellow were nurturing spirits and only belonged to the Laujé. He claimed the sea spirits or foreign ones were red and black and non-hierarchial. This claim avoided including the white/yellow ruler spirit who would obviate his whole logical scheme. It was better to claim no hierarchy and no white/yellow associations with the sea, than to question whether white and yellow were even "pure" Laujé spirits in the first place.

Another logical question I had concerned the olongian. Sumpitan claimed the olongian was a powerful Laujé figure with great political and religious influence. Sumpitan also said the olongian was "pure." His ethnic status was Laujé. But the olongian played a very minor role in the whole rite. The wife of the olongian was much more active throughout every stage of the momasoro, yet she was always possessed by a "foreign," Kaili-speaking, spirit. If the Laujé hated the foreign spirits and thought they were inferior to the Laujé as a whole, how could this "foreign spirit" possess the wife of the olongian and play such a major role in the rite?

It was not until the next momasoro, after Sumpitan's death, that other interpreters explained these discrepancies by refuting Sumpitan's evaluation of foreigners as pestilent. Sumpitan's death was proof to many people that his interpretation had been wrong. Moreover, several of Sumpitan's relatives, who had participated in the momasoro of 1985, followed him to the grave in quick succession. Sumpitan's sister died a few days after he did. She had a mild attack of malaria, "something which rarely leads to death." Also, Sumpitan's cousin died after he was bitten by a rabid dog. These odd deaths further undermined

Sumpitan's standing in the community. The Laujé community regarded them as ominous signs; Sumpitan's way of organizing the momasoro had angered the spirits. To prevent more retaliation by angry spirits, sando and mediums began to discuss the next momasoro long before it was time. They planned to honor all spirits—sea, land, and river—equally; they would not focus primarily on the umputé, of land and rivers, while rejecting the sea umputé as Sumpitan had. Surely, they hoped, this would prevent any unnecessary deaths of future participants.

6

MARRYING THE FOREIGNERS
Erasing Sumpitan's Momasoro

I deeply mourned Sumpitan's death, for I was emotionally and intellectually dependent upon him. I had met no one else who was as articulate about the meaning of umputé and the symbolic relevance of the momasoro. When I was a guest of Sumpitan at the 1985 momasoro and had queried people about the significance of various offerings, no one had explained themselves as eloquently as Sumpitan had. Yet as the weeks passed and mourning for Sumpitan subsided, people began to drop subtle and then not-so-subtle hints that they too would like to talk to me about the momasoro. I learned that it was respect for Sumpitan's interpretation that had kept people silent, not an unwillingness to articulate ideas about the rite. Now that the "spirits" had "proved his interpretation wrong," people were no longer hesitant to disagree with Sumpitan.

People came to me individually and in groups to tell me their version of how umputé spirits were guiding the momasoro. As the variety of interpretations successively accumulated, I found myself confused and frustrated. None of the interpretations fit into a neat, coherent package the way Sumpitan's had. In general, though, the new interpretations did have one cohesive theme: Sumpitan was wrong. Some people, mostly commoners, contradicted Sumpitan by emphasizing accommodation and marriage of the spirits. Others, elites like the Haji and the wife of the olongian, emphasized joining on a different level. These elites referred to literal marriages between foreign men and elite Laujé women. They advocated worshipping foreign umputé more than Laujé umputé.

The competing voices, the dissonance, and the discord are what led me to describe the rite in postmodern theoretical terms. I began to analyze each interpretive stance from the perspective of multiple, often conflicting views of hegemony and powerlessness. I came, simultaneously, I believed, to have a deeper understanding of the Laujé spiritual and social worlds, looking at each individual's perspective as a reflection of their personal histories, their status, their age, and the place from which their ideas sprang.

The competing voices can be roughly diagrammed as follows:

Elites vs.	Commoners
(1) Sea Spirit, Sawerigading, is supreme in myth	(1) Sea Spirits equal to land spirits as in recumbent woman and man myth
(2) Sawerigading predates Mohammed, so Sawerigading is supreme	(2) Recumbent woman and man appear at same time in myth, so neither is supreme

Youth vs.	Elders
(1) Reform Islam is Allah's most recent revelation, so it is supreme.	(1) Ancestral belief in spirits precedes Islam, so adat is supreme.
(2) Religion mixed with Adat is satanism	(2) Adat is the root (so most important); religion is a branch of the tree.

Events Leading Up to the 1986 Momasoro

The olongian and his wife were the first people to openly criticize Sumpitan's handling of the momasoro of 1985. They asserted, as did others, that Sumpitan's message of separation from foreigners was wrong. The elderly olongian and his wife claimed that all spirits were equal, all should be honored. The message of the momasoro should be one of accommodation, of joining, and not of separation. Just a few weeks after Sumpitan's funeral, the olongian hinted that it was the sea spirits who had caused Sumpitan's death. "Those spirits from the sea were insulted by Sumpitan's treatment" and had retaliated by killing him. The olongian believed Sumpitan had wrongly placed the land/river spirits in a superior position to the sea spirits. This had angered the "neglected ones." Proof of Sumpitan's tendency to distinguish between spirits was evident in the way he had erected various colored flags symbolizing the rank of each spirit. He had placed the yellow and white flags representing the spirit of the land and rivers higher than all others. As the olongian said: "These flags were too proud. He [Sumpitan] should have only placed a yellow and white flag to signify surrender [to the spirits]. He said the yellow and white were the flags of our kingdom and he placed those above the red, the black, the green, and the blue, the flags of the other spirits. That was too arrogant." The olongian's opinion was echoed by others who emphasized that the categories of spirits should be recognized as complements to one another—"no higher, no lower."

The wife of the olongian also objected to the sharp distinction Sumpitan had drawn between Laujé and foreigner in the last momasoro. She argued that Sumpitan's sociological facts were wrong. He had insulted the "foreign" spirits by casting them as the evil others in his two-dimensional play pitting foreign/sea spirits against native/land spirits: "For many generations we here in the lowlands, we have all been mixed and multicolored like a speckled hen. From the very first, our ancestors married outsiders. They married Kaili. Other foreigners settled here too." In asserting that the lowlanders were "like the speckled hen," the wife of the olongian was insistent that all parts of Laujé ancestry be recognized. One category should not be favored over another. Of course she had a personal stake in this, since her father had been an immigrant man, a Bugis. She had plans to rectify Sumpitan's mistake. She told me that when the next momasoro was performed, the big house would not be the house of poison, the house of foreigners. As the wife of the olongian put it: "The big house is not just for the sea spirits. It is for all spirits. The big house is not just for the spirits of illness. It is for the spirits of poison and cure. We are all one. The spirits are our bodies." Other people in the community, commoners like the boliang Siinai Samaliu, and the sando Siamae Asarima, repeated the same phrase. "The spirits are our bodies." In making such a statement, people were contravening Sumpitan's attempt to characterize some spirits as poisonous and some as cure. They shifted the emphasis from the momasoro as a curing rite in which the Laujé body needed to be purged of poisonous illness to one in which the fertility of the sea and the land were much like the fertility of male and female bodies, ebbing and flowing with seasonal productivity.[1]

Commoners like Siinai Samaliu and Siamae Asarima told me that one of the "hidden secrets" or "reasons" for performing the momasoro was to bring together the spirits of the land and the sea. These spirits represented the bodies of one male and one female who procreate once a year. Siamae Asarima likened the land/river spirit to a giant recumbent woman—an earth mother. When the recumbent woman urinated, the Tinombo River flowed, engorged with water. When the woman/spirit perspired, the little rivulets and streams high in the hills filled with water. The "secret" was that the giant recumbent woman (a female umputé spirit) was married to the giant recumbent man (a male umputé) spirit who resided at the center of the sea. The woman/spirit's body continually exuded liquids because the man/spirit of the sea continually replenished them. The woman's fluids flowed downward filling the sea. Simultaneously and invisibly the man's liquids flowed upward from the sea through the river to the mountaintops where the rivers flowed down again as female fluid.[2] Thus, the earth and the sea were in a complementary sexual relationship, one that Siamae Asarima regarded as unhierarchical. When he spoke about "our body," those who knew the secret of the recumbent woman knew "our body" implied complementarity and accommodation.

Complementarity: The Momaang *Ompogang* and the Monganjul Poyoan

The recumbent woman was never directly invoked or mentioned at the preliminary momaang and monganjul poyoan rites, but her presence was implied by sando like Siamae Asarima. Rather than follow Sumpitan's interpretation from last year and characterize the two preliminary rites as separating poison from cure, Siamae Asarima said that this was a harvest rite to honor the spirits who gave rice to human beings, honoring the male spirit from the sea who fertilized the soil and the female spirit from the land who made plants grow. He said, "just as the outer covering of rice is husked and thrown into the river, so in this rite is the outer covering of the consumed rice packets thrown into the river." This act "returns to the source" what was "taken from the source." In order to let the spirits "know" that the rice had been eaten and more should be grown, the "skins" have to be returned to the source of the spirits—the river that flows into the sea. The offering trays to the sea spirits, and the land and river spirits, are given, said Siamae Asarima, to honor their "exhaustion" *(ongkolé)* in producing the bountiful harvest. Both spirits are equally responsible for this growth, thus both trays are equally filled as representations of "our body." Each tray serves as a simulacrum of certain parts of the human body created by the spirits. The combined trays comprise a whole body. By giving the tray to the spirits, people are giving "our body" back to its creator—umputé.

When Siamae Asarima told me the offering trays represented "our body," his words triggered a memory involving Sumpitan the year before. Though Sumpitan had choreographed the preliminary rites the year before and Siamae Asarima had followed his orders, there was one point when Siamae Asarima had just finished filling the downstream tray and no one else was around. I asked him what the colored rice offerings meant. Siamae Asarima said, "this is our body." Sumpitan came up to us just as Siamae Asarima spoke. He didn't say anything else. Later Sumpitan had said to me, "Don't listen to him [Siamae Asarima]. The trays are not our body. He's a commoner, he doesn't know anything." The memory was especially poignant this year, as I listened to Siamae Asarima quite eloquently articulate what part of the body each color of rice represented. I realized that his emphasis on "our body" avoided the explicit ranking Sumpitan had made of the spirits and their trays. Moreover, I began to see how intimately intertwined Siamae Asarima's interpretation was with his own status as a commoner. On the cosmological level he saw spirits as complements to one another, both necessary for the whole. I realized that this was analogically related to his and other commoners' views of the social world; just as spirit communities could not function without their complements, neither could human communities. Elites needed commoners and vice versa. They were all equal. Siamae Asarima's interpretation emphasizing "our body" made perfect sense from the perspective of a commoner and little sense from the perspective of an elite man like Sumpitan.

The Momasoro Proper: Joining Sumpitan's Divisions

Not all elites, however, were opposed to the "our body" interpretation. The wife of the olongian had been one of its most vocal supporters. To her, though, the "our body" philosophy implied that the Laujé "body" was married to the foreign "body." Foreigners were no different from elite Laujé because all had intermarried. For the wife of the olongian, the "our body" metaphor was an elite message. Thus, as the time for the momasoro proper neared, her rhetoric espousing complementarity, accommodation, and joining gave way to more elitist ideology. On the one hand, the wife of the olongian publicly espoused the idea that the divisions created by Sumpitan should be joined. On the other hand, she and a few other elite Laujé, like a man I call the Haji, sought to obviate Sumpitan's interpretation by showing how one spiritual half, the sea with its elite foreigners, was superior to another—the land/river with its commoner Laujé.

The wife of the olongian had to be careful. She was an elite woman who worked with spirit mediums who were commoners. In public, the wife of the olongian had to espouse the complementarity line favored by commoners, but in private, among elites, she expressed the philosophy of superiority. When the momasoro began, it was possible for her to walk both sides of the interpretive fence because there was no assertive master of ceremonies, no sando, available to choreograph the whole rite, as Sumpitan had. The wife of the olongian was the only elite spirit medium who participated in this momasoro, since Sumpitan's sister had died the year before. Spirit mediums were almost always of commoner status. Thus, when the wife of the olongian was with spirit mediums like Siinai Samaliu and Siinai Alasan, the wife of the olongian asserted that spirits were equal and complements to one another. Everyone reiterated "the spirits have come to join one another." The divisions Sumpitan had made between good and bad, Laujé and foreign spirits, should be erased. Every night before going into trance, the wife of the olongian, the boliang (Siinai Samaliu), and several other mediums would confer and say "the spirits," which under Sumpitan's direction had remained segregated, "would be welcome in either the little or the big house." Thus, publicly the wife of the olongian worked to erase any elitist tensions that may have been created by Sumpitan's divisions the year before.

In the little house, the wife of the olongian made sure that the separate male and female sides of the little house shrine disappeared. The space where Sumpitan had created a "male altar" now contained, under her direction, both male and female clothing. The wife of the olongian explained "this is not a male altar." She pointed to the male and female clothing to indicate that the shrine represented marriage and accommodation. She laid out items that commoners would use in bridewealth prestations—batik, gold jewelry, a machete, betel nut, and tobacco. In front of the other mediums in the little house, the wife of the olongian told me "this is the request for forgiveness (notitisalah) from all spirits for past wrongs. We wish to join all spirits, to accommodate, marry, and join them."

Her message, I'm sure, was sincere, but she was the wife of the most highly ranked aristocrat in the Laujé community. Elite philosophy surrounding the olongian was too ingrained to gloss over with commoner-oriented rhetoric about joining and accommodation. As soon as the Haji, an elite sando, came into the little house, the wife of the olongian began to agree with his more elitist interpretation of the rite.

Joining the Sea and the Land: The Haji and Sawerigading

The Haji acted as chief sando in the little house two nights in a row during 1986. Occasionally, he would interrupt his sando role to act as a spirit medium. All the other mediums resented his presence and his interpretation of the spirit world. The wife of the olongian was the only medium who agreed with the Haji, probably because they both shared an elitist perspective. The Haji was from a relatively wealthy family, the son of a Bugis man and a Laujé mother who did not live in Dusunan with other Laujé, but in Tinombo with the immigrants. The wife of the olongian also had Kaili and Bugis ancestry, so their similar backgrounds could have influenced their similar interpretations. The Haji, though, had made the pilgrimage to Mecca while still a boy, and he wore a white cap *(songko)* to signal his status. He had not participated in the last momasoro. I suspect this lack of participation was because Sumpitan would not have welcomed such a "foreigner" into the little house.

The controversial and elitist perspective that the Haji brought to the momasoro revolved around a spirit named Sawerigading. The Haji said that Sawerigading, the spirit possessing him, was the supreme sea spirit. He brought that spirit into the little house and claimed that even though it was a sea spirit, it was Laujé. Everyone listening knew that Sawerigading was the name of a famous protagonist in epic myths called I La Galigo, which originated among the Bugis.[3] In the Bugis I La Galigo myth, Sawerigading was an Odyssean hero who wandered the islands introducing Bugis culture to elites in small kingdoms. Though the Haji never said so, his point about Sawerigading was fairly clear to the participants in the little house. It was the opposite of Sumpitan's point. For the Haji, the momasoro was an exclusive rite. It was for those who have intermarried with foreigners, for people who recognize Sawerigading as an ancestral hero. The Sawerigading story told by the Haji is as follows:

Sawerigading, the son of the Voracious Boy and a foreign mother, a Kaili woman, came back to the Laujé land, where his father had been born. By this time, Sawerigading had become a powerful sando in his own land. He had inherited some of the talisman and ritual objects from his father and this gave him power. Sawerigading returned to the Laujé land, bringing these objects of power with him.

During the time between the departure of Sawerigading's father and Sawerigading's own return, though, another person of power, a foreigner from Mecca, the prophet Mohammed, had become Lord of the Laujé Land.

Mohammed challenged Sawerigading to a duel of magic. They were to stack the eggs of a bush turkey *(mamua)* seven layers high on the beach, one on top of the other, without having them break or fall.

Sawerigading used his magic. He was able to stack the eggs seven layers high. But Nabi Mohammed stacked them with a space of air remaining between each egg. Mohammed won. Sawerigading and his magic were banished to the sea. Mohammed became the ruler of the things of the earth, Sawerigading of procreation and death.

The Haji explained that Sawerigading was the first Laujé sando and continued to be the "Lord of the sea spirits." The Haji's aim in invoking the sea spirit Sawerigading was to honor Sawerigading because he had been neglected. Sawerigading had taken his "traditional powers" with him to the sea because the Muslims who remained on shore had neglected tradition. The purpose of the momasoro was to honor this "tradition" and reunite it with "the younger sibling," Mohammed, and Islam.[4]

The Haji used the tale of Sawerigading to assert that the land and sea were separate, just as religion and custom were. This separation between sea and land, however, was not the same separation Sumpitan had made. Sumpitan had marked the sea as a pejorative category associated with foreigners. By contrast, the Haji had evoked an image that at once commented on the superiority of Mohammed in magical and earthly matters, and the superiority of Sawerigading in the more permanent matters of life and death.

The Haji's portrayal of Sawerigading evoked the myth of the recumbent woman and her male consort at the sea, implying that the male was more important than the female. To honor these spirits, the Haji reinstated a crucial "forgotten" offering made for Sawerigading. The offering associated Sawerigading with the fecund powers of the sea spirits. It used an egg from a rare species of bush turkey, the mamua (*maleo* in Indonesian). This was the same type of egg that had been used in the contest between Sawerigading and Mohammed.[5] The turkey egg was placed in front of the altar in the little house, so it could be blessed before it was sent on the boat to the sea.

The egg represented the connection between sea and land. The maleo fowls laid their eggs during the dry season at the end of the monsoon when the rice was about to be harvested. Thus, they were important icons of fecundity and rejuvenation.[6] Because these birds lived in both the realm of the sea and the land, they represented the joining of land and sea, and the female and male fluids needed for fertilizing rice. The Haji also used the egg to talk about the joining of two domains, religion and custom, Mohammed and Sawerigading. By conflating Sawerigading, the bush turkey egg, and the "characters" of the body given by the umputé spirits, the Haji was making a radical claim in the face of Islam: Ultimately it was the "banished" Sawerigading—and not Mohammed, the ruler of the earth—who engendered life. The Haji said:

> Too many of you followers of Mohammed—and I don't wish to belittle you, I only honor you from the tips of my toes to the tops of the hairs on my head—too many of you followers of Mohammed misunderstand if you think that what is done here is to honor Satan. For I say from the depths of my soul that there was not a beginning and will not be an end without our older sibling.

In the Haji's depiction, Sawerigading was the "Lord" of umputé, dividing the world with Mohammed. But, according to the Haji, Sawerigading had been "forgotten, just as the birth fluids of umputé were inadvertently neglected. He said:

> Those spirits are what orders things well for us. For all is from them; they are that which engendered us and made us the younger sibling. We were bespattered and drenched with the liquid of birth, and it was as if the world had opened and we had squirted out, one human. That is, one who was made to live. Later, after we had been squeezed out, we humans, from the womb of the mother, then it was known that this umputé is what we should honor. Some human beings have not opened their eyes and looked. For there are some who say that to honor the umputé spirits here in this place is to worship the devil. But from what do we originate if not from this?

In associating neglected umputé spirits with the banished Sawerigading, the Haji did not differentiate between neglected and nurtured categories of umputé. One kind of umputé did not go to the sea, another to the earth, but all the kinds of umputé—white, black, red, and yellow—were conceptualized as neglected and opposed to religion. The Haji proposed that the banishment of umputé and its customs to the sea was improper. The Haji wanted to honor the sea and the neglected umputé by asserting that customs associated with umputé were the prior and powerful complement of religion or Islam. Like the wife of the olongian, the Haji tried to convince the other participants in the rite, by using the rhetoric of accommodation, complementarity, and marriage.

Underneath his rhetoric about equality was an elitism. Sawerigading and ideas about him were part of an elite esoterica that divided commoners and elites. One elite man listening to the Haji and the wife of the olongian told me that "the commoners only know that the shrine (ginaling) holds a piece of the original tree, but there are other pieces of wood inside it too." These include, he said, "seven types of wood." One type of wood was for the "common people."[7] This "wood of the commoners" was female and could be used to heal commoners of illness. Its "male" counterpart was the olongian's tree, which was used to cure only the aristocrats. This tree was known as the "staff or lance of Sawerigading." He told me that "the olongian ruled the Laujé because of a secret alliance with Sawerigading"—an alliance about which the commoners did not know.

Elites learned about Sawerigading through Sufi methods. This knowledge came from the Kaili and the Bugis whom elite Laujé married. Commoners knew nothing about this. The momasoro was really a rite for elites. The wife of the olongian said that when she was young, there was a Bugis curing rite *(masarungé)* that elite Laujé performed. It was much like the momasoro, but no commoners could attend. This rite was an offering to Sawerigading who sat on the golden throne in the center of the sea. She said that in this rite, the sick person must step on the head of a goat (just as the olongian does on the last night of the momasoro). Then the person must say the name of the puangé or raja, Sawerigading: "He is the first, before all the other spirits. All the others from the sea, the traders, those that ride the waves, the red and the black, they all came later. Sawerigading was there from the first, sitting on the golden throne." According to the wife of the olongian, only people who were descendants of the puangé, the foreign raja, were allowed to invoke Sawerigading. These were the Laujé aristocrats, the descendants of the olongian and the tadulako. She said "the people of the mountains and the commoners do not know Sawerigading." He was at the apex of a pantheon of lesser spirits who served him. The momasoro, then, from the elite perspective, honored Sawerigading more than the other umputé spirits. This was the true "secret" of the rite. Though the wife of the olongian and other elites asserted that the momasoro and its ancillary rites were for all Laujé, in fact, they were not.

The Theme of Joining Is Obviated: Commoners vs. Elites

In many ways this exclusivity had determined how the 1986 momasoro had been orchestrated. The olongian and other elites had differentiated the high-ranking white and yellow spirits from the lower-ranking black and red spirits. The yellow and white were allowed in the little house, the red and black in the big house. Though they promised to erase the divisions Sumpitan had made, these elites merely created new divisions. Such elitism led to resentment.

The resentment was not without a historical precedent. In the pre-reform Islamic days, esoteric Islamic secrets were more or less the exclusive property of lowland elites. In order to gain this knowledge an acolyte had to "pay" the "owner" of the secret with items such as a white cloth, a machete, and a porcelain plate or set of plates. One man described his father's Sufi teachings thusly: "It was in secret. One learned inside a closed tent and one had to pay. To learn to pray, for example, one paid seven palm-lengths of coins. Islam was secret and for the privileged. . . . It wasn't until the Raja Kuti came to Tinombo that Islam became more modern." Many of the secrets elites taught each other were also the secrets revealed in chants and blessings at the momasoro. The momasoro's little house was the exclusive domain of the Laujé aristocracy and their esoteric Sufi secrets. Many of the ancillary ceremonies, such as the headhunting and the banana cutting rites, were imbued with Sufi esoterica, Arabic prayers, and the like. They made explicit distinctions between commoners and elites.

Several commoner women who served as spirit mediums in the momasoro of 1985 complained that the olongian and his wife were selfish and greedy, using the office for their own monetary gains at the expense of poor common folk. Some of the gossip centered on the olongian's now dead mother, Siinai Alo, who had been olongian in the 1950s during the dramatic social upheavals of the postindependence period. Siinai Alo, said the commoners, had "broken the customs." Siinai Alo "had sold the Laujé's sacred regalia (including various implements made of gold)" and pocketed the money for herself. These implements were central to the momasoro rite, they said, and once she sold them the rite was "empty." Other commoners claimed Siinai Alo had begun selling bananas from the courtyard of her house, violating a taboo that the olongian, as ultimate guarantor of agricultural fertility, could never sell the fruits of the soil.

More resentful commoners complained about the present wife of the olongian, who, they said, had "spent the coins of the souls *(doi nu nyaa),"* the antique coins that each Laujé gave at the momasoro at least once in their lives. The "coins of the souls" were blessed during the rite and kept as a sacred and immutable pledge, guaranteeing the safety and long life of each and every Laujé. To spend them was to sell Laujé souls.[8] The gossiping commoners blamed the olongian for misfortunes like the smallpox epidemic in the 1950s and the present-day decline in dry rice productivity. (Highland commoners believed this as well.)

To compensate for this perceived elitist corruption, some of the Laujé spirit mediums and other commoners created a "secret" rite to precede each evening performance of the momasoro of 1986. In this rite, commoner spirit mediums blessed the "coins of the souls" the participants brought. Spirit mediums were possessed by spirits and chanted, just as they did in the momasoro proper. Though there was not much difference between this secret rite and the momasoro proper, it served as a protest against the authority of the Laujé aristocracy. It also chipped away at the unified portrayal Sumpitan had given of the Laujé community.[9]

Of course, it is not all elite lowlanders who are making distinctions. The wife of the olongian believes the commoners and the imams have divided the community. She said:

> When my mother-in-law was still olongian [in the 1950s], she was the focus of Islam. It began to weaken here for us Laujé people when she died. The imam wouldn't let us have a proper funeral for an olongian. The old olongians' bodies were left for weeks before they were buried.[10] The imam buried her that day. The imams, our own people, tried to break our customs!

Islam did drive a wedge among people in the community. The wife of the olongian resented the reform Islam adopted by many Lauje commoners and elites because it necessitated a hatred for traditional custom and the olongian.

Throughout Indonesia, since the colonial period, religious loyalty, especially to Islam, became "somewhat antagonistic to local ethnic customs" (Kipp and Rodgers 1987:25). Much of this antagonism was created by fundamentalist efforts to purify Islam of admixtures. Fundamentalists in control of religious education in the public schools taught that "religion *(agama)* is progressive and a requisite of good citizenship" and that "those persons who do not (strictly) follow religion, [those who follow adat or tradition] appear to be disloyal national citizens, uncommitted to the values of the Indonesian constitution, not to mention intellectually and morally backward" (Atkinson 1987:23). Thus, in Dusunan, government schools brought to the area in the 1970s were teaching young people reform Islam. The young people were learning to regard their own local traditions, some of which had been the exclusive property of elites, as repulsive and "primitive," even "satanic."

Consequently, many of the community's factions divided along the lines of age. Young people came to mock the proceedings in the momasoro, treating the performance in the big house as a masquerade. The year after Sumpitan's death, ironically enough, the olongian's own son went to a fundamentalist "protest ritual" planned by the Muhammadiyah imam. On the third night of the momasoro, while his parents were hosting the 1986 rite at their house, their son crossed the street to attend the "Islamic event." This "event" was in direct competition for the spectators who were expected to attend the momasoro. People, like the youngest son of the olongian, who was educated in fundamentalist Islam, met to read "6,666 verses *(ayat)* of the Qur'an." They read until dawn on the third night of the momasoro and the next day met again to share in the fellowship and feast of a slaughtered goat. The marathon reading in Arabic was an endurance contest in which the words of the Qur'an were melodiously repeated without insight.[11] "The purpose," said one man, "was to ask Allah to protect faithful people from evil spirits" conjured up at the momasoro.

Though young people like the olongian's son were attracted to these meetings because they had been educated in reform Islam at school, some of the older people attending the Qur'an reading were Laujé commoners. They had adopted reformism in protest against the elitism of the "traditional" rites such as the momasoro. The commoners resented the Sufi Islam that was practiced by elites and syncretised into the momasoro.[12] Older commoners who had tried in the past to learn mystical secrets—interpretations of certain passages in the Qur'an, Sufi numerology, and arcane concepts about the Arabic alphabet—had been rejected by elites. Elites had claimed this knowledge was not to be shared. It would "ruin its efficacy if spirit names were known by everyone [such as commoners]." Because elites had refused in the past to teach them Islamic secrets, once reformism came to the Laujé area, its egalitarian appeal attracted many commoners.

Thus, the issue of religion was on the minds of those who participated in the momasoro. Commoners like Siinai Alasan and even devout elites like the Haji were more willing to openly discuss the relationship between Islam and custom. Part of this had to do with the presence of the Islamic protest rite and part had to do with the fact that they were more educated in and about the different kinds of Islam. On the surface Siinai Alasan and the Haji agreed. Both used umputé to talk about religion and custom. Siinai Alasan, however, had a particular perspective that reflected her commoner status and thus her views about Islam. She was a woman in her forties, fairly well educated in Islam, but also a sando in her own right. She took the issue head on.

On the third night of the momasoro, soon after a spirit entered Siinai Alasan, the spirit publicly argued that fundamentalist and reform Islam had no right to claim superiority over custom/tradition because custom came first and thus was superior. Of course, such arguments fell on the ears of the converted, since the protest rite had captured most of the audience for whom the sermon was intended. Siinai Alasan did not like the way the Haji had used umputé to discuss the relationship between Islam and custom. The Haji had associated umputé with the sea and the banished Sawerigading. Siinai Alasan associated umputé with the image of the original Laujé tree. Recalling Laujé origin myths in which the separation of earth from sky began when a tree grew up between them, Siinai Alasan likened umputé and Laujé custom to the tap-root of this tree and religion to the branches. During possession her spirit said:

Custom, adat, was made first here. Before there were humans there was already custom, adat. If there was no custom, there would be no religion. If there was no religion, there would be no custom. We were born with what and how? Wasn't it together with the placenta? If you recognize this, you must believe in the custom. For umputé is with us. We must respect umputé.

Later religion came to us. What is the road for religion? Religion gives meaning to the doctrines in the book. . . . If the doctrines of religion are not put into practice, then certainly Allah's back will be turned to us. If one does not follow the fasting month for thirty days and thirty nights and pray those evenings, one will not receive a guaranteed entrance to heaven. That is religion. And if that religion is not followed, what will happen to your bodies?

Well, the same applies to the custom here [in this ceremony]. Yet, nowadays, it is as if religion is honored, while customs, traditions, have been neglected. This is not right. Tradition, custom, is first. Tradition is . . . the substance which wraps and protects the child.

Later in another conversation, Siinai Alasan likened umputé and Laujé tradition or customs to the tap-root of the tree of life. She equated religion to the branches that grow after the root is firmly established in the ground, saying:

Custom is the root of the tree.
It is that which wraps and protects the tree.
It surrounds its roots.
Pull out a root and look up at the branches.
They will rot and wither.
Custom which is let go, rots bit by bit until the tree dies.
Follow the customs, the chants. Don't stop.
Follow the customs, the rites. Don't stop.
Carry it with religion.

In Siinai Alasan's soliloquy, custom (adat) was called the "older sibling," the "placenta," "that which wrapped and protected." She equated custom not with the neglected umputé, but with the encompassing entity, the placenta. In her scheme, custom remained associated with the earth—rooted and wrapped. Though she granted that God gave the initial gift of life and received the final things of death, she implored the audience to recognize a closer relationship to custom, one which was more personal, like the older sibling who nurtured one. She did not imply that true Laujé "traditions" belonged only to elites like Sawerigading. Siinai Alasan's metaphor avoided suggestions of elitism and "foreign" spirits by simply imploring people to worship both a "traditional" deity and a religious deity. Her tree metaphor eloquently emphasized that umputé and customs were equal to religion.

In some respects, Siinai Alasan's tree metaphor was like the "our body" metaphor. Both had implications for the meaning of the whole rite—the branches of a tree separate, but remain part of one trunk. All the tree's parts are interdependent, part of a whole body. The "our body" metaphor makes the same point: The body or a person ideally matures through her life cycle in the same way that the momasoro cycle develops. Just as an infant gestates in the womb, so too the preliminary harvest rites emphasize new growth and fertile substances. Just as young newlyweds meet, fall in love, and unite, so too the seven-night fete at the momasoro emphasizes marriage. And just as later a body matures, but does battle with sickness and the aging process, so too the spirit mediums engage in mock battles with one another. And, finally, at the end of life, just as one hopes to enter into the kingdom of heaven, after friends and family have said their funereal good-byes, so too spirit mediums clad in mourning clothes cast off a boat with a sail made of white funeral cloth.

The "our body" metaphor, like the "tree metaphor," sends the ultimate egalitarian message: Whether one is high status or low, one is born, matures, ages, and dies. This ritual-as-our-body-in-the-life-cycle idea, however, came from my own extrapolations gleaned from various individuals, elite and commoners. Never did anyone tell me this. Never would the various factions actually agree on much at all.

In sum, then, there were many social rifts in the lowland community that translated to a variety of interpretations about the umputé spirits and the momasoro. There was the rift between commoners and elites, between those who married foreigners with elite status and those who did not, and between those who practiced fundamentalist Islam and those who practiced "custom." By emphasizing accommodation, growing trees, and marriage of the spirits' bodies in the momasoro, some people, mostly commoners, were asserting that the ceremony reflects society and its mutually interdependent parts. Others, elites like the Haji and the wife of the olongian, who emphasized joining, were really referring to literal marriages, the marriage of foreigners with Laujé. They worshiped foreign spirits more than local ones. They alluded to a point Sumpitan wanted to play down: The momasoro is for the aristocracy. It involves spirits of which only elites have knowledge. Other people, including the Haji, but also commoners like Siinai Alasan, who were more educated about the relationship between Islam and custom, were more willing than Sumpitan to discuss and confront the conflict between Islam and adat. Sumpitan had tended to avoid this issue. They made the point very clearly: The rite supported Islam, but not at the expense of tradition. The rite, like the umputé older sibling, needed recognition and respect.

Though each person mentioned here differed as to specific details about umputé and the spirits in the momasoro, and each person chose to obviate Sumpitan's message, they all had one thing in common with Sumpitan: They chose to relate the spirits analogically to the social world. As we shall see in the next chapter, not all participants selected this path.

7

DENYING DIFFERENCE
Siamae Balitangan's "Simple" Momasoro

It was not until the fourth night of the 1986 momasoro that a sando arrived who could provide one cohesive interpretation of umputé by speaking in both houses. This cohesive interpretation came from Siamae Balitangan, the sando who accompanied his brother-in-law, Sanji, to Siamae Sanji's funeral. Siamae Balitangan was born in Taipaobal and raised in Dusunan in an elite household. Living in the mountains with his bela wife, Siamae Balitangan was a sando whose knowledge and experience spanned the conceptual and geographical territory of Laujé land. He was invited to the 1986 momasoro because the wife of the olongian told me "we need someone knowledgeable about the old ways." I suggested his name, knowing that years before, Siamae Balitangan had blessed the offering trays at the harvest rites upstream, but had not attended the rite since the early 1950s. He had only seen the momasoro as a child and never had been invited to sit next to the olongian. Because of my mountain contacts, the wife of the olongian asked me to invite Siamae Balitangan. He was more than happy to accept and be treated as an honored guest.

When Siamae Balitangan came, the spirit mediums were initially ecstatic over his arrival. They hoped Siamae Balitangan would reinvigorate them and the audience. The night before Siamae Balitangan's arrival, the possessed mediums mournfully sang ballads of loss and death. The mediums lamented that so few humans nowadays knew the ancient truths of the rite and seemed uninterested in learning those truths. The Islamic protest rite had attracted audience members away from the momasoro, and there was no dominant master of ceremonies to stir up the audience in the big house. The boliang complained out loud that the audience had dwindled, saying: "The young people don't come. They don't act afraid when I wave my machete at them. They laugh. This never would have happened in the old days." One spirit even incorporated this problem into her chant at the shrine in the big house:

I came here to ask for blessing	*Noduaé mai momongi*
but there are not enough Laujé	*No kura nokurang Laujé*
We are lonesome for the crowds	*Ooniang ite sanu maramé*
Sad for happiness	*Oondongé mesanang*
We just sit in this place	*Ma neduduangé*
It is our duty to have come	*E saba lieté nai notiloa*
To witness and give counsel	*Mai mopogulalangé*
We have no more elders here	*Laumé a sanu mogulanga Ité*
Who listen to what we say	*Lai mongembé amé mongembé*
Our hearts and souls are sad	*Oondongé até nu nyaé*
No one is left to listen to us	*Laumé mai mopoolong*
Our united voice, our single tongue, friends	*Suara songkolog u sanganga*
Is half sad, half happy	*Moondong masanangé tegalangé*

Other spirits sang similar laments. Thus, when Siamae Balitangan first arrived, the mediums enthusiastically welcomed him, hoping, because he still wore the "traditional" Laujé head-wrap *(banto)* (see Figure 7.1) and still knew how to recite the versified Laujé histories *(balagé)*, that this genuine rustic from another era would also be able to reveal forgotten secrets.[1] He relished the attention from the olongian and spirit mediums.

Soon, however, he "wore out" his welcome. As he listened to the spirits chant, he noted that they were "naming" spirits of which he had never heard. He found them to be false names or inappropriate for a ritual that ostensibly honored umputé. Of course, he knew little of the momasoro and was interpreting the proliferation of spirits from his highlands perspective. Nevertheless, there was an abundance of spirits without any seeming order to them. Many of the so-called red and black spirits possessing people in the big house seemed unconcerned with their connection to the overarching issues of umputé and the sea and land spirits. When they talked about themselves, they claimed to be the spirits of human beings with specific and individual life histories, much like Sawerigading was a spirit who had once been human. There were spirits who claimed to be manifestations of warrior ancestors—sometimes foreign, sometimes local. They were guar-

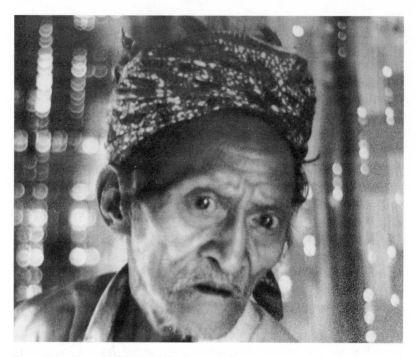

Figure 7.1.   Siamae Balitangan in his brown turban

dians of the "borders" of the Laujé lands. Some claimed to be the spirits of long forgotten hajjis who had been among the first to go on the pilgrimage to Mecca. In addition to these spirits with particular life histories, there were spirits of particular wind directions, spirits from the center of the sun, from the seventh layer of the earth, from the rising sun, the setting sun. In short, it was as if this momasoro had opened up a Pandora's box releasing multitudinous spirits. Their sheer number and diversity threatened to overwhelm the concept of umputé as a simple yet all encompassing outgrowth of procreation and birth.

The proliferation of spirits seemingly distinct from umputé caused Siamae Balitangan to react by attacking first the spirits with their "many names," then the mediums who were "wrongly naming" spirits. For instance, the second day after his arrival, Siamae Balitangan began to loudly criticize the spirit possessing the boliang Siinai Samaliu. He listened to her womb-of-the-world chant and then said to me so all could overhear:

Child, that one there, she sings of "O Yelé Ijati'é, O Elé Gandisié." I say, child, there is no such spirit. That is all bent talk, child.[2] I say, I know the names for the spirit at the womb of the world, and the spirits at the four corner posts. These are the umputé. All that is needed, I know, child. Anything else is false.

These comments continued. The spirits seethed with resentment at his criticisms. Many of the mediums, once out of trance, began to mock him when he turned his back. They moved their heads in a rapid jerky manner, extended their jaws, and barely moved their lips so they could mime Siamae Balitangan's deformity from a childhood illness. Normally, Laujé women would never be so publicly cruel, nor so petty, but Siamae Balitangan's comments and arrogance embittered them.

It soon became clear that even as Siamae Balitangan cast aspersions on the lowland ritualists, so they too found reason to doubt his integrity. When he first had come, some of the participants looked to him to find out secret names of the umputé spirits, or names of place spirits along the Tinombo River and its branches. For instance, on the third night, when another sando quietly asked him the name of the spirit at the mouth of the river, Siamae Balitangan very ceremoniously replied, "later, when there aren't so many people around I'll tell you." The next day the man, the olongian and wife, and several other sando gathered and waited for Siamae Balitangan to whisper the secret name. With great ceremony he loudly whispered "Raja Dunia, the Raja of the World." I had to bite my lip to keep from laughing out loud. The sound of the commonly used Indonesian words seemed so obviously contrived and unspiritual.[3] Almost everyone in this lowland community spoke Indonesian, so Siamae Balitangan's Indonesian name for the spirit seemed too ordinary, not exotic and otherworldly enough. I later found out others agreed with me. The sando who had questioned Siamae Balitangan told me later that he suspected that Siamae Balitangan had tried to give him "false names" in order to protect his own sources of power. The same words could have awed some of the less acculturated Laujé in the mountains, but not these lowlanders. "He's a liar," said the sando. The sando had reason to complain. Siamae Balitangan tried to appear knowledgeable, when he was not. But he was no liar.

Siamae Balitangan's arrogance led him to accuse certain mediums of fakery. "I can tell, child, who is a real umputé spirit and who is not," he said to me, "when I shake their hands. If they have the power,

it flows through their hands to me." Angered at this opened-faced judg-
ment of her fellow lowland healers, the wife of the olongian insinuated
the next day (out of the context of the momasoro ceremony) that Siamae Balitangan was making more of himself than he should have:

> He says he is ninety years old. Well, if he is ninety, then that makes me a
> hundred and ten! [And she was seventy-five.] I remember him when he was
> a child. He had a disease that made his jaw unable to move up and down
> much. I know that because I went with my mother to the house where he
> was a servant. His master had asked my mother to cure him. Ninety years
> old, he says. He's sixty if that![4]

Comments like these about his low status were made within earshot of
Siamae Balitangan. The comments and the cruel miming of his odd
speech patterns, however, did not silence Siamae Balitangan, who was
convinced he knew the right way, the truth about umputé, and the
purpose of the momasoro. He blundered along, bobbing his turbaned
head, interrupting possessed mediums singing their tap-rooting song
as he sang his own blessing for umputé. He repeated the blessing over
and over again. It was the only blessing he knew. It sounded remotely
similar to some of the songs sung by the spirits. He would chant the
blessing loudly, trying to drown out the other spirits. He had borrowed the blessing from an upstream harvest rite to the umputé spirit.
It was out of place at the momasoro.

Siamae Balitangan's persistent and loud recitations drowned out the
others' blessings, almost as if he were attempting an exorcism. Siamae
Balitangan was a simple mountaineer and he found himself in the
company of people whom highlanders would characterize as witches
(pongko), as people possessed by demons or, as corrupt people ("those
who had chosen a crooked path"). As such, he evinced an attitude typical of highlanders.[5] Highlanders trusted the raja, but did not trust the
syncretist lowlanders associated with the olongian. Siamae Balitangan's
persistently inappropriate blessing and his refusal to listen to some of
the spirits' words at the momasoro revealed his blatant distrust.

For mountaineers like Siamae Balitangan, prayers were supposed to
be short, "four or five phrases." His interpretation of umputé was one
that was stripped of any elaborations. Siamae Balitangan wanted to
shut the Pandora's box of the momasoro and reassert a simple ritual
based on submission to umputé as a whole. As he spoke of his and
other highlanders' umputé beliefs in terms like "simple," "straight,"

"a few words needed," he contrasted this with the lowlanders' interpretations. He spoke as a fundamentalist would, focusing on the one
true deity. He reiterated, "Carry the simple customs, carry them but
once every three or seven years and that is enough."

Siamae Balitangan believed the momasoro should honor the
umputé spirits that created the universe before any of the parts had
been differentiated. Thus, he preached against hierarchy, against the
differentiation between poison and cure, and the differentiation between the male sea and the female land. He said any mention of the different parts or characteristics of umputé avoided the ultimate purpose
of the momasoro—to submit to the supreme being. For him umputé
was a simple concept that should be worshiped as a whole, not divided
into a series of entities that were somehow related to the social world.

On one level, his perspective could be generalized as that of all
Laujé highlanders in comparison to lowlanders. Many scholars had
drawn similar conclusions about elites in the courts, and commoners
on the periphery, in other parts of Indonesia. Those in the court elaborate, those on the periphery simplify (see Becker 1979; Anderson
1972; Geertz 1980). Those on the periphery embrace outsiders and external forces, those in the court reject outsiders and their ideas. Thus,
my initial take on Siamae Balitangan's interpretive perspective at the
momasoro was that his place, on the periphery, determined his anti-
metaphoric, anti-elaboration stance.

I concluded that upland commoners like Siamae Balitangan tended
to see the rite and umputé in holistic and minimalist terms. Commoners disagreed with the others who were interpreting umputé from their
higher-status perspective. I concluded that the tendency to symbolize,
differentiate, elaborate, and relate the spiritual to the social was more
of an aristocratic than a commoner practice. Lowland elites tended
to use many symbols and metaphors to explain umputé. Thus, I used
my knowledge about higher-status domination, or hegemony, to assess
the words of Siamae Balitangan and the antisymbolic advocates as
antihegemonic agendas that were filtered through their anti-elite
perspectives.

Healers versus Mediums: Status/Gender Resistance or Something Else?

To conclude that Siamae Balitangan's statements at the momasoro reflect his status as a commoner would be correct, but only one part of

a more complex picture. Siamae Balitangan's way of interacting with the boliang and the to pensio (mediums) was very similar to Sumpitan's way of interacting with them. This became especially clear to me when I was transcribing tapes from the 1986 momasoro and needed to return to a 1985 tape to see if the boliang's song was the same as that of the year before. I happened upon a portion of the tape with Sumpitan's voice. I was shocked at how similar it was to Balitangan's. Both talked to the boliang and the to pensio with the same arrogant, inquisitorial tone. While Sumpitan never openly accused mediums of fakery, he did ignore their comments and assert that his own knowledge was superior. I wondered how these two men from such different social, geographical, and religious backgrounds could adopt the same mannerisms, the same tone and attitude when others like them differed in notable ways? I realized that status, place, and religious knowledge were not the only factors involved here. Gender was a significant element bringing Siamae Balitangan and Sumpitan together against the female mediums. Another indicative factor was that both men were sando.

I began to investigate how men were trained to be sando and women were trained to be mediums, knowing that not all sando were men and not all mediums were women. I found that in the lowlands sando training was inextricably intertwined with Sufi mystical philosophy. The tendency to test spirits and to name them, as Siamae Balitangan and Sumpitan did, was fundamental to Sufi mystic philosophy. Moreover, Sufi mysticism was oddly similar to more general Laujé notions about umputé. Mystics believed that a fetus in the womb was in the most desirable state of being. The child's soul was connected or undifferentiated from the umputé spirits. Once the child was born, though, it was separated from the spirits and continued in this state until it died. When the soul went to heaven, the umputé and the soul were reunited and returned to the most desirable state of being. Sando learn about this mystic state so they can cure people. The most important training they receive is in names of spirits. By learning names, they can call upon the umputé spirits that have separated from the soul during life. Then they can momentarily reunite the soul and spirit, thus creating the most desirable conditions for a cure. Sando say each disease results from either a particular umputé spirit that has separated too far or one that is too close (recall Sumpitan's father-daughter incest story). Additionally, sando increase their knowledge of curing by asking spirits possessing mediums what their names are. Once sando know key names for umputé, they can cure more effectively by calling upon those named spirits for specific cures. They can also tap into the undifferentiated quality of umputé, as it was prior to birth. This gives them intensified healing powers.

Thus, sando use ceremonies like the momasoro as opportunities to complete their quest for secret names of umputé spirits. If sando frame their questions properly (showing respect for the spirit possessing a medium), the spirit may cooperate and tell them its name.[6] Yet, the quest is not easy. Spirits are reluctant to reveal answers to people they feel are testing them. The questers can retaliate, though. Occasionally, a refusal to reveal names is construed as proof that the person who claims to be possessed by a spirit is a fake. When the sando asking a question compares what the spirit has told him against his own knowledge and finds the medium's response inadequate, here too the sando can denounce the medium as fake. This is what Siamae Balitangan did in the 1986 momasoro when he accused some mediums of using "false names." As one can imagine, mediums resent this kind of public interrogation and accusation.

Mediums, outside of the trance state, do not hesitate to turn the tables on their inquisitors. Mediums do this by questioning whether or not sando are ethically motivated. Although the quest for power is a noble enterprise, mediums say it can be self-serving and instill greed. Sando often quest after names "to benefit themselves, not to help others." The sando, say mediums, can use their knowledge to destroy as well as heal. They can become involved in sorcery, "using their powers to vindictively harm" others in acts of revenge. Or they can "take money" in exchange for knowledge of how to seek revenge on enemies. Because of such negative rumors associated with secret names, mediums are disdainful of those who quest for secret knowledge. Siinai Alasan's spirit told Siamae Balitangan he should not be concerned with names, or with weeding out true from false spirits, but Siamae Balitangan persisted, galvanized in the belief he was right. Siamae Balitangan bragged in front of one possessed medium that he knew all the "true names" of spirits that were needed. Such arrogance was typical of sando. Siinai Alasan's spirit warned him:

> We spirits who gather jointly to bless cannot compete with one another as to who is on top. . . . There cannot be one sando on top. We have been

drawn together, yet here comes the enemy. . . . I say you are a new one here.
. . . We spirits cross over to the world of humans . . . to educate and inform.
. . . Long blessings are not allowed. There cannot be one sando on top.

Mediums such as Siinai Alasan did not approve of sando arrogance.
Part of this was due to the difference between medium and sando
training. Mediums did not actively seek their roles. They did not study
with a renowned expert as sando did. The women who became mediums often did so during an extreme illness. When their fever was especially high or when the illness had been extended for a long period
of time, a spirit would often enter the woman's body, making her
speak in a different language or in a tone much lower or higher than
normal. The spirit would tell family members how to cure her, what
foods to feed her and what ritual to perform. The spirit would also tell
relatives to make sure the woman came to the upcoming momasoro to
reunite with the spirit and pay respect to it. From this time forward,
the woman would be a medium. The spirit that had cured her now
possessed her regularly to cure others. Mediums believed the spirits
had honored them by selecting their human bodies as vessels for the
spirit voice. Indeed mediums were often called vessels *(pomalembangané)* or riders *(pesabean),* and the spirits were called winds *(bayalé).*
This is because the spirit is said to take over or "sit in front of" the human body and to use the body as a vessel in which the spirit sails or
rides. The spirit is only effective, though, when many mediums, and
thus many spirits, are present.

Siinai Alasan's spirit explained the boat metaphor to Siamae Balitangan after he had rather rudely called one of her fellow mediums a
fake: "We are like a boat carrying mankind's wishes. If the boat is not
paddled forcefully, if there is only one, it will not arrive at the shore.
We are called the winds. The winds push the boat. The winds carry
rotten smells as they carry fragrant breezes."

Siinai Alasan's spirit reminded Siamae Balitangan that spirits and
mediums were not to be belittled. While they could effect a cure—
bring "fragrant breezes" to humans—they could also bring the "rotten
smells" of illness and death.[7] Thus, in answering Siamae Balitangan,
this spirit, as others, asserted at once that they were powerful and that
there must be many spirits present for the rite to be effective. Many refractions of umputé must possess human bodies so all the other aspects of umputé may be heard.

Sando, however, are not without their own moral reactions to mediums' claims. Siamae Balitangan's answer was to tell Siinai Alasan's spirit "too many spirits confuse the issue." For Siamae Balitangan, the essence of life and creation, umputé, was a unified whole. For him, the spirits should all be one entity. In many respects, then, Siamae Balitangan's stance was similar to that of the spirit possessing Siinai Alasan who saw the spirit refractions as one undifferentiated whole— the winds. But Siamae Balitangan did not regard all the spirits equally. Initially he was antagonistic toward Siinai Alasan and the other mediums. He only became obsequious if he believed the spirit embodying the medium was truly real.

Such a paradoxical tension between sando like Siamae Balitangan and to pensio like Siinai Alasan was not unusual. Sando like Sumpitan and Balitangan were often more allied, despite their other differences, than fellow elite mediums were to Sumpitan, or than fellow commoner mediums were to Siamae Balitangan. No matter what the rank of a sando or his place of origin, he always sought to weed out the false from the true medium and to find the secret names of umputé. An example follows, in a long dialogue between Siinai Alasan's spirit and Sumpitan. Sumpitan sought knowledge while testing Siinai Alasan's spirit. On the one hand, Sumpitan flattered the spirit so he could tease out secret names from her, trusting that all spirits would tell the truth. At the same time, though, he cajoled the spirit possessing Siinai Alasan to reveal secrets that could confirm or deny that the spirit was "true." Siinai Alasan's spirit avoided answering Sumpitan in the direct way he wished. She admonished him for seeking names in the first place. Siinai Alasan regarded the quest for names of the various manifestations of umputé as a misguided venture that distracted the quester from the real issue of the momasoro. The momasoro's purpose, as she saw it, was to invoke the aspects of umputé that were complements to Islam. Their dialogue is as follows:

Sumpitan:
The spirit which you carry is certain. We are all here as one in this house. All joined here in this house. So what is your worry about revealing secrets here? Everything that was protecting and covering the world is here. Is there anything which is not in its place? It is only left for you to give us understanding because we don't know.

Siinai Alasan/The Spirit from the Womb of the World:
Because we believe in our bodies, we also believe in the prayer and in
turn we believe in our body, which means that one believes in God. . . .
But come on now, you there, all this secret stuff. We don't know any of
this deep dark secret stuff you are talking of.

Sumpitan:
So, we each don't know the secret. Huh? So, you spirit, you say I
don't know. Maybe it's that the secret I know can't be told to these
people because that which is on top and that which is below, the deep,
the surface, all is known by you spirits. For example, you spirit, what
is known by you?

Siinai Alasan/The Spirit from the Womb of the World:
You humans, whether you who walk the earth hidden or whether those
of you who are in this generation, these secrets are not to be known by
you. Just we who carry the spirit.

Sumpitan:
Whatever has appeared and developed on earth, that which moves,
that which does not, all comes from the ancestors. We disciples try to
follow what is honest and straight. It is only left for you to give us
understanding because we don't know.

Siinai Alasan/The Spirit from the Womb of the World:
The spirit will be stormy . . . it will capsize the vessel. For you people
just as with the olongian, you must turn your palms up in submission,
so with this secret you must just submit turning your palms up. That is
the knowledge of Allah. This is all Allah needs from you, to turn your
palms up. By that gesture will come a response from Allah.

Sumpitan starts to interrupt.

Siinai Alasan/The Spirit from the Womb of the World:
NO SPEAKING I SAY. There will be no mutual goodwill if there is
no giving of praise. No competition, no games, no testing. That
is it!
    What you see here before you with your eyes is that which has pos-
sessed this body. That is not the sacred thing of which I speak. Only
this ceremony is sacred.

Sumpitan persists in probing for answers to the secrets:
You are probably the male spirit of the seven levels? Not so? So how
about it?

In this interaction between Sumpitan and Siinai Alasan, Siinai Alasan
refused to articulate and describe what umputé meant. She admonished Sumpitan that spirits "don't know this deep dark secret stuff."
The next year, in a conversation with the Haji, she reiterated her dis-
dain for such quests:

> Hey! What is the real origin? That which goes too far away from the real
> origin is this that you do. What we mediums who follow the original ways
> do is to massage the chest, call the ancestors, ask forgiveness. We grand-
> children cure simply. We sing the song to the tree until you humans are
> standing straight, your palms opened in submission to the ancestors.
> We should come here to gain strength for us all. We should come here so
> we cure us all. We should not come and make meaningful words for a few.

Her warning went unheeded. The Haji persisted in his quest as did
Sumpitan. Like Balitangan, they all antagonized the spirits. The men
used the momasoro as an event for which they could learn secret
names from the possessed spirits, and/or show off the knowledge they
already had. When Sumpitan died six months after the 1985 momasoro, women who worked as mediums said it was because of his rude-
ness toward the spirit possessing Siinai Alasan that he died. He was
disrespectful *(mobotong)*[8] to the spirit, continually asking questions
until the spirit was forced to reprimand him. A few women who
worked as mediums said Sumpitan kept proposing riddles for which
he already knew the answer.[9]

The crucial point here about Sumpitan's (and the Haji's) interaction
with Siinai Alasan is it followed the same pattern as Siamae Balitangan's interaction with mediums. In all of the cases, mediums argued
that the sando should give up their aggressive search for names. All
mediums wished to do was speak as a collectivity with "one voice, one
tongue." In this case, mediums were not just defending themselves
against aggressive sando who wanted to gain glory by exposing the
mediums as fakes.[10] Rather, the mediums in their trances were
genuinely articulating a particular moral and religious vision of life.
By submerging multiple identities into a single collectivity, spirits-

speaking-through-mediums portrayed the manifold spirits as a unified essence—a congeries of refractions of a single spirit, umputé. Possessed mediums enacted that congeries, becoming "one voice" in front of a Laujé audience.

For spirits or mediums to argue for a more general notion of submission—that all spirits speak with "one tongue, one voice"—is to make the experiential fact of possession into a consciously expressed ideology. This ideology implies a certain "selflessness" and it contrasts strongly to the self-aggrandizing stance sando such as Sumpitan and Siamae Balitangan, on occasion, take.

Thus there are many patterns of which these interactions between sando and mediums can be expressions. On one level, we may have women resisting or denouncing male assertiveness, but on another level, we may also have commoners contesting the individuating powers associated with elite Islam. When Siamae Balitangan called the multitude of names for the spirit entity "bent talk," on the one hand, he was attacking the mediums' use of spirit names in the prayers, but on the other hand, he was tentatively aligning himself ideologically with mediums as commoners. At this level, then, status and gender issues were at play. Female mediums resisted male sando, but quasi-lowland commoners like Siamae Balitangan aligned with other commoners to contest the elite Sufi's tendency to name the refractions of umputé.[11] At one level Siamae Balitangan was interacting with the mediums as a highlander would, arguing for simplification of umputé. At another level, he was arguing as any sando would, saying that he knew what was best. Status, place, and gender were the lines of resistance that split the community.

Nevertheless, status, place, and gender are not the whole answer to this puzzle. Possession does not involve a covert appropriation of individual power by the powerless. The female mediums are not claiming that they are individually powerful because they are spirits. They do not aggrandize the [spirit] self. Rather, the spirits who speak through them are making an overt claim that selfishly individuating and naming the spirits is immoral. Siamae Balitangan at times is making this claim too. For the mediums (and possibly all commoners as well) collective holism is moral. The "vessel" makes it to its destination if all paddle in unison, if all mediums deny their own selves, if all the refractions of the spirit work together.

The Islamic Context

These professional ideologies in which sando promote themselves and mediums deny themselves must be considered within the context of the fundamentalist attacks against the rite made by immigrants in official positions of power within the government. These immigrant attacks threatened to fracture the Laujé community from within, for fundamentalist Islam—in particular, teachings of the Muhammadiyah sect—had also become a compelling practice for many Laujé.

Recall that the attacks were twofold. The Muhammadiyah fundamentalists said the momasoro's participants were not Muslims. They worshiped multiple spirits that were satanic. The Laujé participants' answer to this was twofold. The elite sando emphasized and underscored the fact that they were Muslim by drawing upon all the Muslim knowledge they had, their Sufism. Sufism, in its syncretic, mystical way, allowed Islam and spirit possession to coexist, an existence the Muhammadiyah fundamentalists believed was heretical (Peacock 1992). The misguided sando, though, when calling on their Sufist knowledge, believed they had answered the fundamentalists' charge. These sando believed their knowledge of Sufism proved to outsiders that the Laujé and their ceremonies followed Islam.

I believe this is one reason Sumpitan was so anxious to have me tape-record his interpretations of the spirit speeches. He wanted to prove to the "outside world" that the Laujé were not pagan, but Muslim. Likewise the commoners' emphasis on the collective spirit comprising the body, umputé, could be a response to fundamentalists' assertions the ceremony is satanic and not monotheistic.

The whole issue of Islam is crucial here because it, to a very great extent, circumscribes how people view and or discuss umputé. Throughout the ceremony, Siamae Balitangan ranted against the other curers like a fundamentalist cleric, but his message was far from the anti-umputé perspective advocated by the fundamentalists. Siamae Balitangan said: "There is no other, there is only umputé. No higher, no lower. We do not need to say more about it, only to submit and worship it." Though Siamae Balitangan was a Muslim, his religious knowledge was rather shallow. He probably knew that to be Islamic was to recognize that there is no deity but Allah, but little more than that. His words about umputé sound like the Islamic profession of faith. Replace umputé in his statement above with Allah, and one has a forceful declaration of submission to God, a submission that would make any imam proud. Yet, if his vision of umputé reflects Islam, the reflection has been subsumed into the image of umputé itself. Siamae Balitangan does not say umputé is like religion. In Siamae Balitangan's vision of umputé, umputé is a self-contained and indivisible totality. Undivided, it no longer can enter into a referential relationship with other transcendental categories. Undivided, it can stand alone: The monotheism of Islam is an unnecessary elaboration. Thus, to Siamae Balitangan, umputé is not "tradition" separated from, or a complement to, religion. Umputé and religion are indistinguishable.[12]

The way that Siamae Balitangan refuses to define umputé could in some respects be called the most valued level of umputé for the Laujé. It is the mystical, the subjective level, one in which umputé is treated as though it were the same force that created the universe. It is a level in which nothing is distinguished from the subjective self. To avoid treating umputé as a political tool through which certain authors can readjust and objectify the hierarchies of the world, Siamae Balitangan advocates treating umputé as a mystical, subjective, and religious entity that should be worshiped, not dissected and elaborated. His point is against that made by Siinai Alasan in her discussions with sando like the Haji and Sumpitan. These people see a distinction between umputé belief and Islamic religion. Ignorant of Islam, Siamae Balitangan sees umputé and Islam as one and the same thing.

In some respects, this may have been what Siinai Alasan and the others wanted to say. Neither Siinai Alasan, nor Sumpitan, nor the Haji could say publicly that umputé and Islam were identical. They were more cognizant than Siamae Balitangan of the threatening overtones such a statement would make to an Indonesian state that requires its citizens to worship a world religion. Thus, they avoided making such statements. To refer to umputé as a religious entity equivalent to Allah, would have been social and political suicide.

Nevertheless, they did realize the value of regarding umputé as though it were an entity that engenders everything, yet is impossible to objectify or distinguish. Sumpitan once told me that umputé in its original form was "whiter than glass, clearer than water." His words could have been uttered by Siamae Balitangan or by a medium. What he meant, of course, is that the truth of umputé lies beyond objective perception: In essence umputé is invisible and intangible. When Siinai

Alasan described umputé as "beyond the reach of the highest climber, deeper than the deepest water," she also was trying to express in words something that by its very nature is beyond expression.

To a certain extent, then, the spirits', the mediums', and the healers' statements reflect contemporary events. They are filtered through the contexts and personal agendas of the vessels speaking for them and the agents speaking about them. Spirits advocate selflessness, and this ideology contrasts strongly with the self-aggrandizing stance sando such as Sumpitan (all the time) and Siamae Balitangan (some of the time) take. The upshot of the perspective of Siinai Alasan's possessing spirit, and that of others', was to emphasize personal passivity in the face of umputé's agency, to emphasize the underlying unity in the seeming diversity of the refractions of umputé. They remind us that to understand possession, we cannot just focus on the medium as the agent and the sociological factors that influence that medium to say what she does during spirit possession. The content of the spirits' speech, its moral stance, deserves to be given equal standing with the sociological factors impinging upon that stance.

In conclusion then, the particular interpreters like Siinai Alasan, Siamae Balitangan, Sumpitan, the Haji, and the wife of the olongian can be regarded as representatives of a variety of general patterns or as unique individuals. The postmodern approach relies on the particularizing method—analyzing the idiosyncratic experiences that shape people's interpretations and creative responses to events like the Islamic ban and to religious, political, and economic change in the region. Following this theoretical line, I can conclude that Siinai Alasan was a commoner who resented elitist interpretations, but could not make the bold statements equating Islam and umputé that Siamae Balitangan did because she lived in an Islamic community in which such statements were heretical. I can conclude that Sumpitan made his statements as an elite advocate for political sovereignty of the olongian and against immigrants, partly because he was a relative of the olongian and partly because he and his family had a long history of run-ins with the immigrant raja. Sumpitan's interpretation of how to deal with mediums was also like Siamae Balitangan's. Both had Sufi training in which they learned how to increase their own self-worth and power. This contradicted the mediums' more selfless moral stance. The Haji and the wife of the olongian were like Sumpitan in that they used umputé as a symbol or metaphor, but unlike him in that they emphasized connection to immigrants. Both the Haji and the wife of the olongian had immigrant fathers and Laujé mothers, so their personal histories definitely influenced how they interpreted umputé.

Siamae Balitangan was the most idiosyncratic of all people mentioned in this book. He had been born a commoner in Taipaobal, he was raised as a servant in an elite imam's house, and he married a bela woman in the highlands. Thus, he incorporated some Sufi mystic knowledge about secret names from the lowland elites, but he also espoused the more egalitarian philosophy of umputé. He returned to the mountains before fundamentalist Islam began to infiltrate his thinking. Like the mediums, Siamae Balitangan regarded umputé as an undifferentiated whole. But unlike them, he made bold statements equating umputé with Islam.

Some people in the lowlands regarded anything Siamae Balitangan said as representative of the highlands, but not all highlanders agreed with Siamae Balitangan. A week after the momasoro, Siamae Balitangan came up to Taipaobal from Dusunan to pay a visit to Siamae Sanji's children, who were the siblings of his sister's husband, Sanji. Idola, Sair, Larsen, and Zharuddin welcomed him, hoping he would tell them one of the names for umputé that their father, Siamae Sanji, had neglected to give to them. A person could only tell such names if they expected to die soon. Siamae Balitangan claimed he was old and ready to die, so the utterance of such a powerful name would not hurt him. He offered us a creation myth involving the first tree. At the end of the story, with great fanfare, Siamae Balitangan, his head bobbing, leaned into the circle of people sitting around him and whispered a name (which I could not hear). All solemnly shook their heads and grunted in a knowing way. The next day, when Siamae Balitangan left, I was surprised at how quickly the children of Siamae Sanji scoffed. Zharuddin said, "These are not the names our father told us! Siamae Balitangan must be a witch."

Just as before, when Siamae Balitangan contradicted Siamae Sanji's history (see p. 50), Siamae Balitangan contradicted Siamae Sanji's name for umputé. Because Siamae Sanji's children faithfully followed their father's narratives and notions about umputé even after his death, there was no chance that Siamae Balitangan's concepts would be accepted in Taipaobal. By contrast, in the lowlands, where the communities were larger, and people with contradictory philosophies lived within the same household, it was less likely that one person's

Siamae Sanji
Highlander
Commoner
Olongian is bad
Raja is good
Umputé is metaphor
Umputé is gendered
Umputé is simple

Siinai Alasan
Umputé is simple
Commoner
Lowlander
Umputé is undifferentiated whole
Umputé is *not* a metaphor
Female medium
Umputé is our body
Tradition is good

Siamae Balitangan
Highlander
Commoner
Lived as lowlander
Umputé is simple
Umputé is undifferentiated whole
Umputé is *not* metaphor
Male sando
Sufi training
Umputé through secret names
Good sando expose fake mediums

Wife of Olongian
Umputé is metaphor
Umputé is connection/marriage
Lowlander
Elite
Female medium
Immigrant
Olongian is good
Secret of Sawerigading

Haji
Lowlander
Elite
Immigrant
Olongian is good
Secret of Sawerigading
Umputé is connection/marriage
Umputé is a metaphor

Sumpitan
Elite
Lowlander
Olongian is good
Good sando expose fake mediums
Umputé through secret names
Sufi training
Male sando
Umputé is a metaphor
Umputé has ethnic identity

Figure 7.2. Schematic outline of different Laujé ideas

view would remain popular after they died. This was Sumpitan's sad fate. As long as he was alive, people agreed with him. As soon as "the spirits proved him wrong by taking him before his time," alternative interpretations sprang up. Moreover, because Sumpitan had no children of his own, there was no one left to protect his interests. Of course, in the lowlands, having a child of one's own does not preclude disagreement. Recall that even the olongian's own son rejected the momasoro and the philosophy embedded in it. He went to the Islamic reading of the Qur'an rather than attend the momasoro. He refused to learn the secret names his parents thought so crucial and instead focused on the "secret names" in the Qur'an, as though they had power to heal all. In sum, then, he and others have diverse backgrounds and opinions that fit well with postmodern theory about the way local philosophies are constructed.

There are many ways, however, to draw conclusions about Laujé philosophy, umputé, and Islam. If I characterized the Laujé only from different individuals' perspectives, I would show the richness and diversity of Laujé life. Yet, this would imply there is little agreement about, or pattern for, the way in which people talk about umputé. Instead, I believe there is a systematic correlation between the way people discuss umputé and the kinds of social positions they occupy—their status, gender, and place positions. The patterned responses, in turn, are reflections of contemporary events, and partial answers to them. For a clear summary of these patterned positions, see Figure 7.2.

It is the overlaps, the patterned responses, and the systematic correlations that social-cultural anthropology traditionally writes about. And it is the individual, idiosyncratic, responses that postmodernists tend to write about. Here I have combined these two approaches: (1) dialogues by particular individuals with personal histories that explain, to a certain extent, why individuals are motivated to speak as they do, and (2) similar responses to the same issues, which reveal general patterns and trends throughout the community. It is only through this combination of theoretical approaches that one can reach a relatively thorough understanding of Laujé life and the individuals who are actors in creating concepts that divide and unite their community.

Four

CONCEIVING THEORY A DECADE LATER

8

PARTIAL TRUTHS
AND LAYERED
REPRESENTATIONS

In demonstrating the particulars of Laujé perceptions about umputé, I have also been making a point about anthropological theory. I have tried to illustrate the variations and oppositions among Laujé about what they think umputé means and does. Yet I have also suggested that the way individual Laujé talk and disagree about umputé spirits overlaps with the way other Laujé talk about umputé, thus forming layers and patterns of meaning. These patterns may not be visible to anyone other than an anthropologist who is aware of subject positions, class, gender, religion, and place, but they are worth noting. Postmodern theorists like Clifford or Tyler have tended to criticize those anthropologists who have presented the world in patterned, coherent terms, filtered through the lens of the anthropologist's authoritative voice. My point is that the anthropologist's perspective does not have to be the final, authoritative truth, but one among many. My goal has been to create a multifaceted view of the Laujé, layering various representations on top of one another until a more complete, though nonauthoritative picture results. In this way I have combined postmodern anthropological theory with important insights raised in more classic approaches.

As I mentioned in the introduction, it is wrong to presume that all earlier anthropology is completely at odds with postmodernism (see Karp and Kendall 1982). In denying their intellectual heritage, many postmodernists have created, inadvertently, their own set of problems, as I noted in the introduction. In trying to distance themselves from the static, uniform quality of structural approaches to culture, postmodern studies have primarily focused on the people who resist the status quo. Thus, provocative, iconoclastic voices have been favored along with case studies of exploitation, colonization, and subaltern resistance in the face of hegemonic authority. In the process, the impact of status-quo statements have been ignored, downplayed, or deleted.

Certainly this is the way I portrayed people when I first wrote up my material about the Laujé. I selected Sumpitan as the radical, willing to fight the immigrant status quo, and Siamae Sanji, willing to fight the elite status quo in the lowlands.[1] When they died, I placed their critics on equal footing with them. I highlighted the words of Siamae Balitangan and Siinai Alasan because I perceived them as religious rebels resisting elitist Islam (see Scott 1985). Their dogged determination to hang on to what I characterized as anti-elitist mysticism convinced me that their views were just as important as those of Siamae Sanji and Sumpitan. They allowed me to represent the contested terrain of the Laujé world.

In retrospect, however, I realize there is a major difference between Siamae Balitangan's and Siinai Alasan's words and the words of Sumpitan and Siamae Sanji. People in the community *really* listened to the latter, felt compelled to enact Sumpitan's and Siamae Sanji's visions, to follow their lead. Siamae Balitangan and Siinai Alasan, while smart and articulate as far as I was concerned, did not rally whole communities of people in the same way Sumpitan's and Siamae Sanji did. Their interpretations of umputé were more reactions to Sumpitan's interpretation than persuasively unique creations. To a certain extent then, I highlighted these individuals because they fit my preconceived (poststructuralist) notions of what I should find in the field. Siinai Alasan was compelling to me because she was one of the few women who could really effectively argue with Sumpitan. As a representative of all articulate women, she fit with my notion of what a complete picture of the Laujé community should look like. But only a few people, mostly young women who were studying to be healers, really listened to her. Her interpretation did not represent what the Laujé community thought was important, but what I, as a gender-sensitive anthropologist doing research in the 1980s, thought was important.[2] Likewise Siamae Balitangan was a compelling figure to me because he seemed to speak in the voice of pure postmodernism. He advocated no interpretation at all, a point Tyler had advocated in the 1986 Clifford volume. I liked him because he fit my new theoretical model.

Now, however, I realize that the point should not be whose voice is more compelling to the anthropologist, but whose voice is more compelling to the Laujé. Sumpitan's and Siamae Sanji's voices, each in their own way, congealed and motivated whole communities of people to act in certain ways. No one else's voice did, but I made the mistake of giving all of those voices equal weight. Part of this was due to what I explained above, the postmodern tendency to privilege pluralism and to look for the iconoclast. Part of it also had to do with my own romantic tendency to search for mystics.

I recalled that the first time Balitangan visited me, he offered to tell his version of Laujé history, the myth of the beginning of the world. When I asked if I could tape record him, he said I could try, "but, child, this story is really too powerful to be caught on tape." When my tape recorder mysteriously refused to work during the telling of the myth, yet ran perfectly well a while later, I was convinced Balitangan was "a man of power." Later, in the lowlands, when the spirit mediums took the same anti-metaphoric stance as Balitangan, refusing to divide umputé's parts and relate them to social issues, refusing to regard umputé as anything other than itself, I had already decided what this meant. The spirit mediums, like Balitangan, were mystics who refused to see umputé as the means to make political and social commentary. I categorized them all in the same way, never questioning my initial assumption that there would be a mystic among the Laujé. I just assumed some locals were mystics.

Moreover, I realized that the reason I first thought of Siamae Balitangan in mystic terms is that I needed someone to fill the mystic slot left when Siamae Sanji died. I first met Balitangan the day after Siamae Sanji was buried. The morning after the funeral, I was sitting on my porch watching the sun rise when I noticed a rainbow appear over Siamae Sanji's grave. Siamae Sanji had told me months before, that only "men of power" *(kangkai baraka)* grow rainbows over their graves to carry them to heaven. Indeed, the appearance of this rainbow in the middle of the dry season provided the miracle I rather romantically sought. Later, after reading the postmodernists, I reassessed Siamae Sanji's view of umputé to be more politically than mystically motivated. I decided Siamae Sanji was not a mystic, but a powerful healer whose persuasive interpretations of umputé could convince Taipaobalers to resist bela and lowlanders' disruptions of his community. Siamae Balitangan became the mystic I had lost when I categorized Siamae Sanji as a political visionary.

When I "converted" from symbolic anthropology to postmodernism, I assumed I had followed the cutting-edge theory, by presenting competing voices, dividing the Laujé people I had met into two camps: (1) anti-metaphoric interpreters who were the religious rebels, the mystics, the people for whom ritual is sacred, and (2) Sumpitan, Siamae Sanji, the Haji, and the olongian's wife, for whom umputé is the means to metaphorically critique and address the political plight of their people. The people and their voices certainly revealed the variety of contests over what umputé was, as the theory said they should, but I was seeing people in fairly simplistic terms.

Ironically, in the process of fulfilling one aspect of cutting-edge mission—to present the contested nature of society—I refuted two others, to use one or two people to stand for a whole class, gender, or place and to presume, rather romantically (see Rosaldo in Clifford and Marcus 1986) that "natives" would be mystics. In hindsight I now understand why extreme postmodern theorists like Clifford and Tyler claim it is impossible to talk about generalities, to draw authoritative conclusions: In the process we present as much our own presumptions and imaginings about the world as we present the reality. I wanted to find religious rebels, mystics, and I did. I wanted to find political activists and I did. My presentation of the Laujé was only part of the truth, filtered through my own romantic lens. Yet I still do not agree with Tyler's claim that my partial truth should be eradicated because it is biased and thus destroys an understanding of local worldviews.

It was not I who first conceptualized Balitangan as a mystic. I was not completely imagining reality; Siamae Balitangan presented himself in those terms. The original tape-recording from our first meeting said it all:

> I'll tell you all there is to know about the Laujé; there are a few simple things only a man of power can know. I know them. I'll give the ones [secrets] I can to you because I will soon die. If you are here when I am dying I'll tell you the last secret for your book, but if I told you now, I'd fall dead right here [because these secrets are so powerful]. . . . I'm a man of power.

I had not completely constructed the image of Siamae Balitangan as a rebellious mystic. Siamae Balitangan had made a concerted effort to portray himself as a mystic. Likewise, Siamae Sanji's children liked to perpetuate the image of their father as a man of power and a political activist. Sumpitan too preferred to emphasize his own image as a political activist, repeatedly telling me how he had resolved a number of local social problems. He would often order me to write this information down for my book.

After realizing that local people had framed their own self-images for me and that I had merely reproduced them, I worried that I was a weak reed, completely manipulated by the desires of local subjects wishing to characterize themselves in a positive light. If locals manipulate the anthropologist, and the anthropologist projects his or her own romantic notions onto subjects, can there ever be anything more than partial truths in the ethnographic record?

I believe there can be more than partial truths if we carefully outline the anthropologists' motivations in characterizing people, then look at who is persuasive in a local community. This is the major key to getting beyond partial truths and toward some sort of shared notion of what people believe. Sumpitan really did convince others that his view was right. To a certain extent this was because he had the power and position to do so, but other powerfully situated people—the olongian, his wife, the Haji—couldn't sway people in the community that their views of umputé were to be believed. Sumpitan had influenced community members until he died an untimely death, until his persuasive perceptions evaporated along with his voice. Sumpitan, while alive, had charisma, the ability to touch that fundamental cultural chord I spoke about in the introduction. There I mentioned that that chord almost always took a similar form when a charismatic person used it. It always fell into neatly opposed binary structures. Sumpitan understood those structures (and so did Siamae Sanji) and used them in a way that resonated with other people's knowledge.

As I also mentioned in the introduction, the possibilities for someone like Sumpitan to construct a believable interpretation are not limitless. The general Austronesian tendency to divide the world into binary structures limits how people can say something that resonates with other people in the community. It must be expressed in binary terms or it is not part of the shared knowledge that will convince others of its truth. There are more limitations as well. Sumpitan used the concept of umputé in a way no one else had. He divided evil immigrants and foreigners from healing Laujé locals. Sumpitan cobbled together a truth for the Laujé of Dusunan and Lombok that made sense for that moment. It was constructed, self-motivated, subjective truth, but it was created within a framework that was already there.

Writing and perception are not merely constructed, subjective, and therefore imagined fictions. People in particular communities talk about specific, circumscribed topics, and those discussions overlap with one another to reveal general cultural themes and trends. Though Laujé may disagree about what umputé means, it still is the topic they focus on, or at least it was while I was there. And though some people tend to characterize umputé one way, and others have different views, their descriptions are an approximate analysis, a representation that is framed or limited by its inherent qualities.

The point is that abstract ideas about umputé are framed by two sometimes competing tendencies: (1) to categorize ideas, as other Austronesians do, in structurally opposed ways and (2) to compare the spirit world to the concrete qualities of the placenta as a physical entity. The placenta, then, is what anthropologists like Leach call "good to think." It generates ideas. These ideas, however, are constrained by the way locals talk about the finite qualities of the placenta itself. For instance, interpreters like Sumpitan, Siamae Sanji, and most other Laujé tend to focus on the physical qualities inherent in the postnatal placenta. After birth the placenta is physically separated from the womb and the fetus. As blood flows out of it, the placenta "dies" so the fetus can live. The placenta's physical qualities, then are contradictory and divisible, life-giving and life-taking, comprised of placental sac, amniotic fluid, fetus, blood, and umbilicus. These divisible and contradictory qualities form the referential field constraining how people speak about umputé spirits. They say umputé spirits nurture, yet poison, thus some are like nurturing mothers or fathers, others like soldiers who rape, and still others like mothers who abort. No one comparing spirits to the placenta in this referential field speaks about spirits in holistic or indivisible terms. By contrast, interpreters like Siamae Balitangan and Siinai Alasan tend to focus on the qualities of the placenta when it is still hidden inside the womb, nurturing the fetus, connected to the mother through the umbilical cord, encompassed by nurturing fluids. Interpreters with these gestating images in mind conceptualize umputé in ways that fit with the ineffable, invisible, and indivisible qualities of the placenta. They urge others to submit to umputé's mysteries. Balitangan says: "There is no other, there is only umputé. We do not need to say more about it."

For the Laujé as a whole, then, there are at least two distinct referential fields, each describing the placenta's qualities in ways that cannot and should not overlap. For Balitangan the metaphoric references Sumpitan and others use to describe umputé's names and its capacity to harm or kill, not only make little sense, but also seem morally wrong. If one thinks of the placenta within the domain of a healthy gestating womb, images of separation imply premature birth (separating placenta and fetus) and untimely death. Thus Balitangan always and Alasan often steadfastly claim it is morally wrong to speak about umputé in metaphoric terms. For Sumpitan and Siamae Sanji, however, metaphoric comparisons conveying the contradictions of life and death seem especially apt.

In some respects, then umputé, with its range of interpretations, is analogous to the Nuer notion of *kwoth* as described by Evans-Pritchard. Evans-Pritchard's classic work, *Nuer Religion* (1956), highlights the subtleties involved in indigenous understandings of spirits and Nuer use of personal metaphors to explain the spirit world. When a Nuer compares the spirit kwoth to his father, he knows he is speaking metaphorically. When he names kwoth "our father," he believes such a name gives the spirit a personality, a history, and that this provides the means to understand one aspect of kwoth. Ultimately, however, he knows such metaphors give only partial understanding of the concept "kwoth." In effect, it restricts understanding of the spirit world within the familiar world of persons, family members, and individual agents. The Nuer example shows that the metaphor "our father" is merely the means to describe kwoth in an imperfect or inexact way. In such an environment, each individual can emphasize either the oneness of kwoth or the allegories, metaphors, and redactions of kwoth in order to understand and commune with the spirit world.

The point here is that in many religions there are two potential interpretations of the spirit world that can predominate—what could be called the metaphoric and the ineffable. The other more important point, however, is that there is a finite quality, a limited or circumscribed semantic domain from which a concept like kwoth or umputé is drawn. Umputé derives from the experience of birth and its paradoxes. Thus the themes, the semantic domain that limits discussion of umputé, are circumscribed by those experiences—separation and unity, neglect and nurturance, sickness and health, procreation and death. Some people may choose to focus on the differences between aspects of that experience—the difference between neglect and nurturance, sickness and health—opposing each aspect of umputé into separate structural categories. When they focus on difference, they tend, as others in the Austronesian archipelago do, to talk about umputé in pairs, in binary oppositions. Turn-of-the-century anthropologists (Hertz 1907; Mauss 1920; van Wouden 1935) and early missionaries (Adriani and Kruyt 1898) who wrote about binary oppositions throughout the Indonesian archipelago did not do so because they dreamed up those structures. Those structures were what people talked about. The local people as active agents characterized themselves and their beliefs in binary, structuralist terms. The mistake early and later structuralists (Josselin de Jong 1977; Downs 1956; Needham 1979) made (which postmodern critics indirectly pointed out) was to presume this was the only way people in those communities talked about their world.[3] Among the Laujé, for instance, some people, like Sumpitan and Siamae Sanji, may at times have talked about the binary differences, the divisible qualities of umputé. At other times, though, they or others chose to focus on umputé as a whole entity. Their choices, to a certain extent, were finite, confined by the placental images, gestating or postnatal, they chose to refer to umputé. Thus umputé's semantic domain circumscribed how far the discussion could go, in the same way that Nuer discussions of kwoth were limited by how Nuer compared kwoth to sky spirits not earth spirits.

These "givens," these limits on how far people can go to construct their symbolic world, do not explain why those symbols are chosen in the first place and why some interpretations resonate with other people when they are expressed by charismatic spokespersons. For these why-and-how questions we end up resorting to contextualizing strategies: We must put umputé back into history. This is one of the advantages of the new perspective. Unlike Evans-Pritchard's way of discussing kwoth, we cannot relegate umputé to a timeless forever of Laujé tradition. Today umputé is a central concept in the Laujé's rituals, but it was not necessarily always so. If I were to analyze umputé as Evans-Pritchard might have I would regard it as an anachronistic holdover from a time "before religion." This theoretical notion tells only part of the story, but it resonates dangerously closely with state assertions that suku terasing (primitive tribes), like the Laujé, are *belum beragama,* or "not yet religious." There is a dangerous assumption that the Laujé will inevitably embrace religion, that they will shed old superstitions (involving umputé) to become new (religious) citizens. Evans-Pritchard might see umputé as a collective cultural concept and compare it in its entirety to concepts of a monotheistic God gleaned from Islamic "culture." Such an analytical perspective would negate the negotiation that goes on regarding how umputé is defined. It would also imply that umputé as a form of animism will inevitably give way to global Islam. To draw such an old-fashioned conclusion, however, is wrong.

What I have been trying to show throughout this book is that umputé is also a "contemporary" concept, not just a "survival." It takes its current, rigorous, conceptually rich, yet pure shape in an alternative, oppositional, or accomodationist dialogue with the state and with Muslim clergy about religion. By talking about umputé through the perspective of diverse individuals, we also get to glimpse the way this new concept is created in a contemporary context. History enters the picture as it is, filtered through current preoccupations. When we put umputé back into history, we see it develop alongside of, in response to, in accommodation with Laujé political marginality and Islam.

Umputé becomes the answer particular actors use in response to the fundamentalists' ban of Laujé ritual. Sumpitan galvanizes community opinion when he characterizes the spirits in ethnic terms. Others in the community obviously agree with him, though when he dies an untimely death, his followers grow fearful and deny they ever agreed. As an alternative to Sumpitan, Balitangan quite rightly addresses the fundamentalist Muslims' claims that Laujé are not monotheistic by declaring that umputé is the only one. His declarations about umputé are not isolated, but part of a dialogue with Islam. Yet his message does not carry the same weight as Sumpitan's did. Umputé, then, probably became central in a series of sometimes accommodating, sometimes acrimonious conversations various Laujé had with each other and against foreigners about Islam, power, authority, and so forth. The most salient issue for lowlanders, the most culturally resonant note struck about umputé, was Sumpitan's point that ethnic others have victimized the Laujé.

Thus, it is certain individual agents at certain moments (for complex reasons having to do with what the philosophers and literary critics call their "subject positions") who are able to persuade others (and themselves) that their views about umputé are right, apt, appropriate. They do so by taking into account what Muslims say about them, what is going on in the world around them. They become charismatic leaders when they say what everyone else is thinking. This ascendant view, then, generates counterdiscourses, but the counterdiscourses do not compel people to act in the same way as do the resonant themes about evil ethnic others (or in the highlands about evil women). It will take several years before another equally charismatic speaker says something that resonates with what the majority thinks. That something will give an anthropologist the clue as to what is culturally significant.

In conclusion, then, my theoretical stance seems to have come full circle. Rather than embracing all of the questions raised in the 1980s critique of classic anthropology, I seem to have returned to my anthropological roots. I do so, however, with newly inspired insights. When new theorists claim that only they highlight informant diversity, they claim to be reinventing the wheel and only a partial one at that. Sapir recognized way back in 1938 that we need both versions—the different voices and the cultural themes—to do deeply textured and responsible anthropology. Sapir points out that diverse voices, seemingly cacophonous, can carry the same tune. If Sapir via Dorsey could recognize in 1938 that informants contradict others of the same culture, postmodernism's claim to provide this new perspective to anthropology is rather late in coming and shallow at that. In the 1960s Victor Turner gave us a perfect model for what Sapir would call responsible, "respectable ethnography." What is interesting is that "respectable" theory and thus "respectable" anthropology, whatever its origins, always considers the subtleties of voice, the contradictions in perspectives, both between and within individual informants. To conduct respectable and responsible anthropology, then, we need to go beyond looking at the world just from "the native's point of view" (Geertz 1976), beyond even contested, multiple points of view. We also must remember that those indigenous dialogues represent motivations, agendas, and desires, and it is up to the anthropologist to reveal the context in which those desires were made manifest, while also situating indigenous perspectives in broader sociohistorical contexts.

It was the cutting-edge books of the 1980s—Clifford and Marcus's, and Marcus and Fisher's—that made many anthropologists drop the hubris of believing we could explain it all, that the anthropologist had the final and only authoritative voice (despite the fact that other anthropologists had said the same thing long ago). The postmodern anthropologists compelled anthropology to question its long association with colonialism (even though this had been an issue for anthropologists long before postmodernists accented it).[4] Postmodernists compelled anthropologists to listen more carefully to the locals to try to avoid prejudiced, colonialist, and authoritative pronouncements. But they did not address a common anthropological scenario: What if different people say the same thing over and over, or give bits and pieces of the same kinds of information that corroborate what one eloquent person says? What happens if many people say, "I agree with so and so"? What does the anthropologist do if the people who agree have similar backgrounds, for instance, are all of one gender, religious persuasion, or class? Is not omission of this information just as much a distortion of the material as drawing conclusions about it? Doesn't omission misrepresent the context to readers and lead them to draw the wrong conclusion—that the world is more fragmented than it really is?

I believe it does. I believe, as Margery Wolf (1992) does, that we have a moral obligation to present as much data as we can and to use the knowledge we have about society and people to draw conclusions. If we present as many voices as we can and describe which voices inspire others to action, then the reader can accept or reject our (mis)representations.[5] The anthropologist should not be silenced; no matter how culturally circumscribed our own anthropological perceptions are, we need to be heard so we can convey whose voice carries the most weight in the ethnographic context. The trick is *not* to make the anthropologist's view the only or most powerful one, but to direct the reader to the words of the most persuasive local. Moreover, to give a careful and nuanced account of individual differences, the anthropologist should not have to sacrifice a discussion of themes and general influences on people.

This dialectic between providing the anthropologist's view and those of the people studied is the goal I have been trying to reach in the book you have just read. Though I may have represented people like Sumpitan and Siamae Sanji through the lens of my own imagination, I have also represented them as they wanted to be seen, as their words revealed them to be, and as others in the community perceived them. Clifford, Tyler, and other postmodernists claim any anthropological characterizations are fictitious. I disagree. All characterizations are inherently fictitious, and the anthropologist's view is just as constructed as the locals' view. Presenting the "native" voice and not the anthropologist's does not avoid partial truths. The goal should be to gather as many constructed versions, as many partial truths, as we can. Only then can we peel away the interpretive idiosyncracies, reveal overlaps and patterns in a broad range of individual interpretations of reality, and come closer to understanding how complex humans are underneath their masks.

NOTES

Introduction. In the Beginning: Ethnography and Theory

1. In his 1912 book entitled *The Elementary Forms of the Religious Life,* Émile Durkheim argued that symbolic representations and classificatory systems are determined by social realities. He asserted that society is not only perpetuated by means of the symbols people use to represent reality (what he calls symbolic representations), but, he argues, society also precedes, generates, and is the object of those representations. The symbols that perpetuate society are generally agreed upon by everyone and Durkheim calls them collective representations. Durkheim says collective representations "are as concrete representations as an individual could form of his own personal environment; they correspond to the way in which this very special being, society, considers the things of its own proper experience" (1947:483).

2. The point made by my professor Fred Damon was a good, if somewhat cynical, characterization of what many anthropologists tended to do. The first goal was to find a knowledgeable or insightful "informant," take what he or she said that corroborated what the anthropologist already knew, and with minimal checking, let this single voice, commenting from a single subject-position, stand for the whole culture. The tendency, in those days, was to expect unanimity. Individuals generally disappeared from anthropological accounts because individuals became entire societies. When a particular person told an anthropologist something, generally the anthropologist reported the story without identifying the person, or the context in which they revealed the information.

3. As is common in anthropology, I have provided this man with a pseudonym, Sumpitan, to protect his family from repercussions should anyone object to his opinions. Such a practice is different from that mentioned in Note 2, in which an anonymous person's ideas are presented as representative of a whole, collective, culture.

4. The Laujé are not alone in seeing birth spirits as central concepts. The literature on Indonesia alone is extensive, as will be discussed in Chapter 3.

Because the cluster of ideas that the Laujé call umputé is so widespread, I believe it is Austronesian in origin. It exists primarily in the Malayo-Polynesian, or Austronesian-speaking world.

5. In most scholars minds, structuralism is a theoretical perspective inspired by Claude Lévi-Strauss, a French anthropologist who came to prominence in the fifties and remained influential until the eighties. In fact, however, structuralism first began in the thirties under the stewardship of Dutch scholars like J. P. B. de Josselin de Jong and F. A. E. van Wouden who used Eastern Indonesia as the source for data from which they developed their theories. As J. J. Fox noted in Flow of Life (1980), van Wouden's (1935) work can be "seen as an early example of structuralism: one of the first systematic studies of the implications of different rules of cross-cousin marriage and of the patterns of exchange that these rules entail." Other commentators (de Heusch 1982:33–34) have recognized that the Dutch structuralists were clearly precursors to Claude Lévi-Strauss's work in Les Structures Elémentaires de la Parenté (1949) and are thus theoretically related to the ideas of later structuralists like Leach (1954), and Needham (1958).

6. Symbolic anthropology was a quite popular, yet diverse, discipline in the seventies and eighties. Though theorists as disparate in perspective as Sherry Ortner (1973 author of "Key Symbols") and Rodney Needham (1979 author of Symbolic Classifications) claimed to be symbolic anthropologists, their approaches were often at odds with one another. Ortner focused more on a particular symbol's meaning and Needham more on the structure of the categories in which symbols were classified. It is not my purpose here to explain the whole field and its branches, but it is important to note that the overarching gloss "symbolic anthropology" actually encompasses theorists who differ in many respects.

7. When I conducted fieldwork, from 1984 to 1986, the government census listed the Laujé population as 15,000 (Anema 1983). I am not sure, however, which Laujé people this included. In 1995 the census for the Tinombo District listed all the residents of the whole district as 11,000 total. Laujé live not only in the mountains and coasts of the Tinombo District (where I conducted fieldwork), but also in the mountains and coasts of Kecematan Tomini and Kecematan Dondo. If all these people are counted, then the 15,000 sum may be too low. My guess would be 35,000 people could claim they were ethnic Laujé, but I have never conducted a systematic census, nor am I confident it would tell me much. Claiming to "be" Laujé, is an ambiguous status. Depending upon who the questioner was, who was listening, and how close the census was to tax time, the answers could vary considerably. For more on this, see Nourse 1993.

8. Most of the highlanders are regarded by lowlanders as "subjects." They are swidden farmers who also grow cash crops. Though in other areas in In-

donesia, wet rice is cultivated on hillsides and mountains through elaborate irrigation and terracing, here in Central Sulawesi where the population density is comparatively low, wet rice is only cultivated on flat land. It is easier to cultivate dry rice on the hillsides. Thus the wet-rice cultivators live in the lowlands and have traditionally modeled themselves after hierarchical kingdoms in other parts of Sulawesi and beyond. The highlanders only intermittently paid tribute to the lowlanders, who nevertheless continued to regard highlanders as their subjects.

Following Hildred Geertz's 1963 lead, most of the literature on Indonesia tends to regard the wet-rice cultivators as culturally distinct from the dry-rice cultivators. It also tends to separate the hierarchical polities of Sulawesi, Bali, Java, the Malay peninsula, and scattered others, saying they were cousins to Polynesian chiefdoms (see also Palmier 1960). Geertz separates these polities from hill tribes, which she regarded as discrete, egalitarian polities, much like those in Eastern Indonesia and New Guinea. My work denies that distinction (see also Palmier 1960).

9. Indeed, making a radical break with the past is a characteristic of postmodernists who relish and even take "a certain delight—some critics would say nihilistic delight—in the impossibility of any universal understanding, any incontestable truth, any indefeasible argument, any ultimate authority. God is surely dead in the post-modernist world" (Crapanzano 1992:88).

10. In 1985 several graduate students and faculty members at the University of Virginia, where I received my Ph.D., had participated in a seminar with Richard Rorty on postmodernism. Though I was still in the field and thus never participated, they continued to discuss insights from that seminar, which then had a great influence on me.

11. Accusations that anthropological writing had been prejudiced came primarily from outside the discipline through the work of Edward Said (1975, 1978) and Talal Asad (1973) who accused anthropologists of looking at the Other through the lens of colonialists.

12. Said, Asad, Clifford, and Marcus delineate Evans-Pritchard and Malinowski as the most egregiously racist anthropologists. Though Evans-Pritchard and Malinowski have clear colonialist and racist biases, it is also evident that they were trying to present "the natives" in a more favorable light than they had been presented before. In *Nuer Religion* Evans-Pritchard intended to show how similar the Nuer notion of kwoth was to the Christian notion of God (p'Bitek 1970; Mazrui 1970) (see Note 4 in Chapter 8), and Malinowski intended to show how rational the Trobrianders were. Though both perspectives tended to make "the native" like us, they were nevertheless more inclusive and radical than the western audience reading about "the natives" were at the time.

13. Marcus and Fischer's 1986 book quite unfairly criticized the whole

Manchester school, and specifically focused on Max Gluckman's work. I say the criticism was unfair because it refused to recognize Gluckman's legacy to postmodernism. For instance, rather than acknowledging that the Manchester School of Gluckman and Turner was the first to initiate the anthropological focus on dissension and contest, Marcus and Fisher tend to trivialize the analytic depth of the Manchesterian approach by relegating it to legalese, saying Gluckman's and Turner's "use of cases [was] inspired by the case method in law" which meant it was inferior to more scientific analysis (1986:57). Moreover, rather than acknowledging that in the 1940s Godfrey Wilson, Monica Wilson, and Max Gluckman were the first to advocate studying processes of colonialism and the way they channeled labor into towns and plantations, while undermining tribal economic, political, and domestic institutions, Marcus and Fisher accuse these ethnographies of being "locally bounded and relatively ahistoric, to avoid considering the larger system of colonial political economy itself" (1986:84). And in the ultimate case of the pot-calling-the-kettle-black, Marcus and Fisher critique the Manchester school for leaving interpretation to individual readers. They say that a series of different ethnographies of tribal economies and the effects of the colonial system on them that were produced by Gluckman in the 1940s for the Rhodes Livingstone Institute in Northern Rhodesia "proved to be the weak part of the project [because] making systematic connections was left to individual readers of the separate studies (1986:91). Rather than acknowledge that this was an early experiment to avoid the anthropologist's authoritative voice (as Marcus and Clifford applaud in Tyler's hands), Marcus and Fisher choose to critique Gluckman's effort. I believe the rush to embrace literary postmodernism has led anthropologists to ignore sensitive and well-thought-out answers to questions already explored several generations before in our own discipline. So we do not continually reinvent the wheel, we need to construct new questions on the shoulders of others and recognize the value of our own anthropological legacy.

14. Though postmodernists like Derrida (1973) and Foucault (1982) have argued that individual agency is a product of the western philosophical tradition, nevertheless the anthropological focus on agency is often inspired by postmodernists' tendency to look at individuals. More in line with postmodernism, though, is the way in which members of the Manchester school examine the countercultural beliefs.

15. Victor Turner (1957) proposed just such an approach forty years ago in *Schism and Continuity in an African Society*. Turner's key informant, Sandombu, was portrayed as an analogue to the anthropologist, an astute observer and exegete. Griaule in *Conversations with Ogotemmeli* (1948) demonstrates how astute Ogotemmeli is, but does not, like Turner, discuss his own perceptions alongside his informants'. It was in the 1960s, in the Casagrande volume, that this method was confirmed as mainstream.

16. Acciaioli notes (personal communication) that the structuralism found in Austronesian cultures owes as much to the Dutch anthropologists as to the British and French anthropologists.

17. One only has to read any of the C. Geertz (1973) essays, the Anderson essays (1990), Tsing's book (1993), the Kipp and Rodgers collection (1987) or the Atkinson and Errington volume (1990) to get a sense of the way distance from Java and from strongly Islamic communities (like Aceh in North Sumatra) have contributed to locals' sense of marginality and, in turn, helped to define ethnographic practice in Indonesia.

18. *Siamae* means father of, and *Siinai* means mother of. Such teknonyms are common Laujé forms of address.

1. Meeting "The" Laujé

1. Traube's book (*Cosmology and Social Life*, 1986) might nowadays be read as the culmination of a certain era's anthropology (structuralist in orientation) in a certain area of the world (East Timor) where structure, as endlessly transforming binary oppositions and locals questing after meaning, is ubiquitous. Though Traube's key informants seemed ideal to me, I knew it would be difficult to replicate her 1970s fieldwork, which had been conducted prior to the fall of the very distant Portuguese colony and invasion of the very near Indonesian army. The Mambai Traube studied had lived in isolated, remote, and seemingly "traditional" villages.

2. My good friend and colleague Greg Acciaioli was conducting field research in Central Sulawesi in the Lake Lindu region. Greg happened to be in Palu when I came to the area and he kindly introduced me to the regent for the District of Donggala, Bupati Jan Kaleb. I told the regent that I wanted to study autochthonous religion. He recommended I study the tribal people (suku terasing) called the Laujé. The term *suku terasing* literally translates as "the tribes who have become foreign." These people are classified by the government as people who "do not yet have a religion" (belum beragama), yet this government official, ironically enough, recommended them as people who practice autochthonous religion (see Acciaioli 1985; Atkinson 1987). According to Acciaioli, most officials of the Central Sulawesi government define *suku terasing* in rather broad, pejorative terms: "1. Those who continually wander: hunter-gatherers; 2. Those who wander only half the time, that is, those who have no fixed wet-rice fields, but do return periodically to a fixed settlement: have only a meager income: subsistence paddy farmers with no surplus rice production or cash crops" (Acciaioli 1985:165).

3. When I first surveyed the mountain area in 1980, the Laujé were categorized, as I said above, as suku terasing. This is an odd term, for it designates

the indigenous people who have not become westernized, who continue, at least in the minds of the government, to live a "backward" style of life as foreigners. Atkinson (1987) and Acciaioli (1985) have written extensively about this issue. During the 1980s, however, the government began to downplay the mountain Laujé's status as suku terasing, instead emphasizing the mountain people's integration into the world economy (through cash cropping) and religion (Christianity and Islam).

4. From my preliminary 1980 visit, I believed the Laujé fit Hildred Geertz's definition of an animist hill tribe practicing indigenous religion. In her influential article on Indonesian culture and communities, Hildred Geertz divided Indonesian societies into four distinct categories or "sociocultural types," based on ecological adaptation, political structure, religious belief, and social hierarchy. She maintains that "most of these mountain societies remained, at least until the present century, in virtual isolation from the outside world, each developing its own distinctive patterns of life . . . generally left untouched by either Hinduism or Islam" (1963:31). From the sparse preliminary data I found on the highland Laujé, they seemed to fit Geertz's tribal category and be distinct from the lowlanders in Tinombo who fit her *pasisir* or coastal culture category. Pasisir are coastal people of Malay origins who are Islamic. They intermarry locals and are usually petty capitalists. Geertz's ideal types did not reflect the "real" interaction I observed between mountain Laujé and lowlanders.

5. The Laujé refer to anything or any person who is not native or autochthonous to the region as "foreign."

6. Until recently there has been enough land and low enough population density that dry-rice cultivation could prevail on the hillsides. Unfortunately, however, a Canadian development study (Anema 1983) has found that land in the Tinombo area is used to its maximum capacity in dry-rice cultivation. No one, however, is switching to wet-rice cultivation. Rather, Tinombo's landless farmers have moved to transmigration centers 40 to 50 miles north of Tinombo. The remaining coastal dwellers are often forced to eke out a living as part-time wage laborers and wet-rice farmers.

7. During the colonial period, the Dutch began to systematically open up wet-rice fields in every village, including Dusunan, Tinombo, and Lombok. The fields in Dusunan and Lombok frequently flooded because they were on the banks of the Tinombo (formerly named Siavu) River and thus did not prove fruitful. Tinombo began to grow as a business and market center, and thus land there became too scarce to use for wet-rice fields. Consequently, flat land in newly created villages, Baina'a and Sidoan, was opened for wet-rice cultivation. The aristocrats from Tinombo and Dusunan were the main ones who owned these fields, though some poorer Laujé did move to Sidoan to take advantage of the newly cultivated acreage. It is probably due to this that Sidoan today tends to have a per capita income higher than Dusunan.

8. These dates are approximate because the records contradict one another.

9. The ethnicity of this raja is a hotly debated question. For more detail on this please refer to Nourse (1991).

10. At the time of my fieldwork, the former raja's son, known affectionately as Om Yaum Tombolotutu, lived in the palace, but when I returned to the field in 1997, the palace had been turned into a museum and the beautiful bougainvillaea shrubs and potted plants gracing the lawn had been removed. The palace now stands shut, its pristine and rather sterile garden gated to all who pass by.

11. The chief of police had decreed that all mountain Laujé take off their machetes before entering the marketplace. He made this rule some fifteen years before because a cuckolded mountain man had gone berserk in the market, swinging his machete at his wife's lover. In the process of lunging for the adulterous man, the machete-carrying man injured many bystanders. The chief of police presumed all mountain Laujé could run amok in the same way at anytime in the future, so he banned all machetes.

12. The town itself was uninviting. In Dusunan there were no asphalt roads, no electrical poles, just a jumble of bamboo huts on stilts. To me, Dusunan was an invisible, less affluent suburb of Tinombo, its people just like those in Tinombo, only more impoverished and more callous to mountain Laujé. It seemed a dark tangle of old coconut trees, most of which had been pawned and forfeited to Tinombo immigrants. Coconut trees start to produce after about eight years, but they do not produce to their full capacity until after sixteen years. At eight years, though, they are at 15 percent capacity and by twelve years they are at 60 percent capacity. For sixteen to fifty years, a coconut tree can produce at full 100 percent capacity, and for another ten years (in other words, at an age of sixty years) a tree can produce up to 70 percent of its capacity. By the time the tree is over seventy years old, it is down to 20 percent of its capacity. Trees that are over eighty years old can produce little or nothing. Most of the trees in Dusunan are seventy to eighty years old. Many of the Dusunan nobles have had to place their coconut trees as collateral for cash loans. They most often need cash for weddings and funerals. Often these nobles, wanting to "keep up appearances" will borrow more than they should. When they cannot pay back their debts to Tinombo store owners, then the collateral becomes the property of the store owner. Dusunaners blame the store owners for confiscating the property before they have had time to pay back the loan, but the trees provide less and less cash for the owners and thus it takes too long to recoup their losses. Yet this also seems to be an old issue, one that the colonial documents record as far back as 1929, accusing the store owners of underhandedness, by duping innocent peasants into borrowing huge sums so they, the storeowners, can then claim the collateral as their own.

13. Unfortunately, in those first few meetings, I barely understood a word

Sumpitan said to me. We conversed in Indonesian for my benefit, but Sumpitan's Indonesian was not the formal language I had studied. It was colloquial Malay, often called Menadonese slang. Sumpitan's way of speaking showed how isolated he was from the educated speech forms and thus the whole mode of social interaction used in Tinombo, just one kilometer away from his home on the other side of the river. Sumpitan occupied the backwater world of old-style language and an Islam that was so syncretic very few "modern" Muslims accepted it.

14. The term *olongian* is used for the priest-rulers in North Central Sulawesi all the way to Gorontalo and the Tongian Islands. Within the Laujé language, the only indigenous term that seems remotely relevant to the title is the word *olongo,* to hear. Olongian could possibly mean the place of hearing, the place of listening. This would fit with the role of the olongian as a silent figure. Throughout Indonesia, the leaders with the most power are said to be passively silent, for the truly powerful do not have to exert themselves, as a warrior would, but sit quietly while others, less powerful, are attracted to the silent leader like a moth is to a flame (Moertono 1968; Anderson 1972; Geertz 1980; Errington 1989).

The other officers in the court of the olongian, the jogugu and walapuluh, are the spokespersons and the active judges in court cases heard by the olongian. The olongian, in earlier days, would not pronounce decisions, but would leave that up to the jogugu.

15. In 1905, after the major Sulawesi ports of Menado, Gorontalo, and Makassar had been successfully pacified, the Dutch began to concentrate on the Tomini Bay in Central Sulawesi. Colonial documents detailing this expansion describe the selection of immigrants to rule as a matter of expediency rather than the typical "divide and conquer philosophy." Whatever the motivations, the documents state that colonial officials hoped to find local rulers who would be willing to order their subjects to plant cash crops. They needed these local rulers to communicate through the Malay language. Most Laujé were not proficient in Malay, and the Dutch could not communicate with them. The Dutch soon turned to the immigrants who were fluent in Malay and claimed to be aristocrats, descendants of junior lines from the Mandar and Bugis courts in South Sulawesi.

16. It seems as if the first palace for the raja was actually built in the town of Tomini, twenty-five miles north of Tinombo, though documents and oral histories are not clear. The Tomini harbor, say oral histories, proved to be too shallow for the Dutch ships, and thus the whole capital of the kingdom (Swapradja) of Moutong was moved to Tinombo in 1928.

17. Despite the fact that the olongian is one of six Dusunan families who own coconut fields that are four times the average size, there is little surplus for bricks and cement. The olongian, as part of his office, owns a wet-rice field

(in the town of Sidoan) large enough to supply subsistence needs. Additionally, he has coconut fields. When the Dutch first came in the 1910s, all people were required to plant coconut trees. The highlanders were also forced to plant trees. Many of them turned over their parcels of trees to the olongian or to the olongian's family members. But because most of the olongian had large families, these parcels have become smaller through the generations. A parcel of land is passed down (at least until recently when Islamic law has stipulated that only brothers receive inherited property) equally among brothers and sisters. Thus, if there are twelve children in a family, the parcel will be divided into twelve units. Some people rotate these units, letting one sibling take the produce during one harvest (there are three or four harvests per year) and then another sibling at the next harvest. This is only feasible, however, if the siblings are compatible.

18. Each year community members still devoted to the olongian work in the fields "free of charge" and donate the rice produce to the olongian. In the days prior to independence, the rice and copra tribute would have been sufficient for the olongian's subsistence needs and for community feasts and "extras." Now this is not the case. The olongian's wife has to supplement their income selling fruit and vegetables at the market or performing individual curing rites for those afflicted by umputé spirits. Many people in the community gossip about the demise of the olongian's power, saying it is the wife of the olongian's fault. She has transgressed ritual prohibitions by selling in the marketplace and thus has singlehandedly brought on the decline. Some of the gossip, no doubt, is due to jealousy. Many former Laujé aristocrats are not as fortunate as the olongian. They have no one to perform the labor for them in the fields and they did not inherit a particularly large plot with their titles.

19. I have spelled momasoro in other publications as momosoro. When I returned to the field in 1997, the mayor of Lombok, S. Kiango, saw my manuscript and said I had misspelled momasoro. I asked a number of people which way was the best way to spell the ceremony. More people said momasoro than momosoro, so I have spelled it that way here.

20. Sumpitan acted as a jogugu or as a walapuluh would in the former court system. As chief officiant, the jogugu was the active organizer and thus it was appropriate for Sumpitan to invite me as an honored guest. The olongian remained passively quiet as he was expected to do.

21. Kenneth George's book, Showing Signs of Violence: The Cultural Politics of a Twentieth-Century Headhunting Ritual (1996), about the mappurondo communities around Mambi area near the Mandar coastal communities in South Sulawesi, resonates well with the ethnographic and theoretical issues discussed here. The groups in the Mambi area, like the highland and lowland Laujé, are trying to formulate their identities vis-à-vis more Islamic and more cosmopolitan peoples, although in the Mambi case they are in the

hinterland of the homeland of the Mandar, whereas the Laujé are dealing with migrants from Bugis and Mandar regions who have come to dominate the local lowlands. George shows how the performance of *pangngae* headhunting rites, which are conducted without "real heads" and without "real headhunting," serves to congeal a sense of identity in contradistinction to the outsiders. As I show, the momasoro serves in an analogous way to promote lowland Laujé identity in the face of foreign incursions and alien rajas. Moreover, like George's material, a portion of the momasoro, actually includes a headhunting ritual without a "real head." The similarities between the two very distant places are fascinating.

22. When I first arrived in Tinombo I told people I wanted a good language instructor, someone who was bilingual in Laujé and Indonesian. Several people pointed out Pak Husin Makaramah, who had worked as a policeman during the Dutch colonial period, spoke Dutch and later Japanese, in addition to Indonesian and Laujé. He was in his seventies, retired, but well educated and thus able to teach me Laujé, through Indonesian, as quickly as possible. He and his family also became our close friends.

23. The New Tribes Missionaries were members of a nondenominational organization that outlined as their "mission" converting "pagan peoples" who had not been previously contacted by other missionary organizations. This meant New Tribes Missionaries usually worked in very remote regions of the world. I met two New Tribes Mission families, the Whateleys and the Williamsons, in 1980 and it was they who kindly offered their notes so I could write a grant proposal based on recent information. When I returned in 1984, I talked with the Williamsons once more and met a new missionary family, the Lees. I asked them which villages would be best for my research and would not impinge upon their Christianization plans. They suggested Taipaobal. Taipaobal was not converting to Christianity and was possibly the mother village from which many of the other highland communities had fissioned. Moreover, it was only two peaks over from the missionaries and a relatively short hike into the mountains from Tinombo. Thus, when I was alone (Eric planned to leave after a few months to conduct his own fieldwork in West Africa) and possibly ill, the doctor in Tinombo, or the missionaries, two and a half hours away, could be reached. They also suggested Sinalutan, but it was more remote.

24. This grassland is called the "bald" and is considered abandoned because nothing will grow on it. According to Siamae Sanji, Aluban, and Pak Husin, this land used to be very fertile. During the Japanese occupation, however, Taipaobalers were forced to plant tobacco and cotton there, season after season, without leaving any fallow land. This so ruined the fields, said Siamae Sanji, that now nothing can grow there except elephant grass.

25. One scheme was to plant the whole hillside of Taipaobal with clove trees. The problem with the plan was that lowlanders wanted the Taipaoblaers

to do the planting for free. The Taipaobalers figured the lowlanders would get the money from their efforts, so inertia finally let that project die. Another scheme was to start a market in Taipaobal. This worked for a few weeks, but then died as well. Too few products and too much markup made the Taipaobalers resist buying anything. They would prefer to make the eight-hour hike down and back from the Tinombo market so they could save some of their very scarce cash. When I returned in 1997 and 1998, however, a permanent market of sorts was set up by lowland traders working privately rather than under government supervision.

26. Taipaobal has become a bridge between the more isolated highland communities and the Indonesian nation-state. The new school, the mosque, and the occasional development project are evidence of a shift in government policy toward the highland suku terasing, such as the Laujé. Until recently the government tried to encourage such groups to move out of the mountains voluntarily and to settle in the lowlands. That approach, however, has been largely unsuccessful. (To better govern the highlanders, the government at one time planned to resettle highlanders in the lowlands. This plan actually spanned back to the colonial period. When the Dutch first came to the area, they forced the highlanders to relocate in the Lombok area. No highlander relocated permanently, but the colonial Dutch and the postcolonial, independent Indonesian governments have been trying to implement this plan since the 1920s.) (For more information on such plans, see Haba 1998.) In the last few years, the government has undertaken a compromise. They have selected some communities, like Taipaobal, as targets of development. The government hopes Taipaobal will serve as a magnet to attract other more distant highland communities to government projects. To develop their plan further, the government plans to construct a covered marketplace and a clinic in Taipaobal.

This "progress" is not without its negative repercussions. Because Taipaobal acts as a bridge community, it finds itself perched precariously on an economic and ecological fence. For instance, Taipaobalers are Muslim converts, so pigs are rampant. (Pigs are widespread because the newly converted Taipaobal Muslims are so afraid that pork is taboo [haram] that they do not even want to set up traps for them. They are afraid that if a pig is caught in the trap, they would have to touch it when they removed it and that this would pollute them. Thus pigs run wild in the fields, destroying quite a bit of the corn and rice crops.) Goats, central to Muslim feasts, are new to Taipaobal, and they are eating more than their share of the planted crops. Because residence patterns are more stable and the community more concentrated, many swidden fields are overplanted. Some of the land, called the bald, is given over to tall elephant grasses since nothing else can grow there. As erosion and lessened fallow periods take their toll, crop productivity has declined severely.

Taipaobalers still plant a small crop of upland rice once every year, but the yields are meager. Rice is the Laujé prestige crop and the people of Taipaobal used to be able to subsist entirely on the rice they grew. Now the average family only eats upland rice for approximately four months a year. The only predictable food crop is corn. The only cash crops are garlic and shallots. (When I left the field, several people in the highlands had started planting coffee, cloves, and chocolate. No one, to my knowledge, had yet made any money on their new ventures, but according to Tania Li [1996], as of 1995, all of these "new" cash crops had come to fruition.) The cash from shallots and garlic provides them with the funds to buy rice from the lowlands, making highlanders more dependent upon lowlanders and their cash economy.

27. Lowlanders told me, and Siamae Sanji corroborated their story, that the older members of Sinalutan had once lived in Taipaobal and had run into the deep forest to settle Sinalutan, when the Dutch came up the mountains and forced everyone to resettle in present-day Lombok. Some community members just ran away, rather than acquiesce to the Dutch imperative to move below.

28. Acciaioli notes that the root, *bela,* in Bugis means "distant," usually appearing in the adjectival form *mabela.* In Laujé *mabela* means a division, like a "string" of rattan used to divide a field so that different kinds of seeds can be planted in different divided places *(pinobelaang).* Eighteenth-century Dutch documents about the Gorontalo olongian and rajas in nearby Toli-Toli reported the use of the term *bela* to refer to the To Belo, the Moluccan trade partners from Ternate.

29. I could not tell if these tattoos were permanent or not. They looked permanent at the time, but I have not noticed any since then.

30. Sair is implying that the Sinalutan dwellers are merely foragers, not horticulturalists. Though he had no anthropological knowledge of evolutionary theory, his comments implied an indigenous ranking of horticulture above foraging.

31. Eric evokes the Native American reservation here because of the passivity of the mountain Laujé and because of the seeming control the lowlanders have over Taipaobal life.

32. These all-night dances were not autochthonous, but imported from the Poso region. The dances, called *modero,* were circle dances in which boys called girls to come join their "side" of the circle. The songs for the dance were sung only in the Pamona language (see Acciaioli 1985 on the origins of modern modero).

33. The gender of the olongian is much debated. Some people, highlanders such as Siamae Sanji, say that the office of olongian was originally filled by males. The office was handed over to a female when the daughter of a male olongian married a Kaili man, converted to Islam, and moved to Dusunan seven generations ago. (This event will be explained in detail in Chapter 2.) Subsequently only women became olongians. Other people, such as the low-

landers in Dusunan, say that the office of olongian was primarily filled by females, but it depended upon the birth order (oldest sibling was always offered the position first), and willingness of descendants who took the ascribed position whether or not the olongian was actually a male or a female. My records show that from the late eighteenth century until the 1960s the olongian was a female. The last two olongian have been male.

2. Sibling Rivalry: Competing Histories

1. The New Tribes Missionaries began to Christianize the Laujé in the mid-1970s. Before they built a base in the highlands two mountains over from Taipaobal, the missionaries lived in Tinombo and regularly flew their plane up to a small landing strip near their mountain mission. In 1983, as part of the Trans-Sulawesi highway project, a bridge was constructed near the Tinombo airstrip. Since that time, the missionaries have not been able to take off and land in Tinombo. They thus switched their base to Palu.

2. The communitywide rituals practiced with bela in the highlands were once conducted in a manner similar to the first part of the momasoro. These rites, called the mantalapu, no longer are performed, because the pasobo who knew the prayers for the rite died without passing the prayers down to his son. Despite knowing this "fact" Taipaobalers blame the ritual's demise on the bela, who they say refused to attend the rite during the smallpox epidemic and thus destroyed the unity among mountain villages.

3. Lowland Laujé cosmology is roughly divided into three domains—the center of the sea, the center of the earth and the center of water. Each "center" appears to have its own hierarchy or pantheon of spirits and also to have its own physical location. The center of the sea is said to be at the eye of the sun, in Mecca. The center of the earth is sometimes said to be at the olongian's "palace," sometimes at Polu Irandu, and sometimes at Polu Batala. The center of the water is located at the mountain source of the Tinombo River high in the central mountains.

4. Dutch documents (van der Hart 1853; van Hoevell 1892; Riedel 1870) mention that by 1820 the Dutch had recognized a Mandar sovereign in the Tomini Bay. This Mandar ruler lived in Moutong and he claimed that "Tinombo" was a vassal state to his own. In turn, the Mandar ruler was a vassal to the raja of Gorontalo to whom he sent an annual tribute of gold. The Gorontalo raja paid tribute to the Dutch who were based at that time in the city of Gorontalo.

These sources also mentioned that as long ago as 1850 Tinombo was a major marketplace dominated by immigrant traders (van Hoevell 1892). During the nineteenth century, immigrant traders moved to Tinombo to sell their

wares. Most of the early traders in the Tinombo market were from South Sulawesi. The Bugis and Mandar were sailors who brought glassware and manufactured goods such as brass plates to Tinombo via ships that would come
once a month. Riding on horseback across the thin arm of Central Sulawesi,
the Kaili brought silk cloths relatives had woven. The Kaili tended to stay
longer than the sailors from South Sulawesi, but eventually many of the sailors
and the horseback traders settled in what is present day Tinombo (then called
Siavu). Along the southern banks of the Tinombo River, each ethnic group
built its own compound of huts for the immigrant traders. According to descendants of these people, the immigrants usually married Laujé women from
Dusunan who often moved to the compounds to live with their spouses.

5. Dutch sources contradict what Sumpitan says here. It is not my intention, however, to discuss the veracity of one narrative over another. I plan to
detail the differences between colonial records and native views of history in
another book.

6. Dutch documents and oral traditions indicate that the Dutch did indeed
wage war in the region from 1901 to 1904 in their campaign to find, and im-
prison, the man named Tombolotutu, who resisted the Dutch choice of raja
(Mashyuda 1979). The war of 1901 was led by Tombolotutu, a Mandar man
from Moutong, who claimed the Dutch had no right to declare a Bugis man,
Daeng Malino, to be raja. Tombolotutu ran into the mountains to hide from
the Dutch. The soldiers eventually found him, minutes after he had prevented
soldiers from capturing him by using his own sword to take his life.

Siamae Sanji says he served as a water boy in 1905 when Tombolotutu
passed through Laujé territory. Siamae Sanji says that Tombolotutu's grandchildren told him that Tombolotutu's wife was with Tombolotutu when he
died. She was pregnant with Kuti (whose birth name is Datu Pamusu Tombolotutu or the Rebel Raja), but instead of giving birth when she should, she
"held Kuti inside her" until it was safe to stop and give birth. She held on until her husband took his own life. When the baby was born, he was immediately given his father's sacred sword. Baby Kuti was also said to be born with
a full set of teeth. Both the sword and the teeth indicate that he had great spiritual power (baraka).

7. Actually other civil servants, alive at the time, say the palace was moved
first from Moutong to Tomini because the Dutch no longer wanted to house
their offices where they had encountered such strong resistance from locals. A
few years later, however, because the Tomini harbor was so shallow, the palace
was moved to Tinombo.

8. Malay is the original term for the Indonesian language, which was only
officially designated as Indonesian after national independence. Malay was a
market language used as the lingua franca for all those people from other ethnic groups who traded at the Tinombo market.

9. The Dutch were quite sincere about instilling the virtues of honesty and thrift into local government. Thus Sumpitan's story about bribing the Dutch to place Raja Borman in power is highly unlikely. On another issue, according to the Borman family, their father or grandfather was not Mandar, but Bugis. Sumpitan possibly conflated the two ethnicities to make a point. He did not like Borman, and he did not like the Mandar, since few Laujé had married Mandar. Thus he preferred to designate the Borman raja as Mandar, distinct from the Bugis raja he claims the olongian's daughter married. On the one hand this story conveys Sumpitan's rather free interpretation of the past, but on the other hand no one in Dusunan questioned it, even after Sumpitan died. The story also shows how readily locals believe outsiders are able to collude when locals are not, and it also shows that ethnic identity is rather fluidly and freely used as a marker.

10. According to Anderson (1972), there is a fine line between rulers who have power, and leaders who are corrupt and greedy. The rulers who have power do not have to try to gain wealth; it just comes to them as naturally as a moth goes to a flame. Those who try to gain wealth for their own worldly use are leaders who are corrupt. They often dissipate the well-being of the kingdom, and thus their own power, through antics like gambling. Eventually, earthquakes, famine, war, and pestilence besiege such leaders and their subjects.

11. Gambling was prohibited by the colonial government, though it was allowed one day a year on Queen Wilhelmina's birthday.

12. Tombolotutu was the son of the Mandar man who had opposed Daeng Malino as raja and had led the war against the Dutch in 1901. Even more ironic was the fact that Kuti Tombolotutu had studied in reformist Islamic schools, which by the late 1920s were already on the Dutch list of potential insurrectionist centers. Nevertheless, the Dutch selected Kuti to be raja in 1927.

13. The letter states:

With due respect to the honorable President of the Republic of Indonesia, we the people under the jurisdiction of the Raja of Moutong, say he is no longer fit to rule because all of his prohibitions under the name of the Islamic religion . . . destroy the safety and peace of all levels of the Indonesian people in his jurisdiction. He is like a spy for the Dutch, who follows their policies and not those of the people. 1. [This clause is reported in Chapter 2.] 2. Whenever he goes to the villages, he gathers up the girls there so he can fondle their bodies, such as happened to one girl named Itja from Ongka, when she got on an oxcart to go to Dambubu, Kuti sat and "rolled her" (petted her) and then hugged her and kissed her and grabbed her breasts in the cart. 3. Also a married woman in Tada, named Aditasa, he raped her, first in an adulterous manner, then he called the imam of Tada to approve of their marriage, thus blaspheming the Islamic law against bigamy. He behaved as if the people of Tada were not Islamic. During this matter he behaved like an animal, not like a Raja. We ask with respect that the SwapRaja be eradicated and joined with the People's Parliament in Jakarta.

14. According to some Tinomboers, mainly descendants of the raja, the area was free of violence and problems during the 1950s because the raja was friends with the leader of the Darul Islam movement. Others said that it was free of violence because the raja had power (baraka). Several people in Tinombo said that when Kuti toured the local villages, the villagers brought water for him to consecrate. This water—filled with the baraka or spiritual power of his words—would then serve as a panacea. "A sip," as one man put it, "would cure a cold; a drop rubbed into a wound would heal it." Many of these people claimed that the raja was a saint. Not all agree as to why the Swapradja was free of violence and problems during this period. Some say it was because the Haupt Imam was friends with the leader of the Darul Islam movement. According to still others, the Laujé area was free of violence and problems during this period, because the Laujé knew the "magic" to keep their land pure and free of violence.

15. The term *puangé* is used in Ternate. It is not clear whether this term was borrowed from that early spice kingdom, or whether it actually came from the Bugis language. The Bugis were renowned sailors and were said to have reached the Saudi Arabian peninsula in the fifth century. Thus, it is very likely that this term, *puangé,* did come from the Bugis language and had been carried to Ternate years before.

Acciaioli (personal communication) notes that *puang* in Bugis means *lord* and is a term of address for high nobles. The *é* in Bugis functions grammatically as a determiner for a noun phrase, whether a single noun or a more complex phrase: Hence, puangé, roughly "the lord," but also "puang mattinro di Rappangé, the lord who sleeps (i.e., whose corpse is buried) in Rappang." Hence a term like *the puangé* in Bugis sounds a bit overdetermined, with English definite article and detachable Bugis determiner. Usually one would cite the term in Bugis simply as *puang*. It is probably the case that Laujé, not sufficiently familiar with Bugis grammar to take apart phrases, have taken over the whole noun phrase as an inseparable noun rather than retaining the analyzability of the term. This is the same phenomenon that occurs in the term *adaé* which cannot be separated into parts *(ada)*.

Additionally Acciaioli notes that the Bugis term for nobles, *andi,* is a variant form of *anri,* which means "younger sibling." In this case, those higher in social rank are accorded the "younger sibling" term because it connotes their special status as those delicate ones who must be supported and cared for, materially and symbolically, by their lower-status followers, i.e., through support given in agricultural labor, warfare, etc. This point is not lost on Bugis commoners, some of whom are aware of folktales that present the counterdiscourse of the basic superiority of the hardy commoners over nobles, one of which is reported in Acciaioli's 1989 dissertation.

16. For instance, in the seventeenth century, the Dutch monopolized the production of certain spices through Ternate rajas. These Ternate rajas agreed to help the Dutch eradicate independent production on the other islands. Siamae Sanji mentioned two events that obviously referred to this period. The magically productive bush, which the To Belo from Ternate destroyed, referred to the cinnamon trade and the trade items the Laujé received in return. The receding sea indicated the abrupt collapse of the world market and the relegation of the Tomini Bay to the status of a backwater territory once the Dutch eradicated independent production on other islands. (See Vansina 1985 for a discussion of the way metaphors in oral traditions can be read as compact histories.)

More concretely, Siamae Sanji's mention of Cendrana referred to a Mandar kingdom, actually called Cenrana, several hundred kilometers to the south of Taipaobal and far beyond the ken of most Laujé. According to Dutch records for the mid-nineteenth century (Riedel 1870), Mandar lords, or puangé, claimed territory in the Tomini Bay as their own. Mandar vassals collected tribute in the Tomini Bay from "small kingdoms" and sent tribute back to their puangé in Cenrana.

Another detail confirmed by independent sources was Siamae Sanji's mention of the "twenty men panning for gold in Moutong" to the north of Taipaobal. In 1880 a Dutch official, Baron van Hoevell (1892), visited Moutong and noted that the raja there received a tribute from his vassals in Dusunan in the form of corveé labor: They panned gold for the puangé in the Moutong River.

17. The story dovetails with similar narratives collected by Tsing in Kalimantan (1993) and Traube in Timor (1986).

18. Exchange of products is ranked. Though the bela give food to the Taipaobalers, taro gathered from the forest, this is not considered real food. Real food is rice and corn, because these products came from the ancestors. Actually, as legend has it, ancestors sacrificed their bodies so humans could have these foods. Rice first came from the head of an older sibling, while corn came from the navel of the Nabi, or Prophet Mohammed. Raats (1969), who worked in the Philippines, has collected a body of myths concerning the origin of rice from a dismembered woman's body. He cites instances of this myth in Java, Borneo, the Manggasai of Flores, and the Bagobo and Bukidnon of Mindanao (Atkinson and Rosaldo 1975:43).

These Laujé myths are similar to, yet different from, Mambai food myths. Among the Mambai of East Timor, rice is excluded from the annual agricultural cycle because of mythological distinctions between food crops. According to Traube, "unlike all other foods, which originate out of Mother Earth's body, the path of rice is traced back to the upperworld and Father Heaven. Rice is said to be of 'recent' origin in relation to other foods" (Traube 1986:265).

19. Siamae Sanji considered selling corn a transgression of "traditional" taboos," but in the 1950s the Taipaobalers sold corn. It was only after a smallpox epidemic decimated the population that Taipaobalers said they should not sell corn. They said this was because the olongian was not following the taboo against selling food, so they had to follow the taboo. Thus the Taipaobalers became more "traditional" than the "traditional leader, the olongian."

20. The Mambi Mandar in Kenneth George's work assert their priority as "elder siblings," because they are closer to the trunk or source. This contrasts with Acciaioli's (1989) observation that among the Bugis, more often than not, people of superior status are designated as "younger sibling."

3. Gifts to the Older Sibling: Siamae Sanjé on Umputé

1. Siamae Sanji acted as both a sando and a boliang. Both terms referred to people who cured, but in the lowlands a sando was someone, usually a male, who cured and interpreted spirit words, while a boliang was a medium who was possessed by a boliang spirit. In the highlands, people used the terms *sando* and *boliang* interchangeably when referring to Siamae Sanji. When they discussed his role as a midwife, they used either term, rather than the Indonesian term *bidan*. Most of the literature translates *boliang* as shaman. I have kept local terms here because the translations convey many things that do not apply to the Laujé case. A Laujé boliang may be possessed by a spirit, but not engage in a shamanistic journey as Wana do (Atkinson 1989).

2. Siamae Sanji's daughter Idola claims that Taipaobalers have no breech births, only lowlanders and bela do because they do not know the proper magic for birth. As long as I was in Taipaobal, there were no breech births there.

3. The Taipaobalers, like many non-Islamic groups throughout the archipelago, do not see menstruation as polluting. The only time I witnessed anyone behaving differently because they were menstruating, was when Siamae Sanji's granddaughter was cooking for guests at his funeral. She said she could not cook for guests because she was too "dirty," so she went home. When menstruating in other circumstances, however, the women continue to cook for their nuclear family. Appell (1988) notes a similar attitude toward menstruation in Kalimantan.

4. Women are associated with the earth. A woman's grave is deeper in the

ground, the spirit at the center of the earth is said to be female, and the olongian was, until recently, a woman and "of the earth."

5. Once they have left their bodies, their souls are released into the pool of souls waiting to be reincarnated into other bodies, usually those of males. The notion of a finite pool of ancestral souls waiting to be reincarnated, those of "remembered" ancestors, and forgotten ones, too, is reminiscent of how only certain people, overwhelmingly men, attain the status of "named ancestor" by sponsoring stone-dragging rituals in Sumba (Hoskins 1986, 1997).

6. When the male midwife cuts each twig off the sacred tree, he utters a prayer over the twigs at the source or tree where he has found them. In the prayer he promises to return what he has taken, that is, the twig, by placing a sacred coin on the tree's trunk, and asking forgiveness from the tree. As in all the male's actions during the birth scenario, he makes sure he nurtures (through prayer) whenever he separates something.

7. No one says why the father cannot collect the nut and the leaves prior to birth. I presume it has to do with collecting items that are "born" at the same time the child is. The spirit or soul of the nut and the leaves are connected to the spirit or soul of the child, its black blood, and its placental spirit. They are all umputé, for there is an umputé spirit of trees, plants, rocks, and animals. Betel nut is symbolically related with (1) men giving sustenance or producing the child, and (2) notions of the origins of blood as a patrilateral/almost patrilineal marker.

8. In the Philippines among the Tawsug, the umbilical cord is also cut with a bamboo knife (Ewing 1960:130). According to D. Hart, the Caticugan midwife in a Bisayan, Filipino village once used a bamboo knife, but now snips the umbilicus with scissors (1965:59). The Makassae in East Timor still cut with a bamboo knife, and they hang the placenta in a momé tree (Forman 1980:343).

9. Interestingly enough, the Laujé word for iron, pué, is the Kaili word for lord. Perhaps it refers to the first Kaili "lords" who brought iron products to the Laujé. Sumpitan and Siamae Sanji told me, in portions of the history not included here, that it was the Kaili who first came as tadulako, or warriors, to this region. Perhaps they brought to the Laujé their iron swords and knowledge about how to be a noble warrior.

10. The spots on the forehead of the infant are the same three marks given in Hindu-Balinese rites performed throughout the archipelago by non-Islamic people. The marks are also given in the postbirth rites in Bali and Java (Tonjaya 1981; Ossenbruggen 1977). Hence this action represents a pre-Islamic or Hindu influence.

11. This gesture is also used when healing a sick person whose spirit or soul may leave them. It is also used when money is exchanged (see Taussig 1980, 1987).

12. The blessing said aloud is in the Laujé language, but the secret prayer is mixed with Malay. The Laujé, like others throughout the archipelago, borrow outside languages because they think the words spiritually efficacious, though they may not know their meaning (see Tsing 1987).

13. I have only provided the English translations of these and subsequent prayers and blessings because I promised Siamae Sanji, and other sando who told them to me, that I would not distribute them to the general public.

14. *Meloon* and *metedes,* upright and hardy, refer to two terms that are used continually in Laujé prayers. They refer to the first tree of the world, which rose up and separated the earth from the sky. The goal of all human beings is to be as upright and as hard or tough as that first tree and thus to strengthen that tree so that the universe will continue. Thus, the individual body and the universal world are not separate entities, but what is done for one is done for the other. Again we find that boundaries between self and outside world are very blurry for the Laujé (see Errington 1989 on macrocosm/microcosm among the Bugis).

15. I find it intriguing that though it is the father who washes the cloths and hence it is he who carelessly lets the remaining blood, and thus, the umputé of blood spirits run downstream without acknowledging them, the mother is blamed. Never did I hear any informant say that the Taipaobal father neglected the black umputé spirits when he washed the blood downstream. (In the next section on the lowlands, however, I note that it is often said there that lowland Laujé men do neglect the umputé spirit of red blood when the birth cloths are washed.) It is women whom the Siamae Sanji–trained midwives regard as neglecting the black blood spirit. This neglect is possibly related to their view that women neglect their relatives (especially if the women are in-marrying bela and are ashamed of their primitive ancestors). Often the mothers establish a teasing, almost sadistic, relationship with their children. More than once I saw Siamae Sanji's oldest daughter by his second wife intentionally trip her toddlers and then laugh uproariously when the children cried, running to their father for comfort. Other female relatives seemed to enjoy waving knives at young children's fingers, tongues, and genitals, threatening to cut them off. Thus, at least in Siamae Sanji's family, the mothers are neglectful compared to the more nurturing fathers, and this may explain some of the association of neglected black umputé with the female gender.

16. Coconuts are called the nest or womb *(benuo)* in Laujé and are probably significant in this birth scenario because they contain such a large seed, just as the placenta contains such a large seed—the baby. As we shall see in lowland rituals, the coconut is also used to replace heads now that headhunting is no longer allowed (see George 1996). They say that the head or an eye is the first part of a human body to form in the womb, though Siamae Sanji's family

denies this is part of their ideology. Some Taipaobal Laujé do equate the coconut juice with sexual fluid and perhaps this prohibition against consuming
the sexual fluid at this point has to do with birth-control beliefs.

17. When a person dies and the body is cleansed before burial, the corpse
is placed perpendicular to this position, across relatives' shins.

18. This umbilical cord was once used by elders as a medicine for curing
the child from umputé-related sicknesses, but now other rites are used. In this
old rite, though, a bit of the cord was scraped off into water, and the child
stroked, or massaged *(nosaub)*, with the solution. The same was done with
seeds to be planted on certain occasions. Nowadays, though, this packet is just
stored, for the knowledge for curing the children with this umbilical cord has
been replaced by more elaborate offerings first practiced by Siamae Sanji.

19. Thus, it would seem that as others have theorized for Melanesia (e.g.,
Strathern 1987), inside/outside exchanges have to occur at the important
points of reproduction in the life cycles of society and culture.

20. Siamae Sanji blows *(nosumpali)* on the water three times before he
gives it to the afflicted to drink. He says blowing resembles the winds that the
spirits travel on. Laderman (1983, 1988, 1991) discusses the spirit winds and
Malay healers who travel in a very similar manner. Like the Malay healers,
Siamae Sanji "blows" to call the spirits or to send them away. When he finishes the short prayers, he very quietly, almost inaudibly, murmurs "Oa" and
then audibly swallows or gulps air. Siamae Sanji says that when he swallows
air in this fashion, he is swallowing the name of the umputé spirit, or the name
of the place in which umputé spirits live. Unless one knows the spirit's name,
or home, the prayer will not "reach" the spirits, nor will it be heard by them.
If the curer fails to attract the spirits' attention, then the person will remain ill.

21. Taipaobal sando trained by Siamae Sanji used to perform these same
cures for people in lowland villages, or for the bela in their mountain communities, but invariably many of those people would never perform their "payment" offerings. This deplorable actuality, say Siamae Sanji's children, is not
only dangerous to the afflicted, but to the sando as well, because they, their
family, or the whole Taipaobal community can suffer from the wrath of the
unpaid, or unpropitiated, umputé spirits. As a result of these defaults, Taipaobal sando now rarely perform such rites outside their own village. They only
perform them in Taipaobal, where they are sure the recipients will repay them.

22. The sando usually comes alone, but depending on how well off the person who has been cured is, they might invite extended family and neighbors. I
found that when I first came to Taipaobal, very few people could afford to include outsiders like myself in the payment ceremonies. So I volunteered to provide several liters of rice and buy anything else needed. This was greatly ap-
preciated and opened many doors for me.

23. Informants say these trays (selasa) were originally used to dry tobacco

(a product, incidentally, that the Laujé say came from outside the Laujé area and can be traded for cash), but hardly any Laujé in the lowlands and highlands grow tobacco today, so I never saw anyone actually using the trays for drying tobacco. Nevertheless, in island Melanesia, specifically in New Ireland, Roy Wagner (1986b) has found very similar trays to exist as drying platforms for catching the fluids from the body after death. A recent book on the Bugis (Pelras 1996), Volkman's book on the Toraja (1985), Metcalf's on the Berawan of Borneo (1989), and Schiller's on Borneo (1997) all make mention of drying platforms for corpses. Because trays similar to the drying platforms are used in Laujé sacrifices and because the lowland Laujé so adamantly reiterate that the rice offerings on the tray signify the human body, I think the connection between the human drying trays for corpses and these rice offering trays is fairly clear, though no informant actually said this. Laujé are loathe to recall how their own ancestors, and even parents, may have participated in funerals in which the corpse lay on a platform for over 100 days (see Atkinson 1987) because they know Muslims would disapprove. Islam places a premium on quick burial after death.

Likewise, I suspect that the five cylinders hung under the trays were originally used to catch the fluids from a rotting corpse. Roy Wagner finds this to be the case in New Ireland (1986b), and Volkman (1985) finds this among the Toraja. Atkinson notes that among the Wana in Central Sulawesi, cylinders were once used to collect menstrual fluid. That these cylinders hang underneath the tray suggests that they "catch" whatever waste products fall from the platform and thus are structurally opposed to the black blood of childbirth, which is not caught before it drops from the house and falls on the ground. Conversely, the white chicken offering is like the placenta and like the child's body, which are kept above the ground in the house or in a tree.

24. Not all mountain Laujé use cradles to hang their babies from the rafters. Many just hang them in a cloth sarong from one of the roof beams. It looks something like a bundle hanging from a stork's beak. The cradles are probably introductions from the lowlands. Only the Taipaobal Laujé and those Laujé who live closer to the lowlands use the cradle.

25. The language here, *lele'e antuonyé*, translates as "it is said that it means." Though such a phrase is rhetorical, it is also very honorific. The meaning is not considered important in prayers, but the honorific quality of the words shows respect for the spirits. In fact, the less words are understood the more efficacious the Laujé seem to regard them. (See Tsing 1987 for a similar scenario in Kalimantan; also Brenneis and Myers 1984 for wider Austronesian cases.) This phrase also represents an ancient speech pattern no longer used. It is the equivalent of "Our father who art in heaven, hallowed be thy name." Unless Laujé have studied this speech, they do not understand it.

Luckily Sair, Larsen, and Konté had studied antiquated language with their father and were well versed in translating it for me.

26. In other mountain communities, the birds for black chicken offerings must be "wild" and those for white chicken "domesticated." In those white ceremonies, the chicken does not have to be immature.

27. These meals are quite costly for the Laujé, roughly two months wages earned in garlic production. Many people save up their offerings and perform two or three at a time or conduct them with neighbors or relatives (usually one and the same). These meals, though, are not quite as elaborate as the funeral feasts that are given once a year to remember a close and recently deceased relative. In those, often a goat is slaughtered and fifty to sixty people invited (though only a sliver of meat is served to each person, quite a bit of rice is served). They often must buy the rice from the go-between to whom they sell their garlic in Lombok. These meals are comparable to wedding banquets, which often cost as much as a whole year's salary.

28. Jane Atkinson (1984), who worked with the neighboring Wana in Central Sulawesi, says betel nut is the exchange item used between enemies, and between prospective marriage partners, and in-laws. Atkinson's findings dovetail nicely with the Laujé since two realms, spiritual and human, are also being bridged.

29. Taipaobalers practice ritual bleaching or whitening of the bride before marriage. The bride is confined to the "hearth" of the house and covered in a paste for three days. A fire is built underneath the house, and it is frequently fanned so that smoke reaches her room. After three or four days, the black paste is removed. Her skin is said to be "white" and "good enough for marriage." (See Ortner 1981 and Sahlins 1981 for similar practices in Polynesia.)

30. As in the prayer before, the name of the spirit's residence (Dinding Batu) is not a Laujé word, but is borrowed from Malay. This use of "foreign" words in prayer is typical of Laujé and others elsewhere in Indonesia (Metcalf 1989; Tsing 1987). Because they are unintelligible words, they represent independent checks against explicit interpretations.

31. Women are rumored to regularly abort children in the highlands. I know of at least two young, unmarried girls in Taipaobal who were rumored to have aborted their children while I was there. Nevertheless, when I asked people the Laujé word for miscarriage, they told me it was the same as abortion. Thus, I do not know if these rumors were about miscarriages or abortions.

32. After the prayer, the antique coin is also removed from the tray. These coins are scarce and needed for all curing ceremonies involving contact with spirits or curers in which an exchange between the spirit world and humans, or between unlike substances, occurs. Trade between Taipaobalers and bela is

initiated by a Taipaobaler giving the bela one of these coins. Marriage proposals always involve such a coin, because the coin is said to "strengthen the bond." I think they also are such significant icons because they bring together disparate domains. In marriage they bring together two families; in trade relations, they bring together two social groups differentially ranked, and in offerings they bring together the human and the spirit world.

33. Traube writes that "Eastern Indonesian societies are already well known in the ethnographic literature for the pronounced dualistic organization of their categorical schemes, as well as for a tendency to realize symbolic dualisms in social arrangements. Dual classification entails the ordering of symbolic categories into pairs of opposites, such as male/female, heaven/earth, above/below, outside/inside. Sets of dual categories are combined in particular contexts and used to represent diverse realms of experience. Whereas a principle of complementarity is signified by the redundant unions of opposites, an equally important feature of the classifications is categorical asymmetry. Typically, one element in any pair is marked as superior to its complement, and the differential ranking of complementary categories expresses hierarchical relationships" (1986:4).

34. I thank Greg Acciaioli (personal communication) for pointing out the encompassing qualities of white umputé to me.

35. The clothing of these black umputé spirits, say informants, is just like the clothing of the Javanese coolies who worked in the cotton and tobacco fields during the Japanese occupation. Oddly enough, though, it is black clothing that very isolated peoples in Sulawesi, such as the hill communities in Tana Toraja (Volkman 1985), wear. Since Siamae Sanji says black is symbolically associated with the isolated bela, perhaps the informant who referenced the Javanese coolies was wrong.

36. The spirit possessing curers is an ancestral spirit connected to the past, just as the white umputé spirit is. Ancestors who have great spiritual power, who were sando themselves, are called boliang. Before they die they transfer the knowledge of how to contact the spirit familiar to sons, and sometimes, daughters. The boliang spirits are passed down to respected sons and daughters who will continue to create bonds with others through postmarital residence within the community. Because nowadays daughters often marry outside the community, even though they should not, these boliang spirits are usually inherited through patrilineal lines. Sometimes a strong or assertive daughter is chosen to be a recipient. These females, though, usually have familial ties to important male figures in the community. They have not married out of the village and their mothers are usually not the in-marrying bela.

37. For instance, the boliang spirit possessing Siamae Sanji may retrieve a dart that has been lodged in someone's eyebrow. This is the spot that clearly indicates witchcraft has been used. Once the boliang extracts the dart, it cures

the person of listlessness or unwillingness to eat. Sometimes boliang spirits are summoned when a person's crops are afflicted by drought or floods. These white spirits can reverse the trend merely by listening to the needs of the humans and returning to the spirits in heaven to beseech them to stop bothering humans. These boliang spirits are conflated with ancestor spirits. For instance, after Siamae Sanji died, his grave was made into a shrine. If Taipaobalers needed rain or to stop a flood, they would go to his grave and summon his spirit. In the past, when Taipaobalers paid tribute to the olongian, during the community harvest rites, the boliang were possessed by the spirits of various foodstuffs indigenous to the area.

38. I draw much the same conclusion that James Fox (1989) does about strucurally opposed categories: "It is not dualism per se that defines societies with so-called dual organization but rather the use of dualism at a general, systemic, level which thus determines the parameters for other forms of classification" (ibid.:53).

4. Fatal Attractions: Sumpitan on Umputé

1. Traube's work on the black and white rituals of the Mambai of Timor and Weinstock's work on the black and white rites among the Kaharingans of Borneo underline the monochromatic similarities to highland Laujé (Traube 1986; Weinstock 1987). It is often the case in Indonesia that highland or peripheral communities practice rituals in a minimalist fashion, whereas those in the center, in the court areas, have a more elaborate repertoire of colors, symbols, myths, etc. (H. Geertz 1963; Becker 1979).

2. Traube writes that "Fox has claimed there is a fundamental ubiquity of dual classification in eastern Indonesian cultures and the presence in these same cultures of special forms of speech characterized by strict semantic parallelism. These speech forms, or "ritual languages," are used on all formal occasions; they require the linking of lexical elements in pairs determined by a variety of semantic criteria. The phenomenon of semantic parallelism is of widespread occurrence (Jakobson 1966) and provides a potentially productive way of approaching the internal structure of symbolic systems. Fox has pursued this direction in a series of articles on ritual language (1971, 1974, 1975, 1988). Fox claims there is a "fundamental relationship between the ubiquity of dual classification in eastern Indonesian cultures and the presence in these same cultures of special forms of speech characterized by strict semantic parallelism" (Traube 1986:248). More generally, Fox has argued that a "linguistic view holds the key . . . to an understanding of the pervasive dualism that van Wouden noted" (1980:16).

3. A few men like Sumpitan who want very much to prove that they are

Muslim, will embellish this idea about the eye as a fetus by adding some notions about conception derived from Sufi Islam. Sumpitan says that the eye grows and grows until the seventh or eighth month of pregnancy when just before the child is born it is given four more characteristics from the spirit owners of the Earth and Water. The soil creates one's body, which is like a warehouse for storing one's essence; fire creates one's blood, wind creates one's breath, and water creates the rest of those things inside us that move. But the child is not alive until Allah or God gives it its last characteristic, which makes it live and breathe—its soul *(nyaa)*. Four elements, come from the mother, four from the father. Four additional elements, invisible in the clear waters of the womb, come from God. Once the thread forms, this adds the thirteenth element. At the time of birth, seven more elements unite with the child. These last elements are the possible days when one will be born and die. When the body carries all twenty of these elements then the child is born. These ideas, drawn from Sufi traditions, are syncretized to Laujé notions about the fetus and conception. It is important to note here that the salient issues the lowland elites discuss in their ideology of how a child is conceived are not completely centered around the theme of gender.

4. Acciaioli (personal communication) has pointed out that it seems odd that an imam would be present at a traditional (non-Islamic) ceremony. According to the wife of the olongian, until the 1920s or so, many imams were actually relatives of the olongian and would perform traditional and Islamic rites with no questions asked. It was only in the 1980s that fundamentalists began to question whether the Laujé rites were non-Islamic. I believe the presence of the imam in this story, signified a respected authority figure. In both Muslim and "traditional" circles, incest is taboo, so the respected imam is the one who discovers and "prosecutes."

5. Sumpitan says that to this day you know that chickens are actually former humans because chickens are the only animals alive who can tell time. "Listen," he says, "they crow every hour, they can tell time just like humans can."

6. The chicken looks like it is alive because it is whole, but dead because it is brown and desiccated.

7. *Unwi* is not a Laujé word. Typically Laujé prayers incorporate words from neighboring languages that no one understands. Such words are believed to be especially powerful (see Acciaioli 1989; Tsing 1987).

8. The red umputé prayer invokes Raja Tandu. *Tandu* means horns. The sea spirit, Sawerigading, is also called the Raja Tandu. Sawerigading will appear in Chapter 6.

9. Despite their hatred for the raja, all subjects were to respect him and show deference to him. Following Anderson (1972) and Geertz (1980), these rajas had power from the gods and to show them disrespect was a sacrilegious act.

10. Boliang refers not only to the curer who may enter into a shamanic

trance, or may engage in spirit possession, but also refers to the spirit-other, the helper who assists the shaman. Siamae Arbou was probably a man of the mountains because he, like mountain dwellers, used boliang spirits for healing. In the lowlands the term *boliang* usually refers to the lead spirit medium in the momasoro.

11. This dream refers to an actual incident that occurred during the early colonial period in Toli-Toli on the west coast of this long arm of Central Sulawesi. The story is told in Nourse 1984.

12. Some people explain the spirit's wrath as though it was the murderers' fault that they did not show proper respect to superiors like the raja. Of course, Sumpitan would disagree with such an interpretation.

13. The brass trays are probably the most significant items for conveying an image of status. Such trays have been traded among the Laujé since at least the sixteenth century (Dagh Register 1569). They are also the articles given as Laujé bridewealth. Though in today's more commodity-oriented world, lowland Laujé are more interested in cash coconut trees as symbols of wealth for brideprice payments, nevertheless, these brass trays represent the former exchange items that marked a bride's status. The pedestal tray could only be given as bridewealth in a family of elite status associated with an olongian or a tadulako. People of lesser status, but equal wealth, could negotiate for the flat trays. Thus the trays were, at one time, the icons of status and hierarchy in Laujé society. In addition to trays, porcelain plates also served as the "closing gift" presented by the groom's family when he came to the bride's house after the wedding. Both heirloom items are still used as bridewealth and only brought out for ritual occasions such as curing ceremonies, weddings, and funerals.

14. When the red chicken was slaughtered, before it was roasted on the charcoal grill, the blood was saved in a cup (something not usually done because the blood is usually allowed to fall where it will). Now this blood is to be poured over the white rice.

15. Egg symbolism is central in Laujé offerings. The egg is always the focal point of all trays. Sumpitan says an egg is a symbol of fertility and potential life. The world began as an egg. "We and everything we see in the world, the plants, the animals, the rocks, the earth and the sky, all started from the first egg of the universe." Thus, eggs are the perfect icons signifying human and cosmic vitality and fecundity. In addition to their mythic beliefs about eggs, Sumpitan says that humans have eggs within each and every body. In the Laujé language, a man's testicles are referred to as his "eggs" *(golau)*. More significantly, women are believed to have eggs inside them too. A barren woman is said "to have broken her eggs." The first time I realized this egg was not just a symbol for fertility, but was really believed to be inside women's bodies, was when some highland Laujé saw me wear pants. I had never worn pants in the highlands, but all my clothes were soaked when we crossed the

flooded Tinombo and Siavu Rivers. I was cold and wet when I arrived at my mountain home, and the only thing dry was a pair of pants I had stored in a box. One of my close women friends, Siamae Sanji's granddaughter, admonished me when she saw the pants: "Be careful! You'll break your egg [wearing those pants]! Is that the way you Westerners practice family planning? If you aren't careful you'll break your egg and the family planning will be irreversible." Though she was teasing me, I could tell she really was a bit worried. This woman brought home to me how important the intact egg is to the Laujé as a symbol of fertility.

16. One rite, *momantas* or *nobantas,* is very different from the highlands rite and is conducted immediately before the birth of a first child. The parents of the father-to-be provide a black chicken and a knife, which are laid on the stomach of the mother-to-be. The black chicken is later raised by the mother-to-be; the knife is used in the garden by the new mother, ostensibly to provide food for the child. What is so compelling here is that black is associated with the male's family. A young black chicken is given to be nurtured and raised. Instead of associating black with death and females as Taipaobalers do, here black is associated with males and life. Why the contrast? As we shall see, black is not essentially connected with females or death, though it does connote separation. The black chicken gift marks the separation from the husband's or father-to-be's family and the creation of a new nuclear family; it also marks their newly severed relationship. The father in these elite lowland rites plays a more distant role marked by symbols of separation and death.

17. It is possible that this hard coin used to stop the soul from flowing out of the child is also placed on the ground to keep the soul of the child and the "dead" placenta from flowing into the ground again. The lowland elite associate the ground with the source of their souls, the female force of the cosmos, and the olongian. Before these souls can be recycled, they must go to heaven at the center of the sea. This coin ensures that the placental spirit will not enter the earth, but will wait for the human to die and then escort it to heaven.

18. Some informants say that the human extremities—the skin, the hands, and the feet—are like the living buds of a tree and that they represent life separated from its origins. These extremities should not be associated with the place of rejuvenation and decay, the earth, if the father wants the soul of the placenta to wait for the soul of the child. Were he to touch the ground with his extremities, he would mark this as a place of separation.

19. Though some scholars (Barth 1969; Glazer and Moynihan 1975) have argued that ethnicity is really only appropriate as a term in the context of groups defining themselves and struggling for resources, material and symbolic, explicitly in relation to the nation state (see also Keyes 1981), Sumpitan's use of ethnic identity fits this notion as others like Linnekin and Poyer (1990), Handler (1988), Royce (1982), Keyes (1981), and Keesing (1982)

have used it. Ethnic identity goes far beyond simple either/or ascription. The ethnic group is a reference group, invoked by people who identify themselves, and are identified by others, sharing a common historical style. As such, then, it is a local concept that can shift with the context of the speaker. Michael Moerman (1965:200) was one of the first to propose and illustrate in a systematic fashion that every group has its own taxonomy of ethnic labels. Within these systems individuals assign labels to others in response to cues they have learned as diagnostic. Moerman suggests that it would be fruitful to compare the structure of folk systems with the prevailing institutional structure (such as state relations).

In this case, it is important to realize that Sumpitan's notion of Laujé versus Bugis versus Mandar versus Kaili ethnicity is a folk concept that does not necessarily coincide with the technical meaning of ethnicity.

5. Casting Out the Foreigners: Sumpitan's Momasoro

1. Sumpitan and all of the male curers were called sando. The women (and a few men) who were possessed by spirits were also called sando. Both were healers. To avoid confusion, however, I have designated the male curers as sando and the female spirit mediums as to pensio. To pensio can be glossed as "those who are entered." The boliang is also considered a sando and a to pensio, but to distinguish her very specific role from the roles taken by mediums and curers, I have called her a boliang. I have done this for clarity's sake, and it does not reflect how the Laujé designate participants in the momasoro. It is worth noting that the boliang is the term used for shaman in the Laujé highlands, and in Kalimantan (balian) (Tsing 1987; Graham 1987; Scharer 1963; Weinstock 1987). Balian is also used in Bali say Connor, Asch, and Asch (1982:16).

2. Raja Kuti and other Muslims in the Tinombo area first learned Islam informally from Arabs or from Indonesians who had lived in Saudi Arabia. This one-on-one teaching method was replaced later by more formal schooling in Islamic pesantren. In 1950 the first branch of the Alchairat Islamic School of Palu, a pesantren, was set up in Tinombo. The Alchairat originated in 1935 under the guidance of Habib Idrus bin Salim Al Jubri. His mother was a Bugis woman living in Palu and his father was an Arab trader in Palu. His father brought him to the Hadramaat (al-Jafri) area of Saudi Arabia when he was a young boy, and he studied Islam there. When he was in his thirties, he returned and set up the first Muslim school or pesantren in Central Sulawesi, the Alchairat. It now has many branches throughout Indonesia.

3. During the 1950s and 1960s, people from South Sulawesi, trying to escape the wars and separatist movements there, moved to Tinombo, knowing

it was a safe haven from both the Islamic separatists (Dar ul Islam rebels), and the anticommunist, largely Christian separatists (Permesta rebels) (Harvey 1977). These newcomers occupied the lower rungs of the Tinombo hierarchy as petty traders and craftsmen. Many of them were followers of the more "modernist" (whether fundamentalist or reformist) Islamic sects that eventually merged in Tinombo. By 1962 the Muhammadiyah sect controlled the fundamentalist Muslims. The Muhammadiyahs were able to build the second mosque in Tinombo, this one in the Gorontalese neighborhood. Once this mosque was erected, it attracted some Laujé from Lombok and Tivu. Muhammadiyah fundamentalist preachers used their positions to attack religious syncretism. By the 1970s Muhammadijah fundamentalists began to replace the more tolerant Tinombo elite on the board of the Alchairat School. Here the Muhammadiyah fundamentalists also advocated no syncretism in the teachings and ceremonies associated with the schoolchildren.

Attacks on syncretism are a hallmark of Muhammadiyah philosophy. Peacock says, "culturally, Muhammadijah offers an alternative to the rich but confusing mixture of folk beliefs and great religions known as syncretism. Muhammadijah, as a distillation of Islam, provides a single authoritative text, a clear and formalized guide to conduct, and single, all-powerful God" (Peacock 1992:100).

4. One reason the Muhammadiyah imams and followers may have focused so strongly on Laujé rites is that the Laujé were potential Muhammadiyah converts. Similar in socioeconomic status to the Muhammadiyah followers, their paths crossed more readily than with higher-status immigrants from Tinombo. The other reason the Muhammadiyah imams and followers may have focused so heavily on Laujé rites is that imams were hesitant to criticize immigrants of high status who performed Bugis and Mandar rituals. Criticizing Bugis and Mandar rites would mean criticizing the immigrants who wielded local political and economic power. The Laujé, thus, became a less threatening target.

5. The ban was not merely local in scope, but related to a more pervasive conflict with the national government (see Tsing 1987; Weinstock 1987; Bowen 1986, 1987, 1993). As local fundamentalists, primarily Muhammadiyah in orientation, attempted to assert their authority over less acculturated peoples like the Laujé, they subtly critiqued syncretism at the national level, contesting the authority of the syncretic Java-centric Suharto government.

The Muhammadiyah fundamentalists used the first clause of the Pancasila to support their claim that this was an animist rite that did not recognize the existence of one God. The Pancasila, or five principles of civic ideology, states that *Tuhan yang maha esa* means that all citizens must worship a God who is omniscient and omnipotent. If more than one God is recognized within a rite, then the rite is not constitutionally sanctioned; it should be banned.

6. GOLKAR (short for Golongan Karya or functional group) is the na-

tional group that all civil servants are obligated to join. In Suharto's "New Order" only two political parties, PDI (Partai Demokratik Indonesia, or Indonesian Democratic Party) and PPP (Partai Persatuan Perkembangan, or Development Unity Party) were allowed. In an effort to diminish the sectarian dimension of party politics, the Suharto government had banned the original Muslim Party, Masyumi, and instead allowed PPP whose name, Development Unity Party, does not even allude to Islam. Like other parties, PPP could not easily compete with the government party, GOLKAR (Emmerson 1981 cited in Kipp and Rodgers 1987:18). GOLKAR was technically not a party, but all civil servants were required to support it, and it was the "group," read *party,* that elected Suharto for thirty years.

7. Downstream and upstream, of course, are relative terms. The monganjul poyoan was downstream from the momaang, or harvest rites, but upstream from the lowland villages like Dusunan and Lombok.

8. The old site was right next to Border Rock (Polu Batala)—the rock marking the border *(batas)* between lowland Islamic Laujé and animist highland Laujé. Sumpitan said that *batala* means Ata Allah or border of Allah. According to Greg Acciaioli, however, Ata Allah usually means slave of Allah. Sumpitan, uneducated in Islam, believed this term uttered by spirits referred to the boundary between the Laujé who had remained upstream and animist, and those who had moved downstream and become Islamic.

9. Not since the 1950s have any Taipaobalers attended this ceremony, though Sumpitan constantly reiterated that everyone was invited. Actually, in December 1984 the rite was "ordered" by the government to be performed. A Japanese anthropologist, Professor Isamu Kurata, was to be in the district for two days. The Chief of Education and Culture wanted him to see this rite, so it was hastily arranged and Sumpitan was asked to choreograph it. Though he was disgruntled that an immigrant should dictate to him when to organize the rite, Sumpitan was nevertheless so glad to have the chance to perform it at all that he kept his negative opinions in check. He also was able to use the "audience" of a foreign anthropologist to his advantage.

10. It is interesting that most of the lowlanders who are spirit mediums are women. It is the lowland men who analyze what these spirits say and who translate their antiquated speech to the audience.

11. Because it was publicly uttered, I received permission to print the Laujé words here along with the English translation. I did not receive such permission in every case. In those circumstances, the Laujé portion of the prayer is omitted.

12. Sumpitan said the wrapped rice packets symbolize each individual Laujé, the way they are nurtured in the womb and grow and evolve. Different shapes of rice packets represent either different aspects of maturity or the female or male substances that create a fertilized egg in the womb.

13. Local imams were less emphatic about syncretism than were the fundamentalist imams in coastal villages like Tinombo. They saw no contradiction in blessing umputé spirits and in being servants of Allah.

14. Tulabala in Laujé becomes *tolak bala* in Indonesian and Malay. Its English translation is "avoid catastrophe." Laderman mentions tolak bala rituals in Malaysia, which "are listed by the Office of Religious Affairs as examples of the kinds of superstition that must be rooted out" (1991:17).

15. Burning incense logs are something the Muhammadiyah fundamentalists find pagan. In fact, however, incense is an item used in the rituals of the Balinese who pratice a state-recognized religion and not simply a custom or a current of belief *(aliran kepercayaan).*

16. The Laujé shrine, or *ginaling,* is supposedly made from some of the first wood of the first tree of the center of the earth. In the old days (whenever that was) people reportedly shaved off some of the wood from the shrine to immerse in water for healing purposes. Now the ginaling wood is always covered with barkcloth.

17. In 1985 and 1986 this part of the momasoro rite was held in the olongian's parlor, an enclosure without walls. The parlor served as a perfect stage. In earlier years the dancing was held on the cleared space in front of the house. The spirits, however, would retire to a closed parlor after they had danced. There, invisible to the audience members outside, they chanted and made offerings at an altar composed of individual plates containing colored rice placed on pedestal trays. In 1985 and 1986 this altar to the "sea" spirits was located in the back of the parlor of the olongian, but within plain view of the audience. Most of the audience was from Dusunan, Lombok, or other Laujé coastal villages; a few spectators were from Tinombo.

18. Sando and audience members claim they do not understand what the spirits say during their prayers (see Hoskins 1988b). Nevertheless, I found that many people did indeed understand the spirit speeches, but felt it rude to claim to understand them.

19. As mentioned above, most of the mediums are women, while most of those who translate for the masses are men. The mediums tend to memorize songs and chants without analyzing what they mean. The main exception to this case was Siinai Alasan.

20. Sumpitan claimed that both words were ancient and pure Laujé. He said that "the young people outside" would not know such words. In fact, *jati* is not ancient Laujé, but a Malay loan word of Sanskrit origin. In the Indonesian-English dictionary (Echols and Shadily 1978:92), *jati* is defined as "genuine," "true," or as "teakwood." Given the importance of wood and trees to origin myths this could have been an older loan word referring to the first spirit of wood.

21. The seven ethnic groups of the world are the ones that were created

from the travels of the Voracious Boy. The ethnic groups are the Chinese, the Dutch, the Mandar, the Bugis, the Kaili, the Gorontalese, and the Javanese.

22. Metcalf (1994) comments on a similar situation among the Berawan in Northern Borneo. He says, "No one listening, even with half an ear, need be in any doubt as to the thrust of the speaker's intention" (1994:1).

23. Lipat leaves are also placed on top of the rice-packet offerings. Lipat leaves are said to cure itchiness and flaky skin caused by diseases like *po'o*, a disease often contracted as a side effect of trying to seek too much spiritual power by combining the forces that have become separated.

24. The olongian's "empire," says Sumpitan, stretches out to the far reaches of the Laujé kingdom through the agricultural specialist or posobo, whom the olongian assigns to live and perform agricultural rites in villages. Most highland Laujé, though, do not recognize the olongian as their leader.

25. The highlanders in Taipaobal formerly performed a mantalapu rite also. But many of the women who participated in this rite are now too old to continue.

26. This rite compares closely to the headhunting rites discussed in depth by Kenneth George (1996). Not only is there similarity in the way Laujé and the Mambi conduct the rites, but in the way they use them to deal with issues of modernity, memory, and religious identity.

27. Travel over the steep mountains and narrow coastline comprising the Laujé land was, until recently, very arduous. This was especially the case during the rainy season when run-off from the mountains made roads impassable. Now, however, the Trans-Sulawesi highway connects the island from end to end. Prior to the road's completion in the late eighties, however, most foreigners came to the Laujé region via the Tomini Bay, what the Laujé call "the sea."

28. Working and cutting, separating things, or killing animals through fishing or hunting might have attracted the umputé spirits of the sea, because as I will show in Chapter 6 the umputé spirits are also associated with death.

29. Respect for a close relative comes naturally, without gifts. Recall in the highlands how the bela relationship is one in which the bela are ostensibly treated as guests, invited into the parlor, and given gifts. In the end, this marks a difference between bela and Taipaobaler, as much as it marks a bond. By giving food gifts or offerings to umputé of the sea in such a profuse manner, the Laujé marked their relationship to the spirits of the sea as distant, rather than close.

6. Marrying the Foreigners: Erasing Sumpitan's Momasoro

1. By chance, their new interpretations coincided more with Austronesian symbolism that emphasizes male-female complementarity (Fox 1980, 1988, 1989; Hoskins 1997; Traube 1980, 1986; Forth 1985).

2. Robert Hefner uncovered the same esoteric myth among the Tengger—a Hindu refugee community in Java. He noted that the myth of the recumbent woman whose sweat and bodily fluids become a river is also told in India in reference to the source of the Ganges (Hefner 1985:179). Additionally Elizabeth Traube's Mambai research emphasizes a recumbent earth mother (1980, 1986). Among the Mambai "the white underground milk flows down to the sea where the children of the 'inner water/inner sea' . . . nurse on it. [They] . . . are the transformed souls of the dead, returned to the watery world of the first creation, the remnants of the original birth fluid" (1986:310).

3. Sawerigading, as most of the audience members know, is the hero whose epic wanderings are outlined in what has been called "one of the most remarkable works of literature to be found in Indonesia," the Bugis I La Galigo epic cycle (Abidin and MacKnight 1974:161). Captivating wherever he is met and in whatever language he is mentioned, the stories about Sawerigading have traveled as their Bugis hero, Sawerigading has. Throughout Sulawesi and beyond, Sawerigading is acclaimed as the great Bugis prince and hero. In a wonderful article by Andi Zainal Abidin, translated and adapted by C. C. Macknight, the diffusion of the Sawerigading story is discussed. They say, "the names, Sawerigading and I La Galigo, are well known in Central Celebes. This strongly suggests that this area might once have been ruled or come under the aegis of the ancient Buginese Kingdom of Luwu, at the head of the Gulf of Bone. Adriani and Kruyt relate the visit of Sawerigading or Lasaeo To Pamona in the Poso area in which he is depicted as a hero from heaven. They conclude from the folk-tales about him in this East Toraja region that the kings of Luwu, Waibunta, and Pamona shared a common origin" (1974:164). Sawerigading also appears in the Palu Valley on the west coast and in nearby Donggala. No mention is made, however, of Sawerigading in Central Sulawesi communities like Tomini, Tinombo, and Moutong, except in my own work (Nourse 1998).

There are many other works on the I La Galigo. The I La Galigo is known as the longest literary work in the world. According to Tol, "its size is estimated at approximately 6,000 folio-pages. Set in a meter of five and occasionally four syllables, it relates events from pre-Islamic, 14th century Luwu, the cradle of Bugis culture. Consisting of dozens of different episodes, each with its own protagonists, and covering several generations, using a wide range of literary conventions such as flashback and foreshadowing, the epic tells the story of the arrival on earth of the gods and the adventures of their descendants. The main protagonist of the story is Sawerigading, the great Bugis culture hero, who travels to remote places and falls deeply in love with his twin sister. This incestuous love is strictly prohibited and Sawerigading ultimately marries another woman. In the end the whole divine family gathers in

Luwu and all the gods depart from the earth, having lived there for seven generations" (Tol 1990:49).

Other noteworthy articles about, or relevant to, the I La Galigo are by Matthes (1954), Mattulada (1982), Errington (1989), Hamonic (1991), Kern (1939) and Nourse (1998).

4. What this case emphasizes is the belief that seniority, especially in birth order, is a primary model for giving value to people. Thus, in a reversal of most Muslim evaluations, Sawerigading, as the older sibling, is superior to Mohammed, despite Mohammad's status among contemporary Muslims as the most important human being who ever lived. Of course, this tale also reverses some of the other evaluations set up in the momasoro by Sumpitan. Now the sea is regarded as a superior place, the place of tradition, while the land is inferior, the place of Islam.

5. The mamua was known as Sawerigading's "plaything." It was said to perch on the "two-branched tree" on the highest mountain. One branch leaned seaward, the other toward the land. From its perch, the bird could fly in either direction. It left its seaward perch to fly to the coast to deposit its eggs. It returned to roost on the landward branch. The mamua egg is an important ritual object among the people of Banggai who also have a ceremony similar to the momasoro (Kennedy 1953). Also, the Haji said that the mamua eggs for the rite were supposed to be seven in number, just like in the Sawerigading tale, but because these turkey eggs were so difficult to find nowadays, one egg was sufficient for the offering.

6. Though the maleo fowl has become an endangered species, it was once prevalent enough in Sulawesi to allow Alfred Wallace to collect several and describe them (1869:270). Wallace was especially interested in the bird because of its peculiar egg-laying habits. He described its behavior in much the same way as the Haji and others at the momasoro were to talk of the maleo. According to Wallace, the birds laid their eggs in the "loose hot black sand" of the beach. "In the months of August and September, when there is little or no rain they come down from the interior to . . . scratch holes three or four feet deep just above high water mark, where the female deposits a single large egg, which she covers with about a foot of sand and then returns to the forest . . . she comes again to the same spot to lay another egg, and each female bird is supposed to lay six or eight eggs during the season" (ibid.:272). Wallace also described the ways in which the chicks hatched from their shells at the seashore. "The young birds, on breaking the shell, work their way up through the sand and run off at once to the forest . . . they can fly the very day they are hatched" (ibid.:273).

7. According to this elite man, the pieces of wood were taken out of their wrappings and scraped into a bowl of water, and curers then used this potion

to massage the severely ill. I was not able to ascertain whether the "seven trees" were mythical or real. The name for the commoner tree, *Si Omogang,* may be derived from the root *ogang,* or river basin, and refer to the people of a single watershed.

8. These coins were kept on a large tray at the rear of the vunkeng. At the beginning of the momasoro, a community leader from each neighborhood arrived with coins for each newborn child. These were added to the pile. The leader also announced the death of any members of his community. One coin was removed from the tray for every person who died. Such coins were thrown into the river to be washed downstream. These doi nu nyaa, or coins of the souls, were primarily copper "pennies" from the colonial era. Recently, however, the smallest denomination Indonesian coins have been used.

9. Ostensibly, once the momasoro was held in Dusunan, smaller river-mouth communities, such as Dongkas and Mobaloi, would hold similar, but scaled-down, rites. These rites were supposed to follow in sequence: The river mouths closest to Dusunan would begin first, followed by those farther away, and finally reaching the border of the Laujé polity to the north and south. Yet, some of these communities had rebelled against Dusunan, or against the hierarchical order embodied in the sequence by either holding their rites out of sequence or making them more ostentatious than those in Dusunan said they should be. For example, Dongkas, for at least twenty years, had filled and cast off two boats, rather than one, as was supposed to be the rule for the smaller communities. This assertion of ritual equality with Dusunan stemmed from a dispute between aristocrats in the two communities over the olongian's succession in the 1950s.

10. The body lay in state while the relatives of the olongian gathered to select a successor. During this period, the corpse was ritually treated. Four women sat on either side of the corpse. Each held a fan and the two sides fanned in a cycle, moving from the feet to the head, and from the head to the feet. The same ceremonial practice was reported among the Kaili in the late eighteenth century (Woodard 1804:114).

11. Ironically, one of the imams in attendance was a member of the Muhammadiyah sect. One of the Muhammadiyah agendas was to discourage such rote readings of the Qur'an, which are characterized as a "medieval" survival of Islamic practice. Such readings were criticized because they did not promote an understanding of the content or meaning of the Qur'an. As one leader of the Muhammadiyah sect in Tinombo put it, "They recite all night and are too tired the next morning to work. . . . They are not good Muslims because they neither work, nor learn." Nevertheless, such readings are a popular pastime in Sulawesi. They are, in a sense, a form of meditation, much like the Sufi *zikir,* or repetition of Allah's name. They are meant to induce a state of selflessness. The words of the Qur'an endlessly recited empty the mind of

thought and allow the human soul to sense its oneness with Allah (Bowen 1987). Such notions verge on syncretism and are anathema to Muhammadiyah philosophy. I suspect the reason the Muhammadiyah imam attended this protest gathering was to support Islam against very obvious syncretism in the momasoro. I suppose he could rationalize that he could purge the syncretic, rote Qur'anic readings later, but now he had larger issues to deal with. Never, though, did the imam say this to me.

12. In early Islamic states throughout Indonesia, this was a typical pattern. Rajas converted all people. Missionization of the populace at large was often actively discouraged (Bowen 1987).

7. Denying Difference: Siamae Balitangan's "Simple" Momasoro

1. When Siamae Balitangan was still a child, his father was arrested and imprisoned by the Dutch for murdering a neighbor. The Dutch placed Siamae Balitangan in the home of a lowland Laujé mayor of Lombok. He worked several years there as a servant. Later, he returned to the mountains, becoming an important intermediary between the Dutch and the bela communities in the mountains above Mobaloi.

2. Note the analogies with "crooked words" elsewhere in Indonesia and beyond (Brenneis and Myers 1984; Brenneis 1984). Among the Laujé, truth is straight and lies are bent.

3. Tsing (1993) has a similar reaction to the use of Malay words in Meratus prayers. The use of foreign language terms in prayers and in secret names for spirits is common. The use of Indonesian, however, seems ludicrous, since it is not a mysterious foreign language, but one taught to school children. As marginal groups become more integrated into mainstream Indonesian culture where Indonesian language is used, the loan words from Malay or Indonesian that are used in marginal peoples' prayers become less exotic and more laughable because they are so commonplace. This is what made Tsing and I react in a similar way in two different communities.

4. The wife of the olongian was particularly concerned about how old Siamae Balitangan said he was because there was prestige in being the oldest in the community. I suspect she wanted that prestige for herself. It meant that the spirits had favored the older person, that the older individual had acted well, had not brought about their death before their time. The wife of the olongian thus exposed as false Siamae Balitangan's claims to superiority through his age.

5. Taipaobalers, for example, always viewed visits to the lowlands with some trepidation. Men like Siamae Sanji or his sons warned of the dangers there. They often questioned me about how I had learned some of the "secrets" of the lowlands. They warned me never to learn anything from a curer

(sando) who would insist that I sit with him on a pure white cloth to gain secrets. Yet, outside of rituals, this was the only way one could learn secrets in Dusunan (see Acciaioli 1988, 1989, for similar restrictions among the Bugis). Siamae Sanji said that to sit on the white cloth was to "disrespect God" and to invite death. This was probably something he had been told by the Muslims in Tinombo. Reformists like Raja Tombolotutu, whose porch Siamae Sanji often slept on, constantly proselytized the men of the mountains and tried to convince them to drop syncretic practices, like sitting on white cloths to learn prayers. Though the raja and other Tinombo elites were reformist and therefore dedicated to purifying Islam of admixtures, they were not as adamant as the fundamentalist Muhammadiyah were about actively eradicating syncretism from all rituals.

6. What some questers seek, though, is more than just names. They seek myths, answers, and philosophical knowledge about the spirits, which their own ancestors have neglected to tell them. If they hear these answers from a person possessed by a spirit, however, they must decipher the meaning of the words from the obscure discourse.

7. In Malaysia Laderman finds similar metaphors for spirit possession. "Patients in trance feel the inner winds as experiential reality rather than merely metaphor" (1991:75). She also noted that *angin* or wind "is a word with multiple meanings, many of which are connected with notions of sickness and treatment (ibid.:67; 1988).

8. Interestingly enough, this term in Bugis means the swollen belly. It is what happens to those who are disrespectful to others of higher status, whether nobles, spirits, deities, etc. In 1985 the Bugis police chief, who was also Muhammadiyah, and who had originally instigated the ban against the momasoro, contracted the swollen belly disease. I was told he left his post in Tinombo and two years later died of stomach cancer.

9. For example, Sumpitan knew a great deal about the *tarekat* or special Sufi order *(tarikah)* that associates characters of the alphabet with the four elements or "characters that come from the woman and the man at intercourse." Interestingly enough, Sumpitan's equation of the characters of the alphabet with the elements or characteristics that come from the man and woman during intercourse and creation of a child are hauntingly similar to the equations Gayo of Sumatra make, as described in the work of John Bowen (1987:120–25). This would corroborate Siamae Sanji's rendition of Islamic history saying that people in Tinombo were first taught Islam by a Kaili man who had studied with a Sumatran teacher in Palu. This Sufi or tarekat knowledge is, of course, anathema to fundamentalists like Muhammadiyah, because it mixes Islam with various mystical philosophies picked up along the route from Saudi Arabia through Persia, India, Malaysia, Sumatra, and Sulawesi. Tarekat or

Sufi philosophy was taught by wandering teachers who "supplemented the rather arid Qur'anic explanations of what man must do with a richer account, often tied to local custom, of how he might do it" (ibid.:116).

10. In an exploration of a related case of possession among the Karo Batak of Sumatra, this is what Mary Steedly (1993) suggests. She notes that mediums are well aware of the ambiguity of voice that possession entails. According to Steedly, because it is hard to tell who is speaking when a medium opens her mouth, audiences are constantly "looking for definitive answers and singular messages. Official interpretations of the mediums' words seek a determinate identity for that which speaks through her, a name, a history, a simple fixed subject-position . . . and any lapse from this clear determination of voice-identity tends to be interpreted by the audience as a sign of either fraud or incompetence on the mediums' part" (ibid.:197). If one substitutes sando here where Steedly mentions "audience," then we have the Laujé case.

11. When it suited him, Siamae Balitangan used his elite religious knowledge, learned while a servant in the imam's house, to align himself with male sando against female boliang. Just as easily, however, Siamae Balitangan resisted elites' tendency to name and individuate all the spirits. Indeed, two weeks after the momasoro, Siamae Balitangan came to visit me in the mountains and offered, Sufi style, to teach me the names of the four spirits of the corner-posts of the world if I offered him, as is Sufi custom, a white cloth for us to sit on and a machete as a gift (see Acciaioli 1989). This aspect of his Sufi training made Siamae Balitangan like Sumpitan.

12. Roy Wagner (1983, 1986a) and Edith Turner (1992), each in their own way, have written on this topic. Wagner's point is that, when people truly understand a symbol, they don't see it as something that refers to something else. Wagner has also written about Western and non-Western consciousness of the double. He believes that in non-Western cultures neither part of the double is more real than the other. Turner writes about experiencing African religion as it is, not as if it stands for something else.

8. Partial Truths and Layered Representations

1. As I mentioned in note 13 in the Introduction, there is a whole branch of classic anthropology, the Manchester School led by Max Gluckman and initially followed by Victor Turner, that analyzes rebels and rebellions, rather than the status quo. Because I was trained in social as well as cultural anthropology, and because I was a student of Victor Turner's, I was inclined to think in Manchesterian terms, thus leading me to see Sumpitan and Siamae Sanji as political iconoclasts. I now realize that my naive assumptions about the gist of

these and other theories, needed to be "tested," as it were, in fieldwork. It was only after grappling with the fieldwork "data" and the implications of each theory's subtleties, that I recognized how nuanced the earlier theory actually was.

2. For a complete discussion of Siinai Alasan's spirit's speech about the relationship between custom and religion, see Nourse 1994a. For a complete discussion of the pitfalls of anthropological dialogue on resistance, see Nourse 1994b and 1994c.

3. In a review of Rodney Needham's 1974 *Remarks and Inventions: Skeptical Essays about Kinship,* Ivan Karp notes that "it is wrong to presume that Needham (a renowned structuralist) is a naive empiricist who assumes that the consequence of an actor's articulation of a rule is that he must follow it unswervingly." Karp demonstrates that Needham's approach is not rigidly static as many believe. Needham acknowledges that people discriminate among different principles and are affected by contingencies (Karp 1976:152–53). Indeed, James Boon made similar points about the subtlety and fluidity of Lévi-Strauss's structuralism (Boon 1972), the structuralism most postmodernists find so reprehensible. One of the big questions Karp's and Boon's analyses of Needham and Lévi-Strauss, respectively, raise is if all structuralists might have been stereotyped by postmodernists.

4. Actually, Edward Said's book *Orientalism* (1978) is often used as the starting point of anthropology's awareness of its own problems (Marcus and Fisher 1986; Clifford 1988). Said accused anthropology of stereotyping "orientals" as different and inferior. His premise is that anthropology is a white discipline, thus it exoticizes nonwhite others. Africanists, however, preceded Said in their criticisms (p'Bitek 1970; Fanon 1963) and continued to accuse anthropologists of collusion with colonial regimes. In the eighties, anthropologists and cultural studies scholars themselves began to jump on the accusatory bandwagon (Clifford and Marcus 1986; Clifford 1988; Marcus and Fisher 1986) as did historians (Vail and White 1991), but with a twist. The anthropologists and the historians began to point the accusatory finger back at Said, saying he essentialized and stereotyped anthropology at the same time as he accused the discipline of essentializing others with exotic stereotypes.

Wolf finds that the trend to label "fieldwork an act of colonialism is an obvious overstatement," even a double standard. Authors like Said, Clifford, and Marcus aim with such statements "to draw our attention to the ways in which white privilege affects anthropological fieldwork" (Wolf 1992:5). But, notes Wolf, such statements "condemn us for our individual colonialist attitudes," but ignore the fact that "even the most arrogant neocolonialist soon discovers that one cannot order rural people to reveal important thoughts about their culture. . . . Those who carry the culture and those who desperately want to understand it may participate in a minuet of unspoken negotiations that totally reverses the apparent balance of power" (ibid.:134).

Though no one nowadays questions early anthropology's collusion with colonial authorities, some see positive outcomes. For instance, historian Ali Mazrui (1970) noted that Evans-Pritchard and Godfrey Leinhardt personally provided the British colonial regimes in East Africa with detailed ethnographies about "native" political organization. It was that detailed information about the ordered logic of indigenous politics that led colonial authorities to opt for indirect rather than direct rule. Had the ethnographies not been provided, says Mazrui, the colonized would have suffered as they did in French regimes (such as Algeria) where no anthropologists colluded with the colonial governments and no indigenous peoples were allowed to rule themselves through absentee (indirect) colonial government. Obviously, Mazrui's claims are controversial, the relative "freedom" under any colonial regime may be more a figment of colonial rhetoric than a reality. Many scholars argue that colonialism under British or French regimes was equally harsh (Asad 1973; Kuper 1973; Mudimbe 1988; Moore 1994).

5. The term "voice" is problematic, since it disembodies the words and ideas from the complexities of the whole person. I believe it is this term that contributes to our tendency to make the person's voices logical, rational, and uniform, rather than reflections of the inconsistencies and irrationalities of human thought and expression. Nevertheless, it is difficult to find a substitute, so I, like everyone else, tend to refer to people's ideas and emotions as "voices."

GLOSSARY

adat   Indonesian for custom or tradition. It is almost always opposed to religion or agama.

agama   Indonesian for religion, meaning world religions like Islam, Christianity, and the unique combinations of Hinduism and Buddhism in Indonesia called Hindu-Buddhism. Animism is categorized in this scheme as adat.

ampini   Called ketupat in Indonesian, these rice bundles, wrapped in woven banana-leaf squares, triangles, and ovals, are cooked and then opened up to be eaten. They are used as traveling food, or in the monganjul poyoan, because their outer wrapping, skins, can be peeled off and sent downstream.

ampunan   Indonesian noun, the root of which (ampun) means forgiving sins, amnesty. With the suffix *-an* the word changes meaning to refer to unfortunate accidents resulting when one promises something and does not follow through on it.

angin   Indonesian for wind. In Laujé the word is bayalé and is often used as a metaphor for spirits.

aruwa   Muslim funeral dirge.

ayat   Arabic for verses of the Qur'an.

bagis   A kind of tree whose leaves are dried and used as cigarette paper.

balagé   Oral histories, usually chanted by men, often to the accompaniment of a stringed instrument.

banto   The cloth headwrap Laujé men wore before the midcentury ubiquitous *topi* or fez arrived.

baraka   An Arabic word that refers to spiritual power.

baundaké An oblong, phallus-shaped rice packet made in the same way that ampini are made, but shaped much differently.

bayalé Literally, winds. A euphemism for spirits.

bela A Laujé term first translated to me in positive terms as meaning trade partner. Later I learned it meant many pejorative things like hillbilly, animist, uncouth, and primitive.

belum beragama An Indonesian term used to refer to animists. It literally means those who have not yet found religion.

benting From the Indonesian word meaning fortress.

benuo Laujé word for the placenta. It literally means nest.

bidan Indonesian term for trained midwife.

boké A bundle of harvested rice.

boliang In the mountains, the spirit familiar who possesses a sando when a serious cure must be performed. In the lowlands the boliang is the leader of all the other spirit mediums, calling (along with sando) the spirits into the ritual space to possess all the other spirit mediums. The boliang in this case is also the last to be possessed.

boya Cluster of houses; a village.

camat Indonesian for the head of a local county or subdistrict within a kabupaten, or province.

dabang Lowland headhunting rite.

damag Tree resin used in old-fashioned oil lamps. It was once a cash crop bringing a certain amount of wealth to highlanders.

didil A kind of tree, said to be associated with the ancestors, because it is one of the first trees planted in the area.

doi mooas Hard money, coins.

doi nu nyaa Literally, the coins of the souls. Coins that are consecrated by the spirits possessing mediums at each momasoro and stored in the vunkeng in non-ritual times.

donu Bark-cloth.

dulang Brass trays, some flat, some with pedestals, used in marriage exchanges.

gandisé White funeral cloth.

ginaling   The Laujé regalia, consisting of sacred machete, the first wood of the first tree of the center of the earth, and coins of the souls of people who have contributed at past rituals. The regalia is housed inside the vunkeng.

gio   The area preceding the entry to Taipaobal, called the bald. Because the soil's nutrients have been depleted from continual planting during the Japanese period, only grass *(arang)* can now grow there.

golau   Egg, testicles, or ovaries.

GOLKAR   The national "group" to which all civil servants in the Suharto regime were required to belong.

hajj   The Muslim pilgrimage to Mecca.

I La Galigo   The Odyssean epic myth from South Sulawesi that describes the travels of Sawerigading.

ilmu   Literally means knowledge, but it often refers to esoteric knowledge about spirits or about healing.

inalugan   Literally, the carrying down. It refers to the time when the Dutch forced the highland Laujé to move to the lowlands. It also refers to a corpse being carried down to its grave. It implies a tragic event.

jajambo   A red flower used in the white chicken rite in the lowlands to symbolize the hymen.

jati   An Indonesian word borrowed from Sanskrit that means true, genuine, or teakwood.

jogugu   The spokesperson in the Laujé court headed by the olongian.

juu nu niu   Juice of the coconut used to anoint the child and the placenta at birth.

Kabupaten Donggala   Indonesian for the Donggala Province in which Tinombo county is one of forty-three others.

kanda mpat rare   Balinese for placental spirit or umputé.

kapitau dagaté   The captain of the sea in the Laujé court once headed by the olongian. This officer's job was to act as foreign diplomat, conversing with ship captains who docked at Laujé shores.

kongtau   An Indonesian term for martial arts.

kupang   A silver coin from the Dutch colonial era.

lele'e antuonyé   Translated literally as, It is said, it means. A rhetorical, honorific phrase used when spirits possess mediums.

lipat   A vinelike plant, with reddish leaves, that grows in brackish waters.

lontar   Geneaology either memorized or written on bark-cloth.

maleo   Indonesian for mamua, the rare bush turkey.

mamua   A rare bush turkey (maleo in Indonesian) that lays huge eggs in the sands of a beach, but nests in a tree farther inland.

mantalapu   A lowland rite in which three young, phallus-shaped banana trees are cut down by a Laujé spirit medium. See montalapu.

marsaoleh   A noble in the Laujé court of the olongian.

masarungé   The Bugis curing rite performed for elites in Dusunan.

meloon   Upright.

metedes   Strong, long-lasting.

mobotong   Disrespectful in Laujé, but swollen belly in Bugis, a physical consequence of disrespect to those of higher status, human or spirit.

modero   Folk dance from the Pamona area of Lake Poso in Central Sulawesi.

momaang   Describes the act of feeding the child for the first time. It is the same verb used to describe food offerings to the spirit owners of the Land and Water, the global umputé spirits of the momasoro rite.

momasoro   The major Laujé ritual banned by fundamentalist Muslims. Some Laujé defined the rite as a curing rite, and others as a harvest ritual.

monca-pat   Javanese for placental spirit or umputé.

monganjul poyoan   The upstream rite preceding the momasoro which literally means the floating, or casting-adrift-the-outer-covering rite.

montalapu   Mountain harvest rites that once were performed by Taipaobalers in tandem with the bela. Now the knowledge of how to perform these rites is lost.

Muhammadiyah   A fundamentalist reform Muslim sect that believes all syncretic rites and beliefs should be purged from Islam.

nokasiviani   Tribute payment to a raja, olongian, puangé, or spirit.

nosaub   Massage.

nosumpali   To blow on water or an object in a ritual manner for the purpose of curing.

notitisalaḥ   An offering asking spirits for forgiveness for the sins of humans.

nyaa   Soul or breath.

olongian   According to Sumpitan, the Laujé political leader; but according to others, the ritual leader only.

ongkolé   Effort, sweat, or exertion.

pa'an   Oil burned over the graves of respected relatives.

pagoraé   Evil foreign pirates, synonym of pengayo.

pasisir   Indonesian for coastal dwellers.

pasobo   The agricultural specialist in the court of the olongian.

payangan   A boat or vessel. Also a euphemism for mediums possessed by spirits, or for spirits' transportation to meet the humans.

pedagang   Indonesian for traders. Sumpitan's word for the spirits from the sea, possessing mediums in the parlor at the momasoro.

pengayo   Evil foreign pirates, possibly the To Belo from Halmahera.

pepali   That which is forbidden or tabooed.

pesabean   Literally riders, a euphemism for the spirit mediums who ride the spirits possessing their bodies.

Polu Batala   The dividing rock located downstream from Polu Irandu. Polu Batala is said to mark the separation of Islam from animism.

Polu Irandu   The Inscribed Rock located west of Taipaobal in the center of the Inogaat River. It is said to be the Womb of the World, the center of the earth from which all creation formed.

pomalembangané   Literally vessels or boats. A euphemism referring to spirit mediums who power the sails of the boats bringing messages to humans.

pombiriḥ salaḥ   Indonesian for a quasi-Arabic prayer asking forgiveness. Among the Laujé the prayer is said on the wedding night.

pongko   A witch in spirit form, or a living human who takes on spirit form at night to bring harm to people during their dreams.

pontianak   Indonesian and Laujé term for a haunting spirit, a woman who has died in childbirth.

po'o   A skin disease that is said to make the skin shed layers like a snake and to make the afflicted person stink.

popolu pusé   Dried umbilical cord.

puangé   Laujé term for lord or raja. The term is probably borrowed from Bugis or Mandar.

pudung   Leprosy.

pué   The Laujé word for iron and the Kaili word for lord.

rupiah   The Indonesian currency.

sando   Literally means healer. Mediums possessed by spirits are also called sando, but to clarify the difference, I have designated sando as healer/translator here and given the spirit mediums a different name.

selasa   The woven bamboo tray on which the offerings to umputé spirits are placed.

sempaang   The symbolic child offering in which a tray with consecrated rice kernels is hung over a buried coconut shell that looks and is treated like a buried placenta.

Si Omogang   The name of one of the original seven trees of the universe, this one being associated with commoners.

songko   The fez, identifying men who wear them as Muslim. The black velvet topi (Indonesian) is for average men. The white topi is for people who have gone on the Islamic pilgrimage to Mecca.

suku terasing   An Indonesian term that literally translates as tribes who find themselves foreign. It is a Suharto-era designation meant to differentiate animist, swidden agriculturalists as noncitizens.

tabanamé   That part in an Islamic prayer after one has asked Allah for forgiveness with palms open to the sky, and then turns the palms down to the ground to signal that the prayer is finished.

tadeko   A locally made bamboo xylophone.

tadulako   A samurai-like warrior in the court of the olongian who often was from a neighboring non-Laujé ethnic group.

takra   A Southeast Asian kick-ball game, somewhat like hackey-sack, played with woven bamboo balls.

tarekat   A Sufi sect or order that focuses on the mystical relationship with Allah and the "characters" that form the body and the universe.

to pensio   Literally, the person who is entered. It refers to spirit mediums.

Tuhan Yang Maha Esa   Indonesian for God who is omniscient and omnipotent.

tulabala   The prayer means avoid catastrophe. In Indonesian the prayer is called a tolakbala.

umputé   Means connection, birth sibling, illness. It refers to the spirits of the placenta.

vunkeng   The Laujé womblike altar. Triangular in shape and covered with bark-cloth and white cloth, it houses the regalia of the olongian.

vuntuh pusé   Literally, relatives who are connected by the navel. Distant cousins, aunts, and uncles.

walapuluh   The judge in court cases and a member of the Laujé's traditional court system.

REFERENCES

Abidin, Andi Zianal, and C. C. MacKnight
1974   "The I La Galigo Epic Cycle of South Celebes and Its Diffusion."
       Indonesia 17:161–70.

Acciaioli, Greg
1985   "Culture as Art: From Practice to Spectacle in Indonesia." *Canberra
       Anthropology, Special Issue: Minorities and the State* 8 (1–2):
       148–75.
1988   "Exposing Invulnerability: Knowledge, Competition, and Hierarchy
       among the Bugis of Sulawesi, Indonesia." Paper presented at AAA
       Meetings, Phoenix, Arizona.
1989   "Searching for Good Fortune: The Making of a Bugis Shore Com-
       munity at Lake Lindu, Central Sulawesi." Ph.D. diss., Australian
       National University.
1990   "How to Win Friends and Influence Spirits: Propitiation and Partici-
       pation among the Bugis in a Multi-Ethnic Community of Central
       Sulawesi, Indonesia." *Anthropological Forum* 6 (2): 207–35.

Adriani, N., and Albert C. Kruyt
1898   "Overzicht van de Talen van Midden-Celebes." *Mededeeling van
       Wege het Nederlandsche Zendeling Genootschap (Tijdschrift voor
       Zendingswetenschap)* 42 (2): 536–35

Anderson, Benedict R.
1972   "The Idea of Power in Javanese Culture." In *Culture and Politics in
       Indonesia*. Eds. Claire Holt et al. Ithaca: Cornell University Press,
       1–69.
1990   *Language and Power: Exploring Political Cultures in Indonesia.*
       Ithaca: Cornell University Press.

Anema, Frans
1983   *Tinombo-Tomini-Moutong Integrated Area Development Project
       Draft Report: Direktorat Tata Kota dan Tata Daerah Direktorat
       Jenderal.* Jakarta: Cipta Karya Departamen Pekerjaan Umum.

Appell, Laura W. R.
1988   "Menstruation among the Rungus of Borneo: An Unmarked Category." In *Blood Magic: The Anthropology of Menstruation*. Eds. Thomas Buckley and Alma Gottlieb. Berkeley: University of California Press, 94–116.

Asad, Talal
1973   *Anthropology and the Colonial Encounter*. London: Ithaca Press.

Atkinson, Jane Monnig
1984   "'Wrapped Words': Poetry and Politics among the Wana of Central Sulawesi, Indonesia." In *Dangerous Words: Language and Politics in the Pacific*. Eds. Donald L. Brenneis and Fred Myers. New York: New York University Press, 33–68.
1987   "Religions in Dialogue: The Construction of an Indonesian Minority Religion." In *Indonesian Religions in Transition*. Eds. Rita Smith Kipp and Susan Rodgers. Tuscon: University of Arizona Press, 171–86.
1989   *The Art and Politics of Wana Shamanship*. Berkeley: University of California Press.

Atkinson, Jane, and Shelley Errington
1990   *Power and Difference: Gender in Island Southeast Asia*. Stanford: Stanford University Press.

Atkinson, Jane, and Shelley Rosaldo
1975   "Man the Hunter and Woman." In *Interpretation of Symbolism*. Ed. Roy Willis. London: Malaby Press, 43–75.

Bakhtin, Mikhail
1981   "Discourse in the Novel." In *The Dialogic Imagination*. Ed. Michael Holquist. Austin: University of Texas Press, 259–442.

Barth, Frederik
1969   *Ethnic Groups and Boundaries: The Social Orginization of Culture Difference*. London: Allen and Unwin.

Bateson, Gregory
1936   *Naven: A Survey of the Problems Suggested by a Composite Picture of the Culture of a New Guinea Tribe Drawn from Three Points of View*. Cambridge, England: Cambridge University Press.

Becker, A. L.
1979   "Text-Building, Epistemology, and Aesthetics in Javanese Shadow Theater." In *The Imagination of Reality: Essays in Southeast Asian*

Coherence Systems. Eds. A. L. Becker and Aram A. Yengoyam. Norwood, N.J.: Ablex Publishing Corporation, 211–43.

Behar, Ruth
1993 *Translated Woman: Crossing the Border with Esperanza's Story.* Boston: Beacon Press.
1995 "Writing in My Father's Name: A Diary of *Translated Woman*'s First Year." In *Women Writing Culture.* Eds. Ruth Behar and Deborah A. Gordon. Berkeley: University of California Press, 65–83.

Behar, Ruth, and Deborah A. Gordon
1995 *Women Writing Culture.* Berkeley: University of California Press.

Benedict, Ruth
1932 "Configurations of Culture in North America." *American Anthropologist* 34:1–27.
1934 *Patterns of Culture.* Boston: Houghton Mifflin Company.

Boas, Franz
1949 *Race, Language, and Culture (Selected Papers).* New York: Macmillan.

Bohannan, Laura
1954 *Return to Laughter.* London: Victor Golancz. Published under the nom de plume Elenore Smith Bowen.

Boon, James A.
1972 *From Symbolism to Structuralism: Lévi-Strauss in a Literary Tradition.* New York: Harper and Row.

Borofsky, Robert
1994 "Diversity and Divergence within the Anthropological Community." In *Assessing Cultural Anthropology.* Ed. Robert Borofsky. New York: McGraw-Hill, 23–28.

Bowen, John
1986 "On the Political Construction of Tradition: Gotong Royong in Indonesia." *Journal of Asian Studies* 45:545–61.
1987 "Islamic Transformations: From Sufi Poetry to Gayo Ritual." In *Indonesian Religions in Transition.* Eds. Rita Smith Kipp and Susan Rodgers. Tucson: University of Arizona Press, 113–35.
1993 *Muslims through Discourse: Religion and Ritual in Gayo Society.* Princeton: Princeton University Press.

Brenneis, Donald
1984 "Straight Talk and Sweet Talk: Political Discourse in an Occasionally Egalitarian Community." In *Dangerous Words: Language and Politics*

in the Pacific. Eds. Donald Brenneis and Fred Myers. New York: New York University Press, 69–84.

Brenneis, Donald, and Fred Myers
1984   *Dangerous Words: Language and Politics in the Pacific.* Eds. Donald Brenneis and Fred Myers. New York: New York University Press.

Briggs, Jean
1970   *Never in Anger: Portrait of an Eskimo Family.* Cambridge, Mass.: Harvard University Press.

Carrithers, Michael
1990   "Is Anthropology Art or Science?" *Current Anthropology* 31:263–72.

Casagrande, Joseph B.
1960   *In the Company of Man: Twenty Portraits by Anthropologists.* New York: Harper and Brothers.

Certeau, M. de
1984   *The Practice of Everyday Life.* Berkeley: University of California Press.

Clifford, James
1986   "Introduction: Partial Truths." In *Writing Culture: The Poetics and Politics of Ethnography.* Eds. James Clifford and George E. Marcus. Berkeley: University of California Press, 1–26.
1988   "On Ethnographic Authority." In *The Predicament of Culture: Twentieth-Century Ethnography, Literature, and Art.* Ed. James Clifford. Cambridge, Mass.: Harvard University Press, 21–54.
1997   *Routes: Travel and Translation in the Late Twentieth Century.* Cambridge, Mass: Harvard University Press.

Clifford, James, and George Marcus
1986   *Writing Culture: The Poetics and Politics of Ethnography.* Eds. James Clifford and George Marcus. Berkeley: University of California Press.

Connor, Linda
1986   *Jero Tapakan, Balinese Healer: An Ethnographic Film Monography.* Cambridge, England: Cambridge University Press.

Connor, Linda, Timothy Asch, and Patsy Asch.
1982   *Jero Tapakan: Stories in the Life of a Balinese Healer.* Canberra: Australian National University. Research School of Pacific Studies. Department of Anthropology, Documentary Educational Resources.

Coughlin, Richard J.
1965   "Pregnancy and Birth in Vietnam." In *Southeast Asian Birth Customs; Three Studies in Human Reproduction.* Ed. Donn V. Hart. New Haven, Conn.: Human Relations Area Files Press, 205–62.

Crapanzano, Vincent
1980 *Tuhami: Portrait of a Moroccan.* Chicago: University of Chicago Press.
1992 "The Postmodern Crisis: Discourse, Parody, Memory." In *Rereading Cultural Anthropology.* Ed. George E. Marcus. Durham: Duke University Press, 87–102.

Dagh Register
1569 *Dagh Register Gehouden in 't Casteel Batavia, 1568–1601.* Batavia and the Hague, Bataviaasch Genooschap.

D'Andrade, Roy
1988 *The Writing of History.* New York: Columbia University Press.
1995 "Moral Models in Anthropology." *Current Anthropology* 36 (3): 399–408.

Derrida, Jacques
1973 *Speech and Phenomena.* Evanston, Ill.: Northwestern University Press.

Downs, R. E.
1956 *The Religion of the Bare'e-Speaking Toradja of Central Celebes.* The Hague: Uitgeverij Excelsior.

Dumezil, Georges
1970 *Archaic Roman Religion.* Chicago: University of Chicago Press.

Dumont, Louis
1970 *Homo Hierarchicus: The Caste System and Its Implications.* Trans. George Weidenfeld. Chicago: University of Chicago Press.

Durkheim, Émile
1947 *The Elementary Forms of the Religious Life: A Study in Religious Sociology.* Trans. J. W. Swain. New York: Free Press. Originally published as *Les Formes Élementaires de la Vie Religeuse* (Paris: Alcan, 1912).

Echols, J., and H. Shadily
1978 *Kamus Indonesia Inggris: An Indonesian-English Dictionary.* 3rd ed. Jakarta: Penerbit PT Gramedia.

Emmerson, Donald K.
1981 "Islam in Modern Indonesia: Political Impasse, Cultural Opportunity." In *Change and the Muslim World.* Eds. Philip H. Stoddard et al. Syracuse: Syracuse University Press, 156–68.

Errington, James Joseph
1988 *Structure and Style in Javanese: A Semiotic View of Linguistic Etiquette.* Philadelphia: University of Pennsylvania Press.

1989   *Exemplary Centers, Urban Centers, and Language Change in Java.*
        Chicago: Center for Psychosocial Studies.
1998   *Shifting Languages: Interaction and Identity in Javanese Indonesian.*
        New York: Cambridge University Press.

Errington, Shelly
1989   *Meaning and Power in a Southeast Asian Realm.* Princeton: Princeton
        University Press.

Evans-Pritchard, E. E.
1934   "Levy-Bruhl's Theory of Primitive Mentality." *Bulletin of the Faculty
        of Arts* 2. Cairo: Egyptian University.
1940   *The Nuer: A Description of Modes of Livelihood and Political Insti-
        tutions of a Nilotic People.* London: Clarendon Press.
1956   *Nuer Religion.* London: Oxford University Press.

Ewing, Franklin
1960   "Birth Customs of the Tawsug, Compared with Those of Other
        Philippine Groups." *Anthropological Quarterly* 33:129–33.

Ewing, Katherine
1994   "Dreams from a Saint: Anthropological Atheism and the Temptation
        to Believe." *American Anthropologist* 96:571–83.

Fabian, Johannes
1969   "An African Gnosis: For a Reconsideration of an Authoritative
        Definition." *History of Religions* 9:42–58.
1971   "Language, History, and Anthropology." *Philosophy of the Social
        Sciences* 1:19–47.
1983   *Time and the Other: How Anthropology Makes Its Object.* New
        York: Columbia University Press.

Fanon, Franz
1963   *The Wretched of the Earth.* Trans. Constance Farrington. New York:
        Grove Weidenfeld.

Firth, Raymond
1936   *We the Tikopia: A Sociological Study of Kinship in Primitive Polyne-
        sia.* London: C. A. Watts and Company.

Forge, Anthony
1980   "Tooth and Fang in Bali." *Canberra Anthropology* 3 (1): 1–16.

Forman, Shepard
1980   "Descent, Alliance, and Exchange Ideology among the Makassae of
        East Timor." In *The Flow of Life: Essays on Eastern Indonesia.*
        Ed. J. J. Fox. Cambridge, Mass.: Harvard University Press, 152–78.

Forth, Gregory
1981 *Rindi: An Ethnographic Study of a Traditional Domain in Eastern Sumba.* The Hague: Martinus Nijhoff.
1985 "Right and Left as a Hierarchical Opposition: Reflections on Eastern Sumbanese Hairstyles." In *Contexts and Levels: Anthropological Essays on Hierarchy.* Eds. R. H. Barnes, Daniel de Coppet, and R. J. Parkin. Oxford: JASO Occasional Papers, 107–15.
1991 *Place and Space in Eastern Indonesia.* Kent, England: Occasional Papers of the Center for Southeast Asian Studies in the United Kingdom.

Foucault, Michel
1982 "The Subject and Power." In *Michel Foucault: Beyond Structuralism and Hermeneutics.* Eds. Hubert L. Dreyfuss and Paul Rabinow. Chicago: University of Chicago Press, 208–26.

Fox, James J.
1971 "Semantic Parallelism in Rotinese Ritual Language." *Bijdragen tot de Taal-, Land-, en Volkenkunde* 127:215–55.
1974 "Our Ancestors Spoke in Pairs: Rotinese Views of Language, Dialect, and Code." In *Explorations in the Ethnography of Speaking.* Eds. R. Bauman and J. Sherzer. Cambridge, England: Cambridge University Press, 65–85.
1975 "On Binary Categories and Primary Symbols: Some Rotinese Perspectives." In *The Interpretation of Symbolism.* Ed. R. Willis. Association of Social Anthropologists Studies 3. London: Malaby Press, 99–132.
1980 *The Flow of Life: Essays on Eastern Indonesia.* Cambridge, Mass.: Harvard University Press.
1988 *To Speak in Pairs: Essays on the Ritual Languages of Eastern Indonesia.* Cambridge, England: Cambridge University Press.
1989 "Category and Complement: Binary Ideologies and the Organization of Dualism in Eastern Indonesia." In *The Attraction of Opposites: Thought and Society in the Dualistic Mode.* Eds. David Maybury-Lewis and Uri Almagor. Ann Arbor: University of Michigan Press, 33–56.

Francillon, Gerard
1980 "Incursions upon Wehali: A Modern History of an Ancient Empire." In *The Flow of Life: Essays on Eastern Indonesia.* Ed. J. J. Fox. Cambridge, Mass.: Harvard University Press, 248–65.

Friedberg, Claudine
1980 "Boiled Woman and Broiled Man: Myths and Agricultural Rituals of the Bunaq of Central Timor." Trans. Elizabeth Traube. In *The Flow of*

Life: Essays on Eastern Indonesia. Ed. J. J. Fox. Cambridge, Mass.:
Harvard University Press, 266–89.

Geertz, Clifford
1960   *Religion of Java.* Chicago: University of Chicago Press.
1968   "Thinking as a Moral Act: Ethic Dimensions of Anthropological Field
       Work in the New States." *Antioch Review* 28 (2): 139–58.
1973   *The Interpretation of Cultures.* New York: Basic Books.
1976   "From the Native's Point of View: On the Nature of Anthropological
       Understanding." In *Meaning in Anthropology.* Eds. Keith Basso and
       Henry Selby. Albuquerque: University of New Mexico, 221–38.
1980   *Negara: The Theater State in Nineteenth-Century Bali.* Princeton:
       Princeton University Press.
1983   *Local Knowledge: Further Essays in Interpretive Anthropology.* New
       York: Basic Books.
1988   *Works and Lives: The Anthropologist as Author.* Stanford: Stanford
       University Press.
1995   *After the Fact.* Cambridge, Mass.: Harvard University Press.

Geertz, Hildred
1963   "Indonesian Cultures and Communities." In *Indonesia.* Ed. Ruth T.
       McVey. New Haven, Conn.: Human Relations Area Files Press,
       24–96.

George, Kenneth, M.
1996   *Showing Signs of Violence: The Cultural Politics of a Twentieth-
       Century Headhunting Ritual.* Berkeley: University of California Press.

Gibson, Thomas
1995   "Having Your House and Eating It: Houses and Siblings in Ara,
       South Sulawesi." In *About the House: Lévi-Strauss and Beyond.*
       Eds. S. Hugh-Jones and J. Carsten. Cambridge, England: Cambridge
       University Press, 129–48.

Glazer, Nathan, and Daniel P. Moynihan
1975   *Ethnicity: Theory and Experience.* Cambridge, Mass.: Harvard
       University Press.

Gluckman, Max
1940   *Seven-Year Plan.* Rhodesia: Rhodes-Livingstone Institute.
1954   *Rituals of Rebellion in Southeast Africa.* Manchester: Manchester
       University Press.
1963   *Order and Rebellion in an African Society.* New York: The Free Press.
1964   *Closed Systems and Open Minds: The Limits of Naïvety in Social
       Anthropology.* Chicago: Aldine.

1965 *Politics, Law, and Ritual in Tribal Society.* Oxford: Blackwell Press.

Graham, Penelope
1987 *Iban Shamanism: An Analysis of the Ethnographic Literature.* Canberra: Australian National University Press.

Griaule, Marcel
1948 *Conversations with Ogotemmeli.* Trans. R. Butler and A. Richards. London: Oxford University Press.

Haba, Johanis
1998 "Resettlement and Sociocultural Change among the 'Isolated Peoples' in Central Sulawesi, Indonesia: A Study of Three Resettlement Sites." Ph.D. diss., The University of Western Australia.

Hamonic, G.
1991 "God, Divinities, and Ancestors." *Southeast Asian Studies* 29 (1): 3–34.

Handler, Richard
1988 *Nationalism and the Politics of Culture in Quebec.* Madison: University of Wisconsin Press.

Hart, C. van der
1853 *Reize Rondes het Eiland Celebes.* Te's Gravenhage: KITLV Press.

Hart, Donn Vorhis
1965 "From Pregnancy through Birth in a Bisayan Filipino Village." In *Southeast Asian Birth Customs: Three Studies in Human Reproduction.* Ed. D. V. Hart. New Haven, Conn.: Human Relations Area Files Press, 1–114.

Harvey, Barbara Sillars
1977 *Permesta: Half a Rebellion.* Ithaca: Cornell University Press.

Headley, S.
1987 "The Body as a House in Javanese Society." In *De la hutte au palais: Sociétés à maison en Asie du sud-est insulaire.* Ed. C. Macdonald. Paris: CNRS.

Hefner, Robert W.
1985 *Hindu Javanese: Tengger Tradition and Islam.* Princeton: Princeton University Press.

Henley, David
1996 *Nationalism and Regionalism in a Colonial Context: Minahasa in the Dutch East Indies.* Leiden: KITLV Press.

Hertz, Robert
1907   "Contribution à une étude sur la représentation collective de la
       mort." *Année sociologique* 10:48–137.
1960   *Death and the Right Hand*. Trans. Rodney and Claudia Needham.
       New York: Free Press. Originally published as "La Prééminence de la
       main droite: Étude de polarité religieuse." In *Revue philosophique*
       (Paris: Société philosophique, December 1909).

Heusch, Luc de
1982   *The Drunken King, or, The Origin of the State*. Trans. Roy Willis.
       Bloomington: Indiana University Press.

Hicks, David
1972   "Eastern Tetum." In *Ethnic Groups in Insular Southeast Asia*, 1. Ed.
       F. LeBar. New Haven, Conn.: Human Relations Area Files Press.
1973   "The Cairui and Uai Ma'a of Timor." In *Anthropos* 68:479–81.
1978   *Structural Analysis in Anthropology: Case Studies from Indonesia
       and Brazil*. Bonn: Studia Instituti Anthropologs 30, Verlag Des An-
       thropos Institut bei Bonn.

Hocart, A. M.
1927   *Kingship*. London: Oxford University Press.

Hoevell, G. W. W. C. van
1892   "Korte Beschrijving van het Rijkje Moeton." *Tijdschrift van het
       Koninklijk Nederlanden Aardrijkskundig Genootschap* 2 (9): 349–60.

Hooykaas, C.
1974   *Cosmogony and Creation in Balinese Tradition*. The Hague: Martinus
       Nijhoff.

Hoskins, Janet
1986   "So My Name Shall Live: Stone Dragging and Grave-Building in
       Kodi, West Sumba." *Bijdragen to de Taal-, Land- en Volkenkunde*
       142:31–51.
1987   "The Headhunter as Hero: Local Traditions and Their Reinterpreta-
       tion in National History." *American Ethnologist* 14 (4): 605–22.
1988a "Etiquette in Kodi Spirit Communication: The Lips Told to Speak,
       the Mouth Told to Pronounce." In *To Speak in Pairs: Essays on the
       Ritual Languages of Eastern Indonesia*. Ed. J. J. Fox. Cambridge:
       Cambridge Unviersity Press, 29–63.
1988b "The Drum Is the Shaman, the Spear Guides His Voice." *Social
       Science Medicine* 27 (8): 819–28.
1997   *The Play of Time: Kodi Perspectives on Calendars, History, and
       Exchange*. Berkeley: University of California Press.

Howell, Signe
1984 "Relations between the Sexes." In *Society and Cosmos: The Chewong of Peninsular Malaysia.* Oxford: Oxford University Press, 51–57.
1985 "Equality and Hierarchy in Chewong Classification." In *Contexts and Levels: Anthropological Essays on Hierarchy.* Eds. R. H. Barnes, Daniel de Coppet, and R. J. Parkin. Oxford: JASO Occasional Papers, 167–80.

Jakobson, Roman
1966 "Grammatical Parallelism and Its Russian Facet." *Language* 42:399–429.

Jameson, Frederic
1984 "Postmodernism, or the Cultural Logic of Late Capitalism." *New Left Review* 146:53–92.
1989 "Nostalgia for the Present." *South Atlantic Quarterly* 88:517–37.

Josselin de Jong, J. P. B. de
1935 *De Maleische Archipel als Ethnologisch Studieveld.* Leiden: J. Ginsberg.

Josselin de Jong, P. E. de
1965 "An Interpretation of Agricultural Rites in Southeast Asia." In *Journal of Asian Studies* 24:283–91.
1977 "The Malay Archipelago as a Field of Ethnological Study." In *Structural Anthropology in the Netherlands.* Ed. P. E. de Josselin de Jong. The Hague: Martinus Nijhoff, 164–82.

Karp, Ivan
1976 "Review of Remarks and Inventions: Skeptical Essays about Kinship by Rodney Needham." *American Anthropologist* 78:152–53.

Karp, Ivan, and Kent Maynard
1983 "Reading the Nuer." *Current Anthropology* 24 (4): 481–503.

Karp, Ivan, and Martha B. Kendall
1982 "Reflexivity in Field Work." *Explaining Human Behavior: Consciousness, Human Action, and Social Structure.* Ed. Paul F. Secord. Beverly Hills: Sage Publications, 249–73.

Keesing, Roger
1982 "Kastom in Melanesia: An Overview." *Mankind* 13 (4): 357–73.

Kennedy, Raymond
1953 *Field Notes on Indonesia: Celebes and Sunda.* New Haven, Conn.: Human Relations Area Files Press.

Kern, R. A.
1939   Catalogus van de Boegineesche, to den I La Galigo-cyclus behoor-
       dende handschriften der Leidsche Universiteitsbibliotheek alsmede
       van die in andere Europeesche bibliotheken. Leiden: Universiteits-
       bibliotheek.

Keyes, Charles
1981   Ethnic Change. Seattle: University of Washington Press.

Kipp, Rita Smith, and Susan Rodgers
1987   Indonesian Religions in Transition. Tucson: University of Arizona Press.

Kondo, Dorinne
1990   Crafting Selves: Power, Gender, and Discourses of Identity in a Japa-
       nese Workplace. Chicago: University of Chicago Press.

Kroeber, Theodora
1961   Ishi in Two Worlds: A Biography of the Last Wild Indian in North
       America. Berkeley: University of California Press.

Kruyt, Albert C.
1973   "Right and Left in Central Celebes." Trans. Rodney Needham. In
       Right and Left: Essays on Dual Symbolic Classification. Ed. Rodney
       Needham. Chicago: University of Chicago Press, 74–91.

Kuipers, Joel
1990   Power in Performance: The Creation of Textual Authority in Weyewa
       Ritual Speech. Philadelphia: University of Pennsylvania Press.

Kuper, Adam
1973   Anthropologists and Anthropology: The British School, 1922–1972.
       New York: Pica Press.

Lacoste-Dujardin, Camille
1977   Dialogue des femmes en ethnologie. Paris: Maspero.

Laderman, Carol
1983   Wives and Midwives: Childbirth and Nutrition in Rural Malaysia.
       Berkeley: University of California Press.
1988   "Wayward Winds: Malay Archetypes and Theory of Personality in
       the Context of Shamanism." Social Science Medicine 27 (8): 799–811.
1991   Taming the Wind of Desire: Psychology, Medicine, and Aesthetics in
       Malay Shamanistic Performance. Berkeley: University of California
       Press.

Leach, Edmund
1954   Political Systems of Highland Burma. Boston: Beacon Press.

Lévi-Strauss, Claude
1949 *Les Structures élémentaires de la parenté.* Paris: Presses universitaires de France.

Levy-Bruhl, Lucien
1923 *Primitive Mentality.* Oxford: Blackwell Press.
1926 *How Natives Think.* Oxford: Blackwell Press.

Li, Tania
1996 "Images of Community: Discourse and Strategy in Property Relations." *Development and Change* 27 (3): 501–27.

Linnekin, Jocelyn, and Lin Poyer
1990 *Cultural Identity and Ethnicity in the Pacific.* Honolulu: University of Hawaii Press.

Lyotard, Jean-François
1984 *The Postmodern Condition: A Report on Knowledge.* Trans. Geoff Bennington and Brian Massumi. Minneapolis: University of Minnesota Press.

Malinowski, Bronislav
1929 *The Sexual Life of Savages in Northwestern Melanesia: An Ethnographic Account of Courtship, Marriage, and Family Life among the Natives of the Trobriand Islands, British New Guinea.* New York: Harcourt, Brace & World.

Marcus, George, and Michael M. J. Fischer
1986 *Anthropology as Cultural Critique: An Experimental Moment in the Human Sciences.* Chicago: University of Chicago Press.

Mashyuda, M. et al.
1979 *Monographi Daerah Sulawesi Tengah (MDST).* Vol. 2. Jakarta: Departamen Pendidikan dan Kebudayan R.I. Direktorate Jenderal Kebudayaan.

Matthes, B. F.
1954 *Catalogus van de Boeginese, tot de I La Galigo-cyclus behorende handschriften van Jajasan Matthes (Matthesstichting) te Makassar (Indonesie).* Makassar: Jajasan Matthes.

Mattulada
1982 "South Sulawesi: Its Ethnicity and Way of Life." *Southeast Asian Studies* 20 (1): 1–18.

Mauss, Marcel
1920 "L'extension du potlatch en Melanesie." *Anthropologie* 30:396–97.

Maybury-Lewis, David
1989 "The Quest for Harmony." In *The Attraction of Opposites: Thought and Society in the Dualistic Mode*. Eds. D. Maybury-Lewis and U. Almagor. Ann Arbor: University of Michigan Press, 1–18.

Mazrui, Ali
1970 "Epilogue." In *African Religions in Western Scholarship*. Ed. Okot p'Bitek. Nairobi: East African Publishing House, 121–35.

McKinley, R.
1981 "Cain and Abel on the Malay Peninsula." In *Siblingship in Oceania*. Ed. Mac Marshall. Ann Arbor: University of Michigan Press, 335–88.

McKinnon, Susan
1991 *From a Shattered Sun: Hierarchy, Gender, and Allliance in the Tanimbar Islands*. Madison: University of Wisconsin Press.

Mead, Margaret
1928 *Coming of Age in Samoa*. New York: Mentor Books.

Metcalf, Peter
1989 *Where Are You/Spirits? Style and Theme in Berawan Prayer*. Washington, D.C.: Smithsonian Institution Press.
1993 "'That's What I Say': Speech Role Projection in Berawan Prayer." In *Working Papers of the Comparative Indonesian Project*. Canberra: Australian National University Press, 1–35.
1994 "'Voilà ce que je dis': La Projection de la parole dans la prière Berawan." *L'Homme* 132:59–76.

Moerman, Michael
1965 *Being Lue: Uses and Abuses of Ethnic Identification*. Berkeley: Center for Southeast Asia Studies, Institute of International Studies, University of California.

Moertono, Soemarsaid
1968 *State and Statecraft in Old Java: A Study of the Later Mataram Period, Sixteenth to Nineteenth Century*. Ithaca: Cornell University Press.

Moore, Sally Falk
1994 *Anthropology and Africa: Changing Perspectives on a Changing Scene*. Charlottesville: University of Virginia Press.

Mudimbe, V. Y.
1988 *The Invention of Africa*. Bloomington: Indiana University Press.

Myerhoff, Barbara
1978 *Number Our Days*. New York: Simon and Schuster.

Needham, Rodney
1958   "A Structural Analysis of Purum Society." *American Anthropologist* 60:75–101.
1979   *Symbolic Classifications.* Santa Monica, Calif.: Goodyear Publishing Company, Inc.

Nourse, Jennifer Williams
1984   "The Tomini Peoples." In *Muslim Peoples: A World Ethnographic Survey.* Ed. Richard V. Weekes. Westport, Conn.: Greenwood Press, 789–93.
1989   "We Are the Womb of the World: Birth Spirits and the Laujé of Central Sulawesi." Ph.D. diss., University of Virginia.
1991   "Foreign Natives: Negotiating National Identity among the Laujé of Sulawesi, Indonesia." Paper presented at the Ninetieth Annual Meeting of the American Anthropological Association.
1993   "Local Heroes and Corrupt Others: Negotiating Ethnic and National Identity among the Laujé of Sulawesi, Indonesia." Paper presented at the British Association of Social Anthropologists, Oxford University, July.
1994a "Making Monotheism: Global Islam in Local Practice among the Laujé of Indonesia." *Journal of Ritual Studies* 8 (2): 1–18.
1994b "Textbook Heroes and Local Memory: Writing the Right History in Central Sulawesi." *Social Analysis* 35 (2): 102–21.
1994c "Introductory Remarks." *Social Analysis* 35 (2): 3–10.
1996a "The Voice of the Winds versus The Masters of Cure: Contested Notions of Spirit Possession among the Laujé of Sulawesi." *Journal of the Royal Anthropological Institute* (formerly *MAN*) 2 (N.S): 1–18.
1996b "Casting Out the Foreigners: Interpretation of a Curing Rite in Central Sulawesi, Indonesia." *Anthropology and Humanism* 21 (1): 1–15.
1997   "Male Midwives and Macho Mothers: Birth and Pregnancy among the Laujé of Indonesia." Paper presented at the Ninety-Sixth Annual Meeting of the American Anthopological Association.
1998   "Sawerigading in Strange Places: The I La Galigo Myth in Central Sulawesi." In *Collected Papers on South Sulawesi History and Culture.* Eds. Katherine Robinson and Mukhlis Paeni. Canberra, Australia, and Jakarta, Indonesia: Australian National University and Arsip Nasional Indonesia.

Obeyesekere, Gananath
1990   *The Work of Culture: Symbolic Transformation in Psychoanalysis and Anthropology.* Chicago: University of Chicago Press.

Ortner, Sherry B.
1973   "On Key Symbols." *American Anthropologist* 75:1338–46.

1981   "Gender and Sexuality in Hierarchical Societies: The Case of Polyne-
        sia and Some Comparative Implications." In *Sexual Meanings*. Eds.
        S. B. Ortner and H. Whitehead. Cambridge, England: Cambridge
        University Press, 359–409.

Ossenbruggen, F. D. E. van
1977   "Java's Monca-pat: Origins of Primitive Classification Systems." In
        Structural Anthropology in the Netherlands. Ed. P. E. de Josselin de
        Jong. The Hague: Martinus Nijhoff, 32–60. Originally published as
        "De Oorsprong van het Javaansche Begrip Montja-Pat, in Verband
        met Primitieve Classificaties." In *Verslagen en Mededeelingen der
        Koninklijk [Nederlandsche] Akademie van Wetenschappen* (Den
        Hague: Afdeeling Letterkunde, 5–3 [1918]: 6–44).

Palmier, Leslie H.
1960   *Social Status and Power in Java*. London School of Economics Mono-
        graphs on Social Anthropology. No. 20. London: Althone Press.

Parsons, Elsie Clews
1936   *Mitla: Town of the Souls*. Chicago: University of Chicago Press.

p'Bitek, Okot
1970   *African Religions in Western Scholarship*. Nairobi: East African
        Publishing House.

Peacock, James L.
1992   *Purifying the Faith: The Muhammadiyah Movement in Indonesian
        Islam*. Tempe, Ariz.: Monographs in Southeast Asian Studies, Arizona
        State University.

Pelras, Christian
1996   *The Bugis: The Peoples of South-East Asia and the Pacific*. London:
        Blackwell Publishers.

Pemberton, John
1994   *On the Subject of "Java."* Ithaca: Cornell University Press.

Pratt, Mary Louise
1986   "Fieldwork in Common Places." In *Writing Culture: The Poetics and
        Politics of Ethnography*. Eds. James Clifford and George Marcus.
        Berkeley: University of California Press, 27–50.

Raats, P. J.
1969   *A Structural Study of Bagobo Myths and Rites*. Cebu City, Philip-
        pines: University of San Carlos Press.

Rabinow, Paul
1977 *Reflections on Fieldwork in Morocco.* Berkeley: University of California Press.

Radcliffe-Brown, A. R.
1922 *The Andaman Islanders.* Cambridge, England: Cambridge University Press.

Radin, Paul
1926 *Crashing Thunder: The Autobiography of a Winnebago Indian.* New York: Appleton and Company.

Rajadhon, P. Anuman
1961 "Customs Connected with Birth and the Rearing of Children." In *Southeast Asian Birth Customs: Three Studies in Human Reproduction.* Eds. Donn V. Hart et al. New Haven, Conn.: Human Relations Area Files Press, 115–204.

Riedel, J. G. F.
1870 "Devestiging der Mandaren in de Tomini Landen." In *Tijdschrift voor Indische Taal- Land- en Volkenkunde* 29:555–64.

Rorty, Richard
1979 *Philosophy and the Mirror of Nature.* Princeton: Princeton University Press.

Rosaldo, Renato
1989 *Culture and Truth: The Remaking of Social Analysis.* Boston: Beacon Press.

Roscoe, Paul B.
1995 "The Perils of 'Positivism' in Cultural Anthropology." *American Anthropologist* 97 (3): 492–504.

Royce, Anya Petersen
1982 *Ethnic Identity: Strategies of Diversity.* Bloomington: Indiana University Press.

Sahlins, Marshall
1981 *Historical Metaphors and Mythical Realities: Structure in the Early History of the Sandwich Islands Kingdom.* Ann Arbor: University of Michigan Press.

Said, Edward
1975 *Beginnings: Intention and Method.* New York: Basic Books.
1978 *Orientalism.* New York: Pantheon Books.

Sapir, Edward
1924 "Culture, Genuine and Spurious." *American Journal of Sociology* 29:401–29.
1938 "Why Cultural Anthropology Needs the Psychiatrist." *Psychiatry* 1:7–12.

Sapir, J. David, and J. Christopher Crocker
1977 *The Social Use of Metaphor.* Philadelphia: University of Pennsylvania Press.

Scharer, Hans
1963 *Ngaju Religion.* The Hague: KITLV Press.

Scheper-Hughes, Nancy
1995 "The Primacy of the Ethical: Propositions for a Militant Anthropology." *Current Anthropology* 36 (3): 409–20.

Schiller, Anne
1997 *Small Sacrifices: Religious Change and Cultural Identity among the Ngaju of Indonesia.* Oxford: Oxford University Press.

Scott, James C.
1985 *Weapons of the Weak: Everyday Forms of Peasant Resistance.* New Haven, Conn.: Yale University Press.

Shostak, Marjorie
1981 *Nisa: The Life and Words of a !Kung Woman.* Cambridge, Mass.: Harvard University Press.

Steedly, Mary Margaret
1988 "Severing the Bonds of Love: A Case Study in Soul Loss." *Social Science and Medicine* 27(8): 841–56.
1993 *Hanging without a Rope: Narrative Experience in Colonial and Postcolonial Karoland.* Princeton: Princeton University Press.

Stoller, Paul A., and Cheryl Olkes
1987 *In Sorcery's Shadow: A Memoir of Apprenticeship among the Songhay of Niger.* Chicago: University of Chicago Press.

Strathern, Marilyn
1987 *Dealing with Inequality: Analysing Gender Relations in Melanesia and Beyond.* Cambridge, England: Cambridge University Press.

Tambiah, Stanley
1976 *World Conquerer and World Renouncer: A Study of Buddhism and Polity in Thailand against a Historical Background.* Cambridge, England: Cambridge University Press.

Taussig, Michael
1980 *The Devil and Commodity Fetishism in South America.* Chapel Hill: University of North Carolina Press.
1987 *Shamanism, Colonialism, and the Wild Man: A Study of Terror and Healing.* Chicago: University of Chicago Press.
1992 *The Nervous System.* New York: Routledge.

Thornton, Robert J.
1992 "The Rhetoric of Ethnographic Holism." In *Rereading Cultural Anthropology.* Ed. George E. Marcus. Durham: Duke University Press, 15–33.

Tol, Roger
1990 "A Wealth of Idiom and Ideology." In *Sulawesi: Island Crossroads of Indonesia.* Eds. Toby Alice Volkman and Ian Caldwell. Lincolnwood, Ill.: Passport Books, 48–49.

Toland, Judith
1993 *Ethnicity and the State.* New Brunswick, N.J.: Transaction Publishers.

Tonjaya, K.
1981 *Kanda Pat Rare.* Denpasar, Bali: Penerbit Ria.

Traube, Elizabeth G.
1980 "Mambai Rituals of Black and White." In *The Flow of Life: Essays on Eastern Indonesia.* Ed. J. J. Fox. Cambridge, Mass.: Harvard University Press, 290–316.
1986 *Cosmology and Social Life: Ritual Exchange among the Mambai of East Timor.* Chicago: University of Chicago Press.
1989 "Obligations to the Source: Complementarity and Hierarchy in an Eastern Indonesian Society." In *The Attraction of Opposites: Thought and Society in the Dualistic Mode.* Eds. D. Maybury-Lewis and U. Almagor. Ann Arbor: University of Michigan Press, 321–44.

Tsing, Anna Lowenhaupt
1987 "A Rhetoric of Centers in a Religion of the Periphery." In *Indonesian Religions in Transition.* Eds. Rita Smith Kipp and Susan Rodgers. Tucson: University of Arizona Press, 96–125.
1988 "Healing Boundaries in South Kalimantan." *Social Science Medicine* 27 (8): 819–28.
1993 *In the Realm of the Diamond Queen.* Princeton: Princeton University Press.

Turner, Edith, with William Blodgett, Singleton Kahona, and Fideli Benwa
1992 *Experiencing Ritual: A New Interpretation of African Healing.* Philadelphia: University of Pennsylvania Press.

Turner, Victor W.

1957 *Schism and Continuity in an African Society: A Study of Ndembu Village Life.* Manchester: Manchester University Press.

1967 "Muchona the Hornet, Interpreter of Religion." In *The Forest of Symbols: Aspects of Ndembu Ritual.* Ithaca: Cornell University Press, 131–50.

1974 *Dramas, Fields, and Metaphors: Symbolic Action in Human Society.* Ithaca: Cornell University Press.

Tyler, Stephen

1986a "Post-Modern Ethnography: From Document of the Occult to Occult Document." In *Writing Culture: The Poetics and Politics of Ethnography.* Ed. James Clifford. Berkeley: University of California Press, 122–40.

1986b "Post-Modern Ethnography." In *Discourse and the Social Life of Meaning.* Eds. Phyllis Pease Chock and June R. Wyman. Washington, D.C.: Smithsonian Institution Press, 23–50.

1992 "On Being Out of Words." In *Rereading Cultural Anthropology.* Ed. George Marcus. Raleigh: Duke University Press, 1–8.

Tylor, E. B.

1958 *Primitive Culture: Researches into the Development of Mythology, Philosophy, Religion, Language, Art, and Custom.* New York: Harper. Originally published same title, 2 vols., London: John Murray, 1873.

Vail, Leroy, and Landeg White

1991 *Power and the Praise Poem: Southern African Voices in History.* Charlottesville: University of Virginia Press.

Vansina, Jan

1985 *Oral Tradition as History.* London: James Currey and Heinemann.

Volkman, Toby Alice

1985 *Feasts of Honor: Ritual and Change in the Toraja Highlands.* Urbana: University of Illinois Press.

Wagner, Roy

1975 *The Invention of Culture.* Englewood Cliffs, N.J.: Prentice-Hall, Inc.

1983 "Visible Ideas: Toward an Anthropology of Perceptive Values." *South Asian Anthropologist (Essays in Honor of Victor Turner)* 4 (1): 1–8.

1986a *Symbols That Stand for Themselves.* Chicago: University of Chicago Press.

1986b *Asiwinarong: Ethos, Image, and Social Power among the Usen Barok of New Ireland.* Princeton: Princeton University Press.

Wallace, Alfred Russell
1869 *The Malay Archipelago, the Land of the Orangutan, and the Bird of Paradise: A Narrative of Travel with Studies of Man and Nature.* New York: Macmillan.

Warren, Kaye
1992 "Transforming Memories and Histories: The Meanings of Ethnic Resurgence in Mayan Indians." In *Americas: New Interpretive Essays.* Ed. Alfred Stephan. Oxford: Oxford University Press, 31–54.

Weinstock, Joseph A.
1987 "Kaharingan: Life and Death in Southern Borneo." In *Indonesian Religions in Transition.* Eds. S. Rodgers and R. Kipp. Tucson: University of Arizona Press, 71–97.

Wilson, Godfrey and Monica
1945 *The Analysis of Social Change.* Cambridge, England: Cambridge University Press.

Wolf, Margery
1968 *The House of Lim: A Study of a Chinese Farm Family.* New York: Prentice-Hall.
1992 *A Thrice-Told Tale: Feminism, Postmodernism, and Ethnographic Responsibility.* Palo Alto: Stanford University Press.

Woodard, David
1804 *The Narratives of Captain David Woodard and Four Seamen.* Pall Mall, England: Dawson's.

Wouden, F. A. E. van
1935 *Sociale Structuurtypen in de Groote Oost.* Leiden: Ginsberg.

Zerner, Charles, and Toby Alice Volkman
1988 "The Tree of Desire: A Toraja Ritual Poem." In *To Speak in Pairs: Essays on the Ritual Languages of Eastern Indonesia.* Ed. James J. Fox. Cambridge, England: Cambridge University Press, 282–305.

INDEX

abortion, 98, 218, 247n31
Acciaioli, Greg, 105, 229nn16, 2, 3, 236n28, 240n15, 242n20
agnatic kinship bonds, 122
Alasan (Siinai), 7, 51, 155–56, 256n19; dispute with Balitangan, 199–201; on first tree's tap-root and custom, 188–90; on qualities of the placenta, 218–19; on umputé and Islam, 206–9
Alo (Siinai), 185–86
altar. *See* shrine
animism, 7, 30, 230n4
anthropological studies. *See* postmodernist approach
Anthropology as Cultural Critique (Marcus and Fischer), 9–10
Arbou (Siamae), ritual cure for dysentery, 114–17, 250n10
aristocracy. *See* elites
Asarima (Siamae), 141, 143, 144, 177–79, 214
Atkinson, Jane Monnig, 229n3, 245n23, 247n28
audiences, at momasoro rites, 147, 160–61, 192, 256nn17, 18
Austronesian societies: binary opposition concepts, 19, 217, 229n16, 257n1; as origin of *umputé* concept, 105, 225n4
autochthonous religion, 27, 229n2

Bakhtin, Mikhail, 9, 12
Balantak people, religion based on placental amniotic fluids, 104–5
Balitangan (Siamae), 7, 20, 50; version of the creation story, 208, 215; version of the momasoro and conception of Islam, 192–210

bananas: leaves used in black illness ritual, 100; use in momasoro ritual, 143, 185
battles, mock, staged during momasoro rites, 158, 162
bela: black umputé spirits manifesting themselves as, 102; as outsiders converting to world religions, 53, 237n1; pejorative meaning for distant, 41, 42, 236n28; Sanji's views on, 65–69, 241n18
Benedict, Ruth, 10, 13
betel nut: as mild narcotic, 82, 146; use in white illness ritual, 92, 96, 247n28
betel nut, yellow, significance in cutting umbilical cord, 82, 84, 87, 243n7
big house. *See* parlor
binary oppositions, 6, 22, 219–20, 229n1; in Austronesian societies, 19, 217, 229n16, 257n1; Sumpitan's concepts of umputé, 120, 217; symbolism in white and black illness rites, 99–101, 248n33
birth rituals: Sanji's explanation, 1, 2–3, 5–7, 19–20, 77, 80–82; Sumpitan's explanation, 117–21
birth spirits. *See* umputé
"black" illness, diagnosis and ritual treatment, 97–102
black umputé spirit(s), 88; as contrasted to white umputé spirit, 79; as human beings, 102–5, 248n35; relationship to red spirit, 107
blessings. *See* prayer(s), highland *and* lowland
blood, black, significance of fluids during birth process, 76, 78, 80–81, 85, 242n4